DENTAL

DENTAL
EXAMINATION REVIEW

SIXTH EDITION

1267 MULTIPLE CHOICE QUESTIONS AND REFERENCED EXPLANATORY ANSWERS

Alvin F. Gardner, D.D.S., M.S., Ph. D., F.I.C.D.
Silver Spring, Maryland
Formerly Associate Professor
School of Dentistry and Graduate School
University of Maryland
Baltimore, Maryland

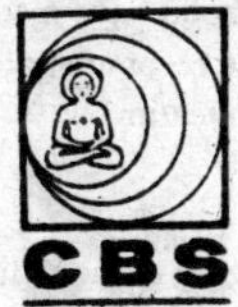

CBS PUBLISHERS & DISTRIBUTORS
4596/1-A, 11 Darya Ganj, New Delhi - 110 002 (India)

ISBN : 81-239-1123-8

First Indian Edition : 1988
Reprint : 2000

Reprinted in India by CBS Publishers & Distributors in arrangement with Elsvier Science Publishing Company, Inc.

Published by S.K. Jain for CBS Publishers & Distributors,
4596/1A, 11 Darya Ganj, New Delhi - 110 002 (India)

Printed at :

Nikunj Print Process, Delhi.

notice

The author and the publisher of this book have made every effort to ensure that all therapeutic modalities that are recommended are in accordance with accepted standards at the time of publication.

The drugs specified within this book may not have specific approval by the Food and Drug Administration in regard to the indications and dosages that are recommended by the author. The manufacturer's package insert is the best source of current prescribing information.

To the memory of
ESTHER VITA GARDNER
1922-1981

In appreciation of her sympathetic assistance and devotion. Without her encouragement this book would not have been written.

Contents

Preface

The variations in test questions are offered to familiarize the dental student with the various types of National Board, State Board, and school examinations in use today. The following test material will give you an opportunity to determine your ability to read, digest, and comprehend the vast accumulation of available knowledge.

Dental students are no doubt aware that the Dental Board Examination represents one of the most important examinations they will ever have to pass. The purpose of this text is to encourage the reader to detect areas of weakness in the understanding of subject matter so that the student may return to textbooks for a more comprehensive review of the subject.

Do not compromise by simply looking up the correct answers. The mature approach is to return to your textbook. The author has provided you with a list of references as a timesaving device to rapidly locate a particular source of information.

The following pages will provide an interesting challenge to the dental student as well as an opportunity to improve skills with multiple-choice examinations.

PART I

BASIC DENTAL SCIENCES

1. ANATOMY

DIRECTIONS: Each of the questions or incomplete statements below is followed by five suggested answers or completions. Select the ONE that is best in each case.

---

1. The cranium includes which of the following?
   A. Crown
   B. Back of the head
   C. Frontal region
   D. Temples and ears
   E. All of the above

2. The face includes the regions of
   A. the eyes
   B. the nose
   C. the mouth
   D. the cheeks and lower jaw
   E. all of the above

3. The thorax consists of which of the following?
   A. Breast
   B. Infraclavicular region
   C. Sternal region
   D. Axilla
   E. All of the above

4. The abdomen is divided into which of the following regions?
   A. Right and left hypochondriac regions
   B. Right and left lumbar regions
   C. Right and left inguinal regions
   D. Epigastric, umbilical, and hypogastric regions
   E. All of the above

5. The upper extremities (members) include which of the following?
   A. Axilla
   B. Shoulder
   C. Deltoid region
   D. Arm, elbow, forearm, and hand
   E. All of the above

6. The lower extremities (members) include which of the following?
   A. Buttocks
   B. Thigh
   C. Knee
   D. Leg and foot
   E. All of the above

7. Fascia is used in anatomy to mean
   A. the anterior crural region
   B. a band, layer, or partition of connective tissue
   C. the posterior antebrachial region
   D. the ligaments
   E. none of the above

8. The curved, bony prominences on either side of the glabella are termed
   A. the superior nuchal lines
   B. the superciliary arches
   C. the mastoid processes
   D. the lambda
   E. none of the above

9. The junction of the coronal and sagittal sutures, and thus the site where both parietal bones meet the frontal bone, is termed
   A. the lambda
   B. the superciliary arches
   C. the bregma
   D. the pterion
   E. none of the above

10. The fontanelles of the fetal cranium correspond to which of the following bony sites of the adult skull?
    A. The bregma, anterior fontanelle
    B. The lambda, posterior fontanelle
    C. The asterion, mastoid fontanelle
    D. The pterion, sphenoid fontanelle
    E. All of the above

11. The auricula is made up of a canal that leads from which of the following structures to the exterior and expanded fleshy part?
    A. The tympanic membrane
    B. The external auditory meatus
    C. The scaphoid fossa
    D. The extrinsic muscles
    E. None of the above

.2. The anterior, exposed portion of the eyeball is covered by
    A. the cornea
    B. the conjunctival sac
    C. the bulbar conjunctiva
    D. the orbital septum
    E. none of the above

13. The nose as an organ has, in addition to its external parts, internal passageways and which of the following structures?
    A. Extrinsic muscles
    B. Accessory nasal sinuses (air cells)
    C. Internal occipital crest
    D. Falx cerebri
    E. None of the above

14. The parotid gland and the masseter muscle contribute to which of the following names for the region which lies external to them?
    A. The parotid region
    B. The mental region
    C. The parotid-masseteric region
    D. The vestibule of the mouth
    E. None of the above

15. Firm pressure with the tip of the finger along a line where the dental arch joins the body of the mandible will reveal a sensitive spot about 2.5 cm lateral to the midline. This is the site of emergence of
    A. the oral vestibule
    B. the mental nerve from the mental foramen
    C. the fauces
    D. the chin
    E. none of the above

16. Which of the following represent triangles of the neck?
 A. The anterior triangle
 B. The submental triangle
 C. The carotid triangle
 D. The muscular triangle
 E. All of the above

17. The neck may be divided into
 A. the right anterolateral region
 B. the left anterolateral region
 C. the right and left anterolateral regions and the posterior or nuchal region
 D. the nuchal region
 E none of the above

18. The seventh cervical vertebra possesses which of the following features characteristic of both cervical and thoracic regions?
 A. Longer spinous process
 B. Vertebra prominens
 C. Massive transverse process
 D. Small transverse foramen
 E. All of the above

19 The skull is the
 A. least complex structure of the skeleton
 B. cerebral cranium
 C. most complex structure of the skeleton
 D. visceral cranium
 E. none of the above

20. The base of the skull is divided for the convenience of description into which of the following portions?
 A. Anterior, middle, and visceral
 B. Suboccipital and anterior
 C. Subcerebral and posterior
 D. Anterior (visceral), middle (subcerebral), and posterior (suboccipital)
 E. None of the above

21. The occipital bone has which of the following anatomic features?
 A. External occipital protuberance
 B. External occipital crest
 C. Superior nuchal line
 D. Supreme nuchal line
 E. All of the above

22. Which of the following muscles are attached to the body of the hyoid bone?
   A. Geniohyoid, genioglossus
   B. Mylohyoid, sternohyoid
   C. Omohyoid, stylohyoid
   D. Thyrohyoid and hyoglossus
   E. All of the above

23. Syndesmosis means
   A. union of the roots of the teeth with the walls of the dental alveoli
   B. a thin layer of fibrous tissue uniting the opposed skeletal parts
   C. serrate suture
   D. ligamentous union with skeletal parts relatively far apart
   E. none of the above

24. Gomphosis means which of the following variety of fibrous joints?
   A. Serrate suture
   B. A thin layer of fibrous tissue uniting the opposed skeletal parts
   C. Union of the roots of the teeth with the walls of the dental alveoli
   D. Ligamentous union with skeletal parts
   E. None of the above

25. The temporomandibular articulation is classified as which of the following?
   A. Simple, synovial, condylar
   B. Simple, synovial, trochoid
   C. Compound, synovial, condylar
   D. Cartilaginous, symphysis
   E. None of the above

26. The articular disk of the temporomandibular joint
   A. is thicker at the center than at the circumference
   B. is thinner posteriorly in relation to the thin bone of the deep part of the mandibular fossa than anteriorly
   C. is an oval plate of dense fibrous tissue which acquires islands of cartilage cells with age
   D. has its inferior surface convex and its superior surface convex anteriorly
   E. is none of the above

27. The muscles of mastication (craniomandibular musculature) include which of the following?
    A. Temporal
    B. Masseter
    C. Medial pterygoids
    D. Lateral pterygoids
    E. All of the above

28. The blood supply to the heart includes which of the following vessels?
    A. The right coronary artery
    B. The artery of the sinoatrial node, canal branch, and preventricular branches of right coronary artery
    C. The left coronary artery
    D. The anterior interventricular branch and circumflex branch of left coronary artery
    E. All of the above

29. The branches of the aortic arch are
    A. the brachiocephalic and left common carotid
    B. the thyroidea ima artery and innominate artery
    C. the aortic spindle and ligamentum arteriosum
    D. the brachiocephalic, left common carotid, and left subclavian arteries
    E. none of the above

30. In the common carotid arteries
    A. each paired vessel has a different origin and different length
    B. the right common carotid arises from the bifurcation of the brachiocephalic trunk
    C. the left common carotid arises from the arch of the aorta as its second branch
    D. the portion of the left common carotid artery that extends from the arch of the aorta lies within the superior mediastinum
    E. all of the above are true

31. The external carotid artery
    A. is the smaller of two branches into which the common carotid divides
    B. is distributed to the anterior part of neck, pharynx, tongue, oral cavity, face, temporal and infratemporal fossae, and nasal cavity
    C. arises from the common carotid at the superior border of thyroid cartilage
    D. has eight independent branches that arise from the external carotid
    E. has all of the above

32. The maxillary artery
   A. is the larger of the two terminal branches of the external carotid
   B. arises deep, opposite the neck of the mandible in the substance of the parotid gland
   C. passes forward between the mandible and the sphenomandibular ligament
   D. is divided for description into three portions: mandibular, pterygoid, and pterygopalatine
   E. has all of the above

33. The internal carotid artery
   A. arises with the external carotid at the bifurcation of common carotid opposite the superior border of the thyroid cartilage
   B. is equal in size to the external carotid in adults but larger than the external carotid in children
   C. has its proximal portion dilated as the carotid sinus
   D. at first has the artery dorsolateral to the external carotid, though it may be dorsal or dorsomedial to it
   E. has all of the above

34. The pulmonary circulation
   A. returns deoxygenated blood to the right atrium
   B. collects blood from the abdomen and transports it to the liver
   C. consists of four short veins which are unique in that they transport oxygenated blood to the left atrium from the lungs
   D. returns blood to systemic circulation by means of hepatic veins
   E. none of the above

35. The portal circulation
   A. is the systemic circulation
   B. returns deoxygenated blood to the right atrium by the superior vena cava
   C. consists of four short veins which transport oxygenated blood to the left atrium from the lungs
   D. collects blood from the capillaries of the abdominal parts of the alimentary tract, spleen, and pancreas and transports it to the liver
   E. does none of the above

36. The external jugular vein
    A. is formed by the confluence of the posterior auricular and posterior division of the retromandibular vein
    B. crosses the external carotid artery
    C. may pass either deep or superficial to the stylohyoid and digastric muscles
    D. passes through the submandibular triangle to the upper border of the hyoid bone
    E. does none of the above

37. The internal jugular vein
    A. begins at the jugular fossa and is the continuation of the sigmoid sinus
    B. passes caudally through the neck, in company first with the internal carotid and then with the common carotid artery, to the inferior border of the sternoclavicular articulation
    C. is at sternoclavicular articulation and bilaterally joins the subclavian to form the brachiocephalic vein
    D. in the larger posterior and lateral part of the jugular foramen is dilated forming the superior bulb of the jugular vein
    E. does all of the above

38. The maxillary sinus (antrum of highmore) is a large pyramidal cavity located in the body of the maxilla. In the articulated skull the nasal wall (an irregular aperture in the disarticulated skull) is partially closed by which of the following bones?
    A. The uncinate process of the ethmoid bone
    B. The ethmoidal process of the inferior nasal concha
    C. The vertical part of the palatine bone
    D. The small part of the lacrimal bone
    E. All of the above

39. Ligaments
    A. are very flattened tendons
    B. are adipose loose fibrous tissue
    C. represent all fibrous connective tissue structures
    D. resist tensions predominantly in one direction with collagen bundles arranged in a parallel fashion
    E. are none of the above

40. The branches of the facial nerve located in the face and neck include which of the following?
   A. The posterior auricular nerve
   B. The posterior auricular nerve, digastric branch, and stylohyoid branch
   C. The digastric branch
   D. The stylohyoid branch
   E. None of the above

41. The subdivisions of the mammalian hypophysis are
   A. pars distalis (anterior lobe of adenohypophysis)
   B. pars tuberalis (anterior lobe of adenohypophysis)
   C. pars intermedia (posterior lobe of neurohypophysis)
   D. pars nervosa (posterior lobe of neurohypophysis)
   E. all of the above

2. MICROBIOLOGY

DIRECTIONS: Each of the questions or incomplete statements below is followed by five suggested answers or completions. Select the ONE that is best in each case.

---

42. Viruses
    A. are sharply differentiated from all cellular organisms (rickettsiae and other bacteria)
    B. consist of a nucleic acid molecule (DNA or RNA)
    C. are enclosed in a protein coat (Capsid)
    D. have an infectious principle, i.e., viral nucleic acid
    E. are all of the above

43. The term algae refers in general to
    A. nonchlorophyll-containing higher protists
    B. Fungi imperfecti
    C. Ascrasiae
    D. chlorophyll containing higher protists
    E. none of the above

44. Which of the following represent major groups of bacteria?
    A. Eubacteria
    B. Spirochetes
    C. Gliding bacteria
    D. Pleuropneumonia-like organisms
    E. All of the above

45. The spirochetes
   A. cell is constructed in a unique fashion, which makes its phylogenetic relationship to other bacteria obscure
   B. spiral cell is intertwined with slimmer filament
   C. filament is difficult to see
   D. mechanism of spirochete motility is not comparable to flagellated eubacteria
   E. are all of the above

46. Sterilization
   A. is spoken of as the process of killing all of the organisms in a preparation
   B. is the process of killing 90% of the organisms in a preparation
   C. is the log of the number of surviving cells per milliliter of a preparation
   D. occurs after 3 hours of any given treatment
   E. is none of the above

47. Septic means
   A. characterized by the absence of pathogenic microbes
   B. killing infectious organisms
   C. characterized by the presence of pathogenic microbes in living tissue
   D. free of life of every kind
   E. none of the above

48. Physical agents producing sterilization are
   A. alcohols
   B. phenol
   C. heat and ultraviolet light
   D. heavy metal ions
   E. none of the above

49. To be a useful chemotherapeutic agent, the compound must be
   A. bacteriostatic and sterile
   B. sterile
   C. either bacteriostatic or bactericidal in vivo
   D. a noncationic agent
   E. none of the above

50. Bacteria are controlled in water by which of the following methods?
   A. Sanitation of drinking water
   B. Sewage purification (screening sludge formation)
   C. Sludge digestion
   D. Disposal of supernatant water
   E. All of the above

51. Food poisoning means
   A. spoilage of food
   B. restricted to infection by enteric pathogens contaminating food or ingestion of food containing exotoxins produced by Micrococcus, staphylococcus, or Clostridium botulinum
   C. food is rendered unfit for human consumption
   D. reductase activity is high
   E. none of the above

52. Control of bacteria in food may occur by which of the following means (preservative measures)?
   A. Irradiation
   B. Low temperature, acids
   C. Drying, chemical preservatives
   D. Heat, salt, sugar, smoking
   E. All of the above

53. Which of the following infectious diseases may be transmitted by food?
   A. Typhoid fever
   B. Salmonella infection
   C. Dysentery
   D. Streptococcic infection
   E. All of the above

54. The fundamental principle of chemotherapy is
   A. restriction
   B. modification
   C. mutation to virulence
   D. selective toxicity
   E. none of the above

55. Tubercle bacilli
   A. have their growth inhibited by para-aminosalicylic acid (PAS)
   B. are inhibited by sulfathiazole
   C. are inhibited markedly by sulfonamides
   D. are inhibited by folic acid
   E. are none of the above

56. Penicillin
   A. is a selective inhibitor of bacterial cell wall synthesis
   B. is a structural analogue of acetylmuramic acid
   C. may be a structural analogue of acyl-D-alanyl-D-alanine
   D. in high concentrations completely blocks cell wall formation and cells may lyse
   E. is all of the above

57. The emergence of drug resistance in an infection may be minimized by which of the following?
   A. Maintaining low levels of the drug
   B. Maintaining sufficiently high levels of the drug, simultaneously administering two drugs which do not give cross-resistance, and avoiding exposure of microorganisms to particularly valuable drugs by restricting its use
   C. Not administering two drugs which do not give cross-resistance
   D. Not restricting use of the drug and avoiding exposure of the microorganism to valuable drugs
   E. None of the above

58. The tetracycline drugs include which of the following?
   A. Chlorotetracycline
   B. Oxytetracycline
   C. Tetracycline
   D. Demethylchlortetracycline
   E. All of the above

59. Facultative parasites
   A. cannot survive with a host
   B. have absolute requirements for a host
   C. stimulate rickettsial growth
   D. live either in relationship to or are completely independent of a host
   E. are none of the above

60. Obligatory parasites
   A. survive without a host
   B. have absolute requirements for a host and cannot survive or propagate without a host
   C. do not have absolute requirements for a host
   D. are commensalism
   E. are none of the above

61. Virulence
   A. denotes toxicity
   B. is the ability of microorganisms to cause disease
   C. introduces the concept of degree, subdivided into toxigenicity and invasiveness
   D. is the ability of microorganisms to result in the production of progressive lesions
   E. is none of the above

62. Exotoxins
   A. are nonantigenic
   B. are specific injurious substances secreted into the environment by certain gram-positive bacteria (rarely by gram-negative)
   C. are not rapidly destroyed by heat (60°C)
   D. are not converted into nonpoisonous toxoids by heat, formalin, or prolonged storage
   E. are none of the above

63. In diphtheria (caused by toxin-producing bacteria)
   A. the toxin is not absorbed
   B. the toxin does not block the synthesis of the cytochrome b enzyme
   C. Corynebacterium diphtheriae usually are limited to the upper respiratory tract
   D. the toxin produces gas in the tissues
   E. none of the above is true

64. Koch's postulates
   A. currently apply to human viral disease
   B. had to be modified extensively for virus diseases
   C. do not apply to diseases caused by toxin-producing bacteria
   D. do not apply to facultative parasite
   E. are none of the above

65. Natural immunity
  A. is passive immunity
  B. is active immunity
  C. is that which is not acquired through previous contact with the infectious agent or a related species
  D. has antigenic specificity
  E. is none of the above

66. Antigens
  A. are species immunity
  B. are substances which, when introduced parenterally into a foreign species, can elicit the formation of antibodies in the living animal
  C. are due to differences in age
  D. depend on hormonal and metabolic influences
  E. are none of the above

67. A hapten
  A. is more susceptible to RBC hemolysis
  B. is a phagocytic compound which by itself can elicit the formation of antibodies
  C. is a compound of low molecular weight which cannot by itself elicit the formation of antibodies but can combine with antibodies elicited by a large molecule with a structure similar to hapten
  D. is a biochemical tissue constituent which by itself can elicit the formation of antibodies
  E. is none of the above

68. Antibodies are
  A. not present in the blood in certain abnormal states
  B. specialized serum proteins (immunoglobulins) which act specifically with the antigen that stimulated their production
  C. three combinations of two antigens present in red cells
  D. four combinations of two antigens present in red cells
  E. are none of the above

69. Immunoglobulins are produced
  A. in the liver
  B. in the reticuloendothelial system (lymphoid cells, plasma cells)
  C. in cardiac cells
  D. in islands of Langerhans
  E. in none of the above

70. Which of the following represent characteristics of exotoxins?
   A. Excreted by living cells; found in high concentration in fluid medium
   B. Highly toxic; fatal for laboratory animals in micrograms or less
   C. Relatively unstable; toxicity usually destroyed rapidly by heat over 60°C
   D. Converted into antigenic, nontoxic toxoids by formalin, storage, etc.; highly antigenic and heat-labile proteins
   E. All of the above

71. Which of the following represent characteristics of endotoxins?
   A. Liberated by microbial cells only upon their disintegration
   B. Weekly toxic; fatal for laboratory animals in milligrams or more
   C. Relatively stable; not converted into toxoids
   D. Do not stimulate the formation of antitoxin, lipopolysaccharide complexes
   E. All of the above

72. Allergy refers (in common usage) to
   A. idiosyncrasy
   B. hyperreactivity and hypersensitivity
   C. a homeostatic function of the animal body
   D. immunologic paralysis
   E. none of the above

73. Which of the following physiologic disturbances may be observed in anaphylaxis?
   A. Leukopenia
   B. Smooth muscle spasm in bronchioles and arterioles
   C. Edema due to injury to vascular endothelium
   D. Liberation of histamine, serotonin, bradykinin, and heparin and fall in normal serum complement
   E. All of the above

74. The arthus reaction
   A. is a delayed reaction resulting in localized tissue damage
   B. is an immediate type of reaction which results in localized tissue damage
   C. is a collagen disease
   D. is a desensitization reaction
   E. is none of the above

75. The staphylococci
   A. are gram-positive spherical cells arranged in clusters
   B. grow readily on a variety of media and are active metabolically
   C when pathogenic often hemolyze blood and coagulate plasma
   D. may be members of the normal flora of the skin and mucous membranes of man; others cause suppuration, abscess formation, and pyogenic infections
   E. are all of the above

76. Streptococci
   A. are spherical microorganisms arranged in chains and widely distributed in nature
   B. may elaborate a capsular polysaccharide
   C. may be members of normal human flora, others are associated with important human diseases
   D. cause human diseases due to sensitization or to infection
   E. are all of the above

77. Diseases attributable to invasion by beta-hemolytic group A streptococci are
   A. streptococcal sore throat
   B. impetigo
   C. acute bacterial endocarditis
   D. erysipelas, puerperal fever, and sepsis
   E. none of the above

78. Neisseriae
   A. are a group of gram-negative cocci, usually occurring in pairs
   B may be normal inhabitants of the human respiratory tract and occur extracellularly
   C. may be human pathogens and occur intracellularly (gonococci, meningococci)
   D. are strict aerobes
   E. are all of the above

79. Clostridium tetani
   A. has a worldwide distribution in the soil and feces of animals
   B. are several types of organisms that can be distinguished by specific flagellar antigens
   C. all share a common 0 (somatic) antigen
   D. all produce the same toxin
   E. are all of the above

80. Corynebacteria
   A. are gram-positive rods, nonmotile and nonspore-forming
   B. often possess club-shaped ends and irregularly staining granules
   C. occur in characteristic arrangements resembling Chinese letters or palisades
   D. form acid but not gas in certain carbohydrates and produce a powerful exotoxin which causes diphtheria in man
   E. are all of the above

81. Mycobacteria
   A. are rod-shaped bacteria which are acid-fast bacilli
   B. have many saprophytic forms
   C. are more resistant to chemical agents than other bacteria because of the hydrophobic nature of the cell surface and clumped growth
   D. are fairly resistant to drying and survive for long periods in dried sputum
   E. are all of the above

82. Candida albicans infection
   A. is communicable
   B. cannot be controlled
   C. cannot be stopped by preventive measures
   D. is not communicable
   E. is none of the above

83. Spirochetes
   A. are a large, heterogeneous group of spiral, motile organisms
   B. treponema causes syphilis, bejel, yaws, and pinta
   C. borrelia causes relapsing fever
   D. leptospira causes systemic infections with fever, jaundice, and meningitis
   E. do all of the above

84. In genetic engineering, plasmids
   A. undergo conjugation
   B. are released from a cell upon forced lysis, are incubated with DNA from an unrelated organism along with enzymes capable of breaking and fusing DNA
   C. and genetic recombination are not severely restricted in range
   D. transformation does not involve the uptake of DNA into a cell
   E. are none of the above

85. Which of the following components of bacterial cells may be identified ultrastructurally?
   A. Ribosomes
   B. Globular proteins
   C. Fibrils
   D. Cell walls
   E. All of the above

86. Humans are the natural host of which of the following herpes viruses?
   A. HSV type 1
   B. HSV type 2
   C. Cytomegalovirus
   D. Varicella-zoster virus and Epstein-Barr virus
   E. All of the above

87. The microscopic flora of the oral cavity contains which of the following species indigenous to the oral tissues?
   A. 30 species
   B. 100 species
   C. No species
   D. 2 species
   E. None of the above

88. Microbially induced oral lesions are caused by which of the following microorganisms?
   A. Bacterial
   B. Rickettsial
   C. Chlamydial
   D. Viral, mycotic, and protozoal (metazoal)
   E. All of the above

89. In planning the treatment of oral infections, which of the following commonly found microorganisms may be present in the oral lesions?
   A. Pyogenic granuloma (gingiva) has an oral flora of low virulence.
   B. Vincent's acute necrotizing ulcerative gingivitis contains Borrelia vincenti, Fusobacterium fusiforme, and Bacteroides melaninogenicus
   C. Herpetic gingivostomatitis contains herpes simplex virus I.
   D. Streptococcal gingivitis contains Streptococcus viridans and rarely beta-hemolytic streptococci
   E All of the above

90. Which of the following are examples of infections encountered in oral surgery?
    A. Herpes simplex infection
    B. Palatal infection
    C. Periorbital space infection
    D. Parotid capsule infection, external perforation through the buccinator muscle, buccal space infection, panfacial infection lateral to the mandible, panfacial infection medial to the mandible, subcutaneous infection, and subcutaneous anaerobic infection
    E. All of the above

91. Which of the following streptococcal microorganisms may cause dental caries?
    A. Streptococcus faecalis
    B. Streptococcus liquefaciens
    C. Streptococcus mitis
    D. Streptococcus salivarius, Streptococcus sanguis, and Streptococcus mutans
    E. All of the above

92. Dextranase is produced by which of the following oral bacteria?
    A. Streptococcus mutans
    B. Actinomyces
    C. Bacteroides
    D. Fusobacterium
    E. All of the above

93. Microorganisms gain entry into the pulp by which of the following routes?
    A. Direct access
    B. Direct access, pulpo-periodontal pathways, and bloodstream
    C. Pulpo-periodontal pathways
    D. Bloodstream
    E. None of the above

94. Which of the following microorganisms have been found in contaminated canals?
    A. Streptococci, Pneumococci, Staphylococci
    B. Gaffkya, Sarcinae, Lactobacilli
    C. Bacillus subtilis (cereus), Diphtheroids
    D. Neisseria, Pseudomonas, Escherichia coli, Veillonella, Bacteroides, Candida (Monilia), Actinomyces, Nocardia
    E. All of the above

95. On the average, a greater success rate of which of the following percentages can be achieved in endodontics when the canals are obturated only after negative cultures?
    A. 50%
    B. 80%
    C. 10%
    D. 1%
    E. None of the above

96. Which of the following represent disadvantages of culturing root canals?
    A. Need to purchase a bacteriologic incubator
    B. Need to purchase and stock culture media
    C. Inconvenience of taking, labeling, and reading cultures
    D. Inconvenience of recording culture results
    E. All of the above

97. Supragingival plaque grows by
    A. the addition of new bacteria
    B. the multiplication of bacteria
    C. the accumulation of bacterial products
    D. variation between individuals, on different teeth in the same mouth, and on different sites of the same tooth
    E. all of the above

98. Dental plaque is a common factor in the etiology of which of the following diseases?
    A. Periodontal disease (periodontitis)
    B. Dental caries
    C. Herpes simplex infection
    D. Periodontal disease (periodontitis) and dental caries
    E. None of the above

99. The incidence of asymptomatic carriage of type B hepatitis is
    A. 5%
    B. 10%
    C. less than 1%
    D. 20%
    E. none of the above

100. The treatment triad for successful endodontics has been
   A. debridement
   B. sterilization
   C. obturation of the root canal system
   D. debridement, sterilization, and obturation of the root canal system
   E. none of the above

101. The minimal acceptable requirements for an aseptic operating technique in endodontics includes which of the following?
   A. Knowledge and adherence to basic principles of surgical asepsis in endodontic treatment
   B. Proper application of the rubber dam
   C. Disinfection of the field of operation
   D. Use of sterile instruments and materials
   E. All of the above

3. PHYSIOLOGY

DIRECTIONS: Each of the questions or incomplete statements below is followed by five suggested answers or completions. Select the ONE that is best in each case.

102. Which of the following represent levels of organization of the human organism?
   A. Atoms
   B. Monomers
   C. Macromolecules
   D. Organelles, cells, tissues, organs, and organism
   E. All of the above

103. Which of the following represent physico-chemical criteria for rates of diffusion across cell membranes?
   A. Lipid solubility
   B. Hydrophilia
   C. Permeability coefficient
   D. Molecular size
   E. All of the above

104. Pinocytosis is
   A. phagocytoses
   B. cell drinking (an active transport process in which the carrier is the unit membrane)
   C. active secretion
   D. reabsorption
   E. none of the above

105. Which of the following are characteristics of the excitatory postsynaptic potential (EPSP)?
   A. Monophasic and nonpropagating
   B. Represents a depolarization which is localized to the soma of the motoneuron
   C. Is a potential which is not all-or-none since it can be augmented by increasing the intensity of the input volley
   D. EPSP's of different inputs can sum on a postsynaptic cell to produce a greater depolarization
   E. All of the above

106. Which of the following represents the results of the role played by acetylcholine in the transmission of nervous effects?
   A. Stimulation of the chorda tympani nerve to the salivary glands
   B. The liberation of acetylcholine from parasympathetic endings in the iris
   C. Acetylcholine as an intermediary of parasympathetic effects to the alimentary tract and bladder
   D. Liberation of acetylcholine from sympathetic preganglionic fibers, acetylcholine liberation during the discharge of adrenaline, and acetylcholine as the transmitter of effects to the sweat glands
   E. All of the above

107. An electromyograph is
   A. a measure of the cell body neuron
   B. a measure of the structure of mitochondria
   C. a measure of energy from high-energy bonds
   D. a high-gain amplifier with a preference of selectivity for frequencies in the range from about 10 to several thousand cps.
   E. None of the above

108. The functions of the body fluids and the requirements of individual cells are
   A. respiratory
   B. nutritive
   C. excretory
   D. maintenance of water content of the tissues and regulation of body temperature
   E. all of the above

109. The chief conditions associated with an elevated nonprotein nitrogen are
   A. adrenal insufficiency, dehydration
   B. infectious fevers, lobar pneumonia
   C. intestinal obstruction
   D. parathyroid intoxication, peritonitis, and renal insufficiency
   E. all of the above

110. The fluid within the cells or intracellular fluid amounts to
   A. 41% of body weight
   B. 50% of body weight
   C. 20% of body weight
   D. 65% of body weight
   E. none of the above

111. Edema has a variety of causes and is associated with which of the following?
   A. Cardiac edema
   B. Mechanical obstruction of veins
   C. Edema due to renal disease
   D. Inflammatory edema
   E. All of the above

112. The blood from different persons is classified into which of the following groups?
   A. A, B, and O
   B. A, B, AB, and O
   C. B, AB, and O
   D. A, AB, and O
   E. None of the above

113. The life span of the majority of lymphocytes is
   A. 50-60 days
   B. 100-120 days
   C. 5-10 days
   D. 200-250 days
   E. none of the above

114. According to the law of Laplace (T = PR) the tension (T) developed in the ventricular wall is
   A. related to the pressure developed within the cavity
   B. related to the circumference of the cavity
   C. related to the pressure developed within the cavity and to the radius of the cavity
   D. related to the diameter of the cavity
   E. none of the above

115. The reserve in heart rate is
   A. 100-110 beats/minute
   B. 60-80 beats/minute
   C. 160-180 beats/minute
   D. 130-140 beats/minute
   E. none of the above

116. The relation of coronary perfusion pressure to coronary flow is generally such that
   A. the calculated coronary resistance increases as the coronary flow rises
   B. the calculated coronary resistance remains unchanged as the coronary flow rises
   C. the calculated coronary resistance decreases as the coronary flow rises
   D. thère is elevation of right atrial pressure
   E. none of the above are true

117. Which of the following cutaneous reactions are believed to be produced by the same humoral mechanism?
   A. Burning and electrical stimulation
   B. Freezing only
   C. Burning, freezing, and electrical stimulation
   D. Burning only
   E. None of the above

118. The splanchnic circulation is represented by
   A. the mesenteric bed supplying the gastrointestinal tract
   B. the splenic bed
   C. the hepatic bed
   D. the mesenteric, splenic, and hepatic beds
   E. none of the above

119. Which of the following drugs have powerful vasoconstrictor effects upon the renal vessels?
   A. Antidiuretic hormone (ADH)
   B. Beta receptors
   C. Atropine and beta receptors
   D. Epinephrine and norepinephrine
   E. None of the above

120. Poisuille's law states
   A. that P = F/R
   B. that R = P/F
   C. that the volume (F) of blood flowing through a circulating system increases with the perfusing pressure (P) and decreases with the resistance (R) so F = P/R
   D. that the volume (F) of blood flowing through a circulating system decreases with the perfusing pressure (P) and increases with the resistance (R)
   E. none of the above

121. Which of the following are affections of rhythm due to impaired conduction through the A-V node and the bundle of HIS?
   A. Delayed conduction
   B. Missed heart beats
   C. Partial heart block
   D. Complete heart block
   E. All of the above

122. The most important measurement in the circulation is that of
   A. vagal tone
   B. volume flow of blood through the aorta or any vital region or organ
   C. extrasystoles
   D. sinus arrhythmia
   E. none of the above

123. Circulation time is
   A. the shortest time which a particle of blood takes to go from one point in the circulation to another
   B. 25 seconds from arm to tongue
   C. 50 seconds from arm to lung
   D. 50 seconds from arm to tongue
   E. none of the above

124. Which of the following indirect methods may be used for measuring human blood pressure?
   A. Palpatory and auscultatory
   B. Palpatory and oscillatory
   C. Oscillatory and auscultatory
   D. Palpatory, oscillatory, and auscultatory
   E. None of the above

125. Which of the following is the sequence of events of a cardiac cycle?
   A. Ventricular contraction, closure of mitral valve, "c" wave in atrial curve
   B. Left ventricular isometric or isovolumic contraction period, ventricle is a closed cavity, ventricular pressure exceeds the aortic pressure
   C. Aortic valves open, ventricle and aorta are common cavities
   D. Ventricular volume decreases, period of maximum ejection, beginning of incisura, end of ejection of blood and of ventricular systole
   E. All of the above

126. The principal factors entering into the production of the first heart sound are
   A. closure of atrioventricular valves and tension set up in the valve leaflets and chordae tendineae as the intraventricular pressure rises
   B. contraction of ventricular muscle
   C. rush of blood from the ventricles
   D. shock transmitted to the walls of the aorta and the pulmonary artery (vascular element)
   E. all of the above

127. With an occluded coronary artery branch
   A. most hearts die
   B. most hearts live 12 hours
   C. most hearts live 1 week
   D. most hearts survive indefinitely
   E. none of the above are true

128. Which of the following factors determine the cerebral blood flow?
   A. Cardiac output and total peripheral resistance
   B. Intracranial pressure
   C. Blood viscosity
   D. Vascular diameter
   E. All of the above

129. The maximum heart rate during maximum exercise is
   A. the same in the aged
   B. higher in the aged (200/minute in the 70-year-old)
   C. lower in the aged (160/minute in the 70-year-old)
   D. higher in the aged (100/minute in the 70-year-old)
   E. none of the above

130. The chief manifestations of chronic congestive heart failure are
   A. increased extracellular fluid volume
   B. increased blood volume
   C. elevated venous pressure
   D. dyspnea, cyanosis, enlargement of liver and spleen
   E. all of the above

131. The major problems of respiratory physiology are
   A. the uptake of oxygen from alveolar air and its delivery to the tissues
   B. the uptake of carbon dioxide from tissues and its delivery to the alveolar air
   C. mechanism of rhythmic inspiration and expiration
   D. the mechanism by means of which the amount of air breathed per minute is adjusted to the needs of the body
   E. all of the above

132. Which of the following laws govern the kinetic theory of gases?
   A. Boyle's law
   B. Avogadro's law
   C. Law of Charles (or Gay-Lussac)
   D. Dalton's law of Partial Pressures and Henry's law
   E. All of the above

133. During voluntary hyperventilation the alveolar tension of carbon dioxide
   A. rises and that of oxygen falls
   B. rises and that of oxygen rises
   C. falls and that of oxygen rises
   D. falls and that of oxygen falls
   E. none of the above are true

134. The oxygen content of blood is dependent upon
   A. gas volume
   B. the oxygen tension, but the relationship between these two variables is not linear (oxygen dissociation curve)
   C. dead space gas
   D. diffusing capacity
   E. none of the above

135. The oxygen dissociation curve describes the equilibrium between
   A. oxygen and carbon dioxide
   B. oxygen and hemoglobin
   C. oxygen and nitrogen
   D. oxygen and electrolytes
   E. none of the above

136. It is customary to refer to airway ventilation as
   A. alveolar spaces
   B. inspired volume
   C. free space
   D. dead space
   E. none of the above

137. Any increase in dead space (physiologic or anatomic dead space)
   A. decreases alveolar ventilation unless total ventilation is increased
   B. increases alveolar ventilation unless total ventilation is increased
   C. decreases alveolar ventilation unless total ventilation is decreased
   D. increases alveolar ventilation unless total ventilation is decreased
   E. is none of the above

138. Alveolar hypoventilation is invariably associated with
   A. resistance to diffusion
   B. elevated arterial and alveolar PCO_2
   C. anatomic shunts
   D. perfusion abnormalities
   E. none of the above

139. The muscles of respiration include
   A. the diaphragm
   B. the intercostal muscles
   C. motion of the ribs increases diameter of the chest
   D. the accessory muscles
   E. all of the above

140. The efficiency of the muscles of respiration can be calculated from
   A. interpleural pressures
   B. the Reynolds number
   C. the viscous resistance of the lungs
   D. the work they perform and the oxygen cost of doing this work
   E. none of the above

141. Dyspnea means
   A. hypernea
   B. increased pulmonary ventilation
   C. difficult breathing
   D. periodic breathing
   E. none of the above

142. Arterial hypoxia is characterized by
   A. a lower than normal PO_2 in arterial blood
   B. a higher than normal PO_2 in arterial blood
   C. a decreased rate of blood flow
   D. a decreased oxygen capacity of the blood
   E. none of the above

143. Asphyxia means
   A. hypoxia
   B. changes associated with acclimatization
   C. hypercapnia
   D. conditions in which hypoxia is combined with hypercapnia
   E. none of the above

4. PATHOLOGY

DIRECTIONS: Each of the questions or incomplete statements below is followed by five suggested answers or completions. Select the ONE that is best in each case.

144. The cardinal signs of inflammation are
   A. tumor, dolor, suppuration, calor, functio lasa
   B. dolor, calor, rubor, functio lasa
   C. tumor, suppuration, dolor, rubor
   D. tumor, dolor, rubor, calor, functio lasa
   E. none of the above

145. Suppuration in acute inflammation is
   A. productive or formative variety
   B. chronic inflammation
   C. softening of the tissues and the formation of pus
   D. subacute inflammation
   E. none of the above

146. Active hyperemia results from
   A. heat in mild degree and action of chemical irritants
   B. phagocytosis
   C. exudation
   D. productive or formative inflammation
   E. none of the above

147. Diapedesis is
   A. passage of red corpuscles through endothelium into tissues (aperture in vessel wall closes immediately)
   B. hemorrhage from vessel wall
   C. passage of fibrin through vessel wall
   D. passage of thromboplastin through vessel wall
   E. none of the above

148. Which of the following are varieties of inflammation?
   A. Catarrhal inflammation
   B. Fibrinous inflammation, suppurative inflammation
   C. Hemorrhagic inflammation, phlegmonous inflammation
   D. Necrotic inflammation, diphtheritic or pseudo-membrane inflammation
   E. All of the above

149. During resolution
   A. retrogression of the phenomena of inflammation occurs
   B. blood flow is not restored
   C. exudate is absorbed by blood vessels
   D. fibrin is not digested by leukocytes and thereafter absorbed
   E. none of the above happens

150. Acute inflammation is characterized by
   A. productive inflammation
   B. exudative inflammation
   C. proliferation of fixed cells of the part
   D. new formation of blood vessels
   E. none of the above

151. In primary tuberculosis
   A. bacilli cause only small lesions where they enter
   B. bacilli spread along the lymphatics draining the portal of entry
   C. regional lymph nodes become enlarged
   D. the focus of infection may be a local ulcer of the mucous membrane where bacilli penetrate into alimentary or respiratory tract
   E. all of the above are true

152. Acute miliary tuberculosis
   A. produces small tubercle nodules throughout the organs
   B. produces one tubercle nodule more fully formed with three giant cells
   C. produces tubercle nodules with caseation
   D. produces one tubercle follicle with giant-cell in process of formation apparently by fusion
   E. none of the above

153. Neoplasia
   A. serves a useful purpose
   B. is not autonomous in nature
   C. obeys the laws governing proliferative growth of cells
   D. is a new growth of tissue, autonomous in nature and serving no useful purpose
   E. is none of the above

154. Cancer
   A. arises de novo
   B. is not the result of a chemical alteration
   C. does not begin from a transformed single cell or small focus of cells
   D. does not arise de novo as a result of magic transformation
   E. is none of the above

155. The characteristics of malignant neoplasia at the tissue level are
   A. altered organization
   B. destructive invasion of adjacent non-neoplastic tissue
   C. heterotopia-reflecting distant metastasis
   D. proneness to necrosis, stimulation of nonseptic inflammatory reaction, and abnormal function
   E. all of the above

156. Pleomorphism means
   A. increased density of staining
   B. displacement from normal position
   C. variation in size and shape
   D. a reversal of the process of differentiation, i. e., dedifferentiation
   E. none of the above

157. Hyperplasia encompasses which of the following characteristics?
   A. occurs in direct response to an extracellular stimulus
   B. regresses when stimulus is removed
   C. cells are typical and organized
   D. involves multiple tissue elements, tends to be diffuse, and does not exhibit heterotopia
   E. all of the above

158. The primary lesion of syphilis or hard chancre appears on the external genitals
   A. without any incubation period
   B. after an incubation period of 3-4 days
   C. after an incubation period of 3-4 weeks
   D. after an incubation period of 3-4 months
   E. none of the above

159. Tertiary lesions of syphilis
   A. appear within the first year
   B. always appear within the first few years
   C. appear only after many years
   D. do not undergo gummatous change
   E. none of the above

160. In actinomycosis
   A. 25% of infection is in the appendix or cecal region
   B. 50% of cases produce lesions in the oral cavity and jaws
   C. in 15%, the initial site is in the lungs
   D. in 5%, the lesion is subcutaneous
   E. all of the above are true

161. Sarcoidosis
   A. is due to tubercle bacilli
   B. includes many clinically distinct conditions of which the underlying pathology appears to be similar
   C. is caseating proliferative tuberculosis
   D. is acute miliary infiltration of the lungs
   E. is none of the above

162. The process of healing begins by
   A. proliferation of cells and new formation of blood vessels
   B. absorption of tissue
   C. callus formation with trabecular woven bone
   D. formation of nervous tissue
   E. none of the above

163. Metaplasia
   A. is undifferentiation of tissues
   B. is anaplasia of cells
   C. is bone formation in organs and tissues
   D. is the transformation of one tissue into another
   E. is none of the above

164. The nutmeg liver indicates
   A. chronic venous congestion
   B. cyanosis
   C. anoxemia
   D. cyanotic induration
   E. none of the above

165. Carcinoma of the lung has which of the following characteristics?
   A. By far it is the most malignant neoplasm arising in the entire respiratory tract
   B. Its incidence has increased almost tenfold in the past 30 years
   C. It is the most common cause of death from cancer in the United States
   D. Death rate from carcinoma of the lung will reach one-quarter of all neoplasms within the next decade
   E. All of the above

166. Carcinoma of the breast usually metastasizes to
   A. brain, suprarenal glands, lung
   B. brain, lungs, liver, skeletal system
   C. brain, liver, suprarenal glands
   D. lungs, bones, suprarenal glands
   E. none of the above

167. Carcinoma of the prostate has which of the following characteristics?
   A. Is present in one of every five men over the age of 60 years
   B. Half of all males over 70 have it
   C. Many prostatic carcinomas in old men are latent
   D. It is curable if it is detected early
   E. All of the above are true

168. The major types of leukemia are
A. lymphocytic, myelocytic, and monocytic leukemia
B. plasma cell leukemia
C. lymphocytic and plasma cell leukemia
D. aleukemic leukemia
E. none of the above

169. Diseases caused by fungi have which of the following general characteristics?
A. Low invasiveness, low virulence, marked chronicity, and slow, indolent progression
B. High invasiveness
C. High virulence
D. Necrotic focus
E. None of the above

170. Malaria is characterized by which of the following?
A. Parasite produces asexually within the red blood cell
B. Parasite uses cellular material for their growth
C. Parasite causes damage by the deleterious effects of their metabolic by-products
D. The malarial by-products are pyrogenic
E. All of the above

171. Pneumoconiosis
A. is an infectious granuloma
B. is due to pathogenic mycobacteriae
C. is not a foreign body reaction
D. is a foreign body reaction due to inhalation of dusts
E. is none of the above

172. The infectious granulomas are dominated by which of the following responses?
A. Exudative response
B. Proliferative response
C. Fibrocaseous response
D. Epithelioid response
E. None of the above

173. Viruses and rickettsiae
A. multiply outside of living cells
B. multiply in necrotic cells
C. multiply intercellularly
D. multiply only within living cells
E. are none of the above

174. Infectious hepatitis
   A. follows parenteral introduction of serum containing type B virus
   B. follows parenteral introduction of serum containing type A virus
   C. follows ingestion of type B organisms
   D. follows ingestion of type A organisms
   E. is none of the above

175. Pyemia is
   A. a condition of bacteria in the blood stream
   B. a particular kind of septicemia with bacterial emboli in many organs and tissues
   C. a disease with bacteria in the blood stream
   D. a harmless bacteremia
   E. none of the above

176. Which of the following represent the collagen diseases?
   A. Polyarteritis nodosa
   B. Disseminated lupus erythematosus
   C. Rheumatic fever, rheumatoid arthritis
   D. Glomerulonephritis, anaphylactoid purpura, scleroderma, and dermatomyositis
   E. All of the above

177. Bronchiectasis means
   A. allergic hypersensitivity to foreign protein
   B. chronic catarrh
   C. a dilatation of the bronchi (generalized or localized)
   D. putrid bronchitis
   E. none of the above

178. Emphysema means
   A. the presence of bullae or abnormal spaces containing air
   B. excess of blood in pulmonary vessels
   C. chronic form of pulmonary edema
   D. hyaline membrane disease
   E. none of the above

179. Anemia, i.e., a reduction in the percentage of hemoglobin, is due to which of the following?
   A. Eosinophilia
   B. Increase of mononuclears, monocytosis
   C. Excessive loss or destruction of blood and failure of output
   D. Leukopenia
   E. None of the above

180. Subacute glomerulonephritis has which of the following characteristics?
   A. An exaggeration of the lesions seen in the acute phase
   B. Kidneys are enlarged, capsule strips easily leaving a smooth surface with irregular congested vessels and minute hemorrhages
   C. Glomeruli are enlarged and glomerular tufts are rich in nuclei, glomeruli have a lobulate or digitate form
   D. Extracapillary proliferation of the capsular epithelium is marked
   E. All of the above

181. Acute osteomyelitis has which of the following characteristics?
   A. Is produced by beta-hemolytic streptococcus and pneumococcus
   B. Necrosis of marrow with cellular reaction occurs
   C. Sequestrum, suppuration
   D. Irregular formation of new bone around the sequestrum
   E. All of the above

182. Ulcerative colitis
   A. has a distinct cause (single)
   B. has two distinct etiologic factors
   C. has no specific cause but it behaves as a distinct clinical and pathological entity
   D. is due only to vegetative amoebas
   E. is none of the above

183. Acute gastritis may be classified as
   A. acute catarrhal gastritis
   B. acute erosive gastritis
   C. membranous gastritis
   D. phlegmonous gastritis
   E. all of the above

184. Peptic ulcers have which of the following characteristics?
   A. Concerned with the action of the gastric juice
   B. Met with in parts exposed to the action of the gastric juice
   C. Are not infrequent in Meckel's diverticulum
   D. Are more common in males than females but the disease has shown a decreased incidence in recent years
   E. All of the above

185. Diverticulitis has which of the following characteristics?
   A. The interior of the diverticula is first affected
   B. General interstitial inflammation in the affected region of the colon develops with overgrowth of fibrofatty tissue
   C. It may cause a considerable segment of the bowel to become stiffened
   D. Ulceration and perforation, diffuse peritonitis, or localized abscesses may result
   E. All of the above

5. ORAL HISTOLOGY AND EMBRYOLOGY

DIRECTIONS: Each of the questions or incomplete statements below is followed by five suggested answers or completions. Select the ONE that is best in each case.

---

186. The primitive endoderm is formed from the
   A. embryonic disc
   B. amniotic cavity
   C. trophoblast
   D. primitive yolk sac
   E. blastocyst

187. The buccopharyngeal membrane is formed
   A. when the stomodeum ectoderm contacts the entoderm of the foregut
   B. from the primitive gut
   C. from the fifth branchial arch
   D. from the tuberculum impar
   E. from none of the above

188. The branchial arches are separated from each other by
   A. the stomodeum
   B. the prosencephalon
   C. the neural groove
   D. the ectodermal and entodermal grooves
   E. none of the above

189. In the development of the face, which of the following play a major role?
A. Lateral nasal process
B. Maxillary process
C. Mandibular process
D. Frontonasal process
E. All of the above

190. Each maxillary process forms a horizontal extension termed
A. the lateral nasal process
B. the internal nares
C. the median nasal septum
D. the palatal process
E. none of the above

191. The anterior two-thirds of the tongue develops from
A. the third arch mesenchyme
B. the copula
C. the hypobranchial eminence
D. the tuberculum impar and adjacent tissue
E. none of the above

192. The salivary glands arise from
A. the ectodermal germ layer
B. the entodermal germ layer
C. the ectodermal and entodermal germ layers
D. the oral mesenchyme
E. none of the above

193. The developing mandible grows backward (not surrounding Meckel's cartilage) to form
A. the incus and malleus
B. the otic capsule
C. the hyoid cartilage
D. the coronoid process
E. none of the above

194. Growth in length of the mandible is accomplished by growth of
A. Meckel's cartilage
B. the coronoid process
C. the temporomandibular joint
D. the condylar cartilage
E. none of the above

195. The beginning of the dental lamina occurs as
   A. a thickening of the oral epithelium
   B. a thickening of the lamina propria
   C. a thickening of the submucosa
   D. a downward growth of oral connective tissue
   E. none of the above

196. The bell stage of tooth development refers to
   A. dental lamina
   B. proliferation
   C. apposition of dental tissues
   D. histodifferentiation and morphodifferentiation
   E. none of the above

197. In the cap stage, which of the following cell types can be recognized in the enamel organ?
   A. Outer enamel epithelium, inner enamel epithelium, and stellate reticulum
   B. Outer enamel epithelium and inner enamel epithelium
   C. Outer enamel epithelium, inner enamel epithelium, and stratum intermedium
   D. Stellate reticulum and dental papilla
   E. None of the above

198. The formation of dentin
   A. is not a necessary stimulus for the formation of enamel
   B. is apparently a necessary stimulus for the formation of enamel
   C. decreases the blood supply
   D. is not based on tissue interdependence
   E. is none of the above

199. The ameloblasts
   A. do not cause the differentiation of odontoblasts
   B. play no role in tissue interdependence
   C. cause the differentiation of dentin-forming cells
   D. cause shrinkage of the stratum reticulum
   E. are none of the above

200. Amelogenesis
   A. requires matrix formation and maturation
   B. requires maturation only
   C. is farthest advanced in the area of the cervical loop
   D. is farthest advanced midway between the incisal edge and cervical loop
   E. is none of the above

201. What percent of the enamel consists of inorganic salts?
   A. 100%
   B. 96-98%
   C. 90-95%
   D. 85-90%
   E. None of the above

202. Predentin is
   A. a thin layer of homogeneous eosinophilic material laid down between odontoblasts and ameloblasts
   B. composed of Korff's fibers
   C. composed of membrana preformativa
   D. composed of the cell-free zone
   E. none of the above

203. After dentin and enamel formation have reached the cementoenamel junction, the cervical loop
   A. degenerates and disappears
   B. becomes transformed into the epithelial sheath of Hertwig
   C. forms the membrana preformativa
   D. forms the cell-free zone
   E. does none of the above

204. When the growing Hertwig's sheath approaches a nerve or blood vessel, the sheath
   A. vessel or nerve degenerates
   B. grows around the vessel or nerve
   C. degenerates and disappears
   D. grows through the center of the vessel or nerve
   E. does none of the above

205. The neonatal line is
   A. the result of reduced rate of formation of calcified tissues in the few days after birth
   B. rapidly erased in the enamel
   C. persistent in bone tissue
   D. the Hunter Schreger bands
   E. none of the above

206. Enamel rods are
   A. composed of one enamel globule
   B. arranged vertically in the cervix of deciduous teeth
   C. composed of 20 micra thick enamel globules
   D. composed of a number of 4 micra thick enamel globules
   E. none of the above

207. Enamel is
A. the only tissue whose formation does not cease
B. made up of 100% inorganic material
C. made up of 20% organic material
D. the only calcified tissue in mammals of epithelial origin
E. none of the above

208. The periodontal ligament arises from the
A. cementum
B. alveolar bone
C. middle portion of the dental follicle
D. secondary cementum
E. none of the above

209. Sharpey's fibers
A. arise from Hertwig's sheath
B. are collagen fibers of the dental follicle embedded in cementum
C. arise from the epithelial diaphragm
D. arise from the epithelial rests of Malassez
E. are none of the above

210. Cementum formation
A. is not a continuous process
B. always results in cellular cementum
C. is present in the dental follicle
D. is a continuous process
E. is none of the above

211. The dentinoenamel junction
A. is smooth
B. is not smooth
C. has an irregular surface which appears scalloped
D. consists of only concavities which face both dentin and enamel
E. is none of the above

212. Nasmyth's membrane
A. is a calcified and keratinized coating covering the enamel prior to eruption
B. contains fermentable carbohydrates and lactic acid
C. is the interprismatic substance
D. remains throughout life as a covering over the enamel surface
E. is none of the above

213. Enamel lamellae are
   A. imperfections filled with inorganic material
   B. enamel imperfections extending from the enamel surface to the dentinoenemal junction and sometimes into the dentin
   C. imperfections confined to the enamel only
   D. imperfections always extending into dentin
   E. none of the above

214. Surface enamel contains
   A. two or three times more zinc than does internal enamel
   B. the same amount of zinc as internal enamel
   C. much less zinc than internal enamel
   D. zinc, most of which is deposited after eruption
   E. none of the above

215. The addition of 1 part/million fluorine (F) to the drinking water causes
   A. an increment of about 300 part/million in surface enamel
   B. a decrement of about 100 part/million in surface enamel
   C. no change in F concentration in surface enamel
   D. an increase in aluminum in the surface enamel
   E. none of the above

216. Dentin consists of
   A. cells
   B. intercellular substances
   C. cementing substance
   D. cells, collagen fibers, and cementing substance
   E. none of the above

217. Tomes' fibers
   A. never produce branching odontoblastic processes
   B. lie without rather than within the dentin
   C. are calcospherites of dentin
   D. are odontoblastic processes which lie in dentinal tubules
   E. are none of the above

DIRECTIONS: Each group of questions below consists of lettered headings followed by a list of numbered words or statements. For EACH numbered word or statement, select the ONE heading that it is most closely associated with. Each lettered heading may be selected once, more than once, or not at all.

A. Calcospherites
B. Dental lymph
C. Sheath of Neumann
D. Odontoblasts
E. Tomes' fibers
F. Neonatal line
G. Cementing substance
H. Incremental lines of Von Ebner

218. Tissue fluid in dentinal tubules and dentin matrix

219. Rest periods between periods of dentin activity

220. Poorly calcified band representing dentin in the process of formation at birth

221. Globules present in interglobular dentin

222. Dentin immediately surrounding the tubules which has a darker staining quality

A. Sharpey's fibers
B. Cementoid
C. Cementicles
D. Acellular cementum
E. Canaliculi
F. Cementocyte
G. Secondary cementum
H. Cementum spikes

223. Is devoid of cells and occurs in the cervical and middle third of the root

224. Contains cells and occurs in the apical third of the root

225. Fiber bundles from periodontal ligament extending into the cementum

226. Fine canals extending from each lacuna in cementum

227. Uncalcified eosinophilic matrix of cementum

6. BIOCHEMISTRY

DIRECTIONS: Each of the questions or incomplete statements below is followed by five suggested answers or completions. Select the ONE that is best in each case.

---

228. Biochemistry for dental students covers which of the following topics?
- A. Chemistry of tissues and foods
- B. Chemistry of digestion and absorption
- C. Chemistry of respiration and tissue metabolism
- D. Chemistry of glands of internal secretion, blood and excretion, and physical chemistry of protoplasm
- E. All of the above

229. At equilibrium, all the components of the heavy phase are in dynamic equilibrium
- A. with weak electrolytes
- B. with all of the components in the light phase
- C. with the mean ionic activity coefficient
- D. with a binary electrolyte
- E. with none of the above

230. According to the mass law, the equilibrium equation for $AgCl \rightleftarrows Ag^+ + Cl^-$ is
- A. $\frac{Ag^+ . K}{Ag} = Cl$
- B. $\frac{Cl^- . K}{Ag} = Ag\ Cl$
- C. $Cl^- . K = Ag\ Cl$
- D. $\frac{[Ag^+].[Cl^-]}{[Ag\ Cl]} = K$
- E. None of the above

231. The new theory of Brönsted defines an acid as
   A. a substance that yields H^+ ions in solution
   B. a substance that yields OH^- ions in solution
   C. a substance that gives off protons (H^+ ions)
   D. a substance that yields NH_2^-
   E. none of the above

232. According to the Henderson-Hasselbach equation
   A. pH = log Ka
   B. pH = 4.73 + log Ka
   C. pH = pKa = log (salt/acid)
   D. $pH = 4.73 + \log \frac{5}{5}$
   E. none of the above are true

233. Buffers are of primary importance in
   A. regulating the pH of the fluids and tissues of living organisms
   B. weakly dissociated solutions
   C. completely dissociated solutions
   D. neutral solutions in water
   E. none of the above

234. A buffer functions efficiently
   A. over a wide pH range
   B. over a rather definite and limited pH range
   C. between pH 2 - 4
   D. between pH 8 - 10
   E. for none of the above

235. Osmotic pressure
   A. is diffusion of water through a membrane
   B. is the same as hydrostatic pressure
   C. is the pressure that must be put upon a solution to keep it in equilibrium with the pure solvent when the two are separated by a semipermeable membrane
   D. is measured by the glass electrodes
   E. is none of the above

236. Van't Hoff's law of osmotic pressure is described by which of the following?
   A. Osmotic pressure of a solution varies indirectly with the absolute temperature
   B. Osmotic pressure is not dependent on the number of dissolved molecules
   C. Osmotic pressure of a solution varies directly with the concentration of the solute in the solution
   D. Osmotic pressure is dependent upon the kind of molecules present
   E. None of the above

237. Viscosity
   A. never varies
   B. is given by a unit termed a dyne
   C. is fluidity
   D. is the resistance experienced by one layer of a liquid in moving over another layer
   E. is none of the above

238. Characteristics of lipids include which of the following?
   A. Solubility in ether (organic solvents)
   B. Solubility in chloroform (organic solvents)
   C. Presence of esterified fatty acids
   D. Utilizability by living organisms
   E. All of the above

239. Fatty acids are classified into
   A. saturated acids
   B. unsaturated acids
   C. branched-chain acids
   D. hydroxy acids and cyclic acids
   E. all of the above

240. The fatty acids of the human body fat are
   A. lauric, myristic
   B. palmitic, stearic
   C. tetradecenoic, hexadecenoic
   D. oleic, octadecadienoic
   E. all of the above

241. Which of the following are physical properties of the fats?
   A. Glycerides of lower fatty acids are somewhat soluble in water
   B. Glycerides of higher fatty acids are insoluble in water
   C. Specific gravity is generally lower than that of water
   D. The melting point of a fat
   E. All of the above

242. Waxes are
   A. esters of higher fatty acids and of higher monohydroxy alcohols
   B. unsaturated aldehyde acrolein
   C. palmito-deunsaturated
   D. glyceryl trioleate
   E. none of the above

243. Which of the following are physical properties of the lecithins?
   A. When purified they are waxy white substances
   B. They are soluble in fat solvents with the exception of acetone
   C. They are hygroscopic and mix well with water to form colloidal solutions
   D. They do not have definite melting points but decompose when heated
   E. They are all of the above

244. Sphingomyelins or phosphosphingosides
   A. yield upon hydrolysis the unsaturated nitrogen-containing alcohol sphingosine
   B. yield upon hydrolysis an aliphatic aldehyde
   C. yield upon hydrolysis a hydroxyproline
   D. yield upon hydrolysis a phosphatidic acid dimethyl ester
   E. do none of the above

245. Gangliosides are
   A. fatty acids
   B. hexoseamine
   C. sphingosine
   D. a class of carbohydrate-rich glycolipids
   E. none of the above

246. Cholesterol
   A. is the most abundant steroid as sterol cholesterol
   B. is found in all animal tissues but not in plant tissue
   C. is usually accompanied by dihydrocholesterol, and 7-dehydrocholesterol
   D. concentrations in tissues range from 0.01 to 10.0%
   E. are all of the above

247. Which of the following represent properties of cholesterol?
   A. When mixed with a fat or oil it enables the fat or oil to absorb relatively large amounts of water
   B. Forms water - in - oil emulsions
   C. Is used as the grease vehicle in preparation of ointments containing water-soluble constituents
   D. Is a poor conductor of electricity and has a high dielectric value; it is a good insulator against electric discharge
   E. All of the above

248. Carbohydrates
   A. are present in all animal tissues and tissue fluids, blood, and milk
   B. such as starch, dextrins, sucrose, and lactose or milk sugar are easily converted to the simple sugar, glucose, which is the primary carbohydrate utilized by body tissues
   C. as starches are abundant and widespread in grain, tubers, and roots
   D. as sucrose are present in nectar of flowers, fruits, and juices of various plants; glucose is the sugar of the blood and body fluids
   E. are all of the above

249. Concerning glucose
   A. muscles and other tissues remove glucose from blood to form glycogen
   B. blood glucose serves as the direct food for brain tissue
   C. other sugars are formed from blood glucose and combine with proteins and other substances to make essential tissue constituents
   D. it is oxidized perferentially by all the tissues of the body to provide energy
   E. all of the above are true

250. Which of the following represent simple sugars or monosaccharides?
   A. Trisaccharide
   B. Phenylhydrazine
   C. Hexoses and pentoses
   D. Compound carbohydrates
   E. None of the above

251. Oligosaccharides are composed of
   A. Monosaccharides
   B. lactose
   C. disaccharides, trisaccharides, and tetrasaccharides
   D. dextrins
   E. none of the above

252. The most important disaccharides are
   A. turanose and melibiose
   B. trehalose, sucrose
   C. fructose and galactose
   D. sucrose, lactose, and maltose
   E. none of the above

253. Concerning polysaccharides
   A. they are hydrolyzed by the group of enzymes called polysaccharidases
   B. some contain units that are derivatives of the monosaccharides
   C. they are readily hydrolyzed by mineral acids but are resistant to alkaline hydrolysis
   D. glycans is another term for polysaccharides
   E. all of the above are true

254. Dextrins
   A. formed from amylose do not have unbranched chains
   B. are not present in the leaves of starch-producing plants
   C. are produced by the partial hydrolysis of starches by acids or alpha- and beta-amylase
   D. are insoluble in water and their solutions gel as starch solutions gel
   E. are none of the above

255. Cellulose
   A. is the chief constituent of the fibrous parts of plants and the most abundant organic material in nature
   B. cereal straws contain 30-43% cellulose
   C. yields D-glucose as the final product of hydrolysis
   D. bacteria and lower forms possess enzymes, cellulases, capable of hydrolyzing cellulose
   E. is all of the above

256. Heparin
   A. is a blood anticoagulant present in liver, lung, thymus, spleen, and blood
   B. is a polymer of D-glucuronic acid and D-glucosamine
   C. has a molecular weight of 17,000-20,000
   D. is strongly acidic due to sulfuric acid groups and readily forms salts
   E. is all of the above

257. Which of the following are general properties of proteins?
   A. All proteins are polymers of amino acids
   B. Some proteins yield only alpha-amino acids when they are hydrolyzed
   C. Protein molecules are large and are often classed among the colloids
   D. All proteins contain C, H, O, N, and generally S
   E. All of the above

258. Which of the following represent physical properties of the amino acids?
   A. They are readily soluble in water and insoluble in alcohol and ether
   B. They are generally soluble in dilute acids and bases, in which they form the amino acid salts
   C. They possess a high melting point
   D. They are either sweet, tasteless, or bitter
   E. All of the above

259. Albumins
   A. are not products of both plants and animals
   B. are soluble in water, coagulated by heat, and usually deficient in glycine
   C. never contain carbohydrate residues
   D. do not have a conjugated nature
   E. are none of the above

260. Globulins
   A. constitute an important and widely distributed group of animal and plant proteins
   B. are soluble in pure water and insoluble in neutral solutions of salts of alkalies and acid
   C. are not precipitated from solution by half saturation with ammonium sulfate
   D. do not generally contain glycine
   E. are none of the above

261. Concerning myoglobin,
   A. the molecule is compact
   B. there are no channels through the molecule
   C. almost all the polar groups are on the surface
   D. the interior of the molecule is made up of nonpolar residues
   E. all of the above are true

262. Hemoglobin
   A. is four times larger than myoglobin
   B. is a spherical molecule formed by four subunits, which are identical in pairs
   C. conformation changes upon oxygenation
   D. conformation closely resembles that of myoglobin
   E. is all of the above

263. Collagen
   A. is a widely distributed connective and supportive protein
   B. appears to be a triple-chain coiled coil
   C. contains unusual links and cross-links such as intermolecular ester cross-links and links with carbohydrate
   D. extra stability and strength are conferred by winding into coiled coils
   E. is all of the above

264. The major types of nucleic acid are
   A. nuclear deoxyribonucleic acids
   B. messenger ribonucleic acids
   C. transfer or soluble ribonucleic acid
   D. ribosomal ribonucleic acids and viral nucleic acids
   E. all of the above

265. Enzymes
   A. are nonprotein substances
   B. are proteins
   C. do not act catalytically
   D. are not hydrolyzed by acid after protracted boiling
   E. are none of the above

266. Saliva
   A. is a secretion of the buccal accessory glands
   B. is a mixture of secretions from the submaxillary, sublingual, parotid glands, and buccal accessory glands
   D. is pure mucin
   E. is none of the above

267. Stimulation of salivary secretion is governed by
   A. reflex stimulation
   B. salivary secretion is not under hormonal control
   C. mechanical stimulation due to the presence of substances in the mouth
   D. chemical stimulation from action of substances on taste buds
   E. all of the above

268. Gastric juice is composed of
   A. 50% water and 50% organic substances
   B. 70% water and 30% inorganic substances
   C. 99.4% water and solids (organic substances and inorganic constituents)
   D. 25% water and 75% organic substances
   E. none of the above

269. The pH of pancreatic juice
   A. is acidic
   B. varies from 7 to 8
   C. is 9.5
   D. is 2.8
   E. is none of the above

270. Concerning bile,
   A. it is secreted continuously by the liver cells and stored in the gall bladder
   B. the ingestion of food and stimulants bring about emptying of the gall bladder into the intestines
   C. it contains liver secretion and constituents added by the mucosa of the gallbladder and biliary passages
   D. in the gall bladder, water and certain inorganic salts are absorbed
   E. all of the above are true

271. Porphyrins
   A. are breakdown products of heme
   B. are active succinate
   C. are glucuronides
   D. are intermediates in the synthesis of protoporphyrin of heme
   E. are none of the above

272. Concerning blood,
   A. it constitutes 6-8% of body weight
   B. it represents 66-78 ml/kg
   C. it represents of 2,000-2,900 ml/sq m
   D. it has a specific gravity of 1.060, viscosity of 3.6-5.3, and pH about 7.4 average
   E. all of the above are true

7. NUTRITION

DIRECTIONS: Each of the questions or incomplete statements below is followed by five suggested answers or completions. Select the ONE that is best in each case.

---

273. Dietary counseling
   - A. is an impractical-objective in a dental office today
   - B. is a practical biological technique that is available in a dental office today
   - C. has not been shown to be effective
   - D. cannot be put into action today
   - E. is none of the above

274. The caloric requirement consists of
   - A. the amount of energy required to maintain the organism in its minimal state
   - B. basal metabolism
   - C. the amount of energy required for the specific dynamic action of foods
   - D. the energy required for growth, repair, and physical activity
   - E. all of the above

275. Carbohydrates
   - A. are a source of dietary energy
   - B. act as starting materials for the synthesis of other compounds
   - C. play a role as part of the structure of other materials
   - D. supply the major portion of the energy of the diet
   - E. are all of the above

276. Glucose
A. is the least common of the carbohydrates
B. is the most common of the carbohydrates
C. is the most familiar sugar in domestic use
D. is the energy stored in most plants and seeds
E. is none of the above

277. The reason that starch may not be very cariogenic is
A. that the small starch molecule does not penetrate through the dental plaque as readily as di- and mono-saccharides
B. that starch remains in the inner layer of plaque
C. that the large starch molecule does not penetrate through the dental plaque as readily as di- and mono-saccharides
D. that starch cannot be washed away and eliminated
E. none of the above

278. Dental caries activity increases
A. with the interrupted consumption of sugar
B. when sweets are withdrawn from between-meal periods
C. indicate that the quantity of sugar consumed is the all-important factor
D. with consumption of sugar in sticky form between meals
E. because of none of the above

279. Lipids
A. are insoluble in water
B. are soluble in ether, chloroform, and benzene
C. contain or are combined with one or more fatty acids in natural state
D. are those compounds utilizable by or occurring in biological systems
E. are all of the above

280. Body protein is constantly being broken down to its constituent
A. carbohydrates
B. fats
C. keratin
D. amino acids
E. none of the above

281. Essential amino acid is defined as
   A. one that can be synthesized by the organism
   B. one that the organism cannot synthesize itself in sufficient quantities
   C. the proteolytic enzyme pepsin
   D. a carboxyl group
   E. none of the above

282. Calcium
   A. controls the permeability of all cell membranes
   B. regulates muscle irritability
   C. regulates nerve irritability
   D. plays a role in kidney function
   E. is all of the above

283. Iron deficiency anemia results in which of the following oral signs?
   A. Amyloid in tongue
   B. White tongue
   C. Fissures in labial commissures and superficial glossitis
   D. Iron storage disease
   E. None of the above

284. Fluoride reacts with the hydroxyapatite of teeth to form
   A. calcium fluoride
   B. potassium fluoride
   C. fluorapatite
   D. magnesium fluoride
   E. none of the above

285. Fluorosis is limited almost exclusively to
   A. the deciduous molars
   B. the permanent teeth
   C. the deciduous cuspids
   D. the deciduous incisors
   E. none of the above

286. The known fat soluble vitamins are
   A. vitamins A and D
   B. vitamins A, D, and K
   C. vitamins D and K
   D. vitamins A, D, E, and K
   E. none of the above

287. Vitamin A deficiency is characterized by
   A. growth failurc only
   B. growth failure, visual defects, inability to maintain the integrity of epithelial structures, and reproductive failure
   C. visual defects only
   D. inability to maintain the integrity of epithelial structures
   E. none of the above

288. In children, vitamin D deficiency
   A. retards the eruption of teeth
   B. causes keratinization of epithelium
   C. causes oral leukoplakia
   D. causes ankylosis of teeth
   E. is none of the above

289. Vitamin K deficiency results in
   A. pigmentation of the incisors
   B. loss of pigmentation of the incisors
   C. metaplasia of epithelial cells
   D. a defect in blood coagulation
   E. none of the above

290. The characteristic lip lesions of ariboflavinosis are
   A. cheilosis or angular stomatitis
   B. gingivitis
   C. stomatitis
   D. glossodynia
   E. none of the above

291. Two-thirds of all patients with pernicious anemia have
   A. microcytic anemia
   B. recurrent attacks of sore tongue
   C. Vincent's infection
   D. dermatitis
   E. none of the above

292. Ascorbic acid deficiency is characterized by
   A. loss of weight and appetite
   B. swollen and tender joints
   C. subperiosteal hemorrhage
   D. brittle bones and fracture
   E. all of the above

293. Which of the following minerals are required in the metabolism of the body?
   A. Calcium, iron, sodium, potassium, and cobalt
   B. Chlorine, phosphorus, sulfur, and molybdenum
   C. Magnesium, copper, iodine, and manganese
   D. Selenium and possibly chromium, bromine, and fluorine
   E. All of the above

294. In old age the caloric needs are
   A. higher than in middle years
   B. the same as in middle years
   C. the same as in childhood
   D. lower than in middle years
   E. none of the above

295. Infancy is
   A. the period of diminution in appetite
   B. the period of slowdown in growth
   C. the period of most rapid growth and development
   D. the period free of mineral requirements
   E. none of the above

296. With the exception of infancy, adolescence is the period of
   A. less rapid growth
   B. low nutritional needs
   C. moderate nutritional needs
   D. most rapid growth
   E. none of the above

297. Fad diets are commonly followed by some teenagers as
   A. nutritionally sound diets
   B. a means of weight control
   C. a means of gaining weight
   D. a means of acquiring mental alertness
   E. none of the above

298. During pregnancy the need for protein, minerals (particularly calcium), and vitamins are
   A. the same as for the nonpregnant woman
   B. decreased
   C. the same as those of infancy
   D. increased
   E. none of the above

299. The recommended dietary allowances during lactation are
   A. the lowest in adult life
   B. the same as for the teen-ager
   C. about the highest in adult life
   D. the average during adult life
   E. none of the above

300. Which of the following factors cause losses in nutrients during home preparation?
   A. Trimming
   B. Chopping
   C. Boiling
   D. Roasting and baking, frying, and leftover foods
   E. All of the above

301. Vitamin A deficiency is suggested by
   A. xerosis of skin and keratomalacia
   B. xerophthalmia
   C. nonpurulent conjunctival infection
   D. photophobia and night blindness
   E. all of the above

302. Clinical signs of protein deficiency are
   A. hair changes (color, texture, easily pluckable) only
   B. angular stomatitis
   C. keratomalacia
   D. papillary atrophy of the tongue
   E. none of the above

303. The most constant and significant consequence of infection is
   A. increased appetite
   B. decreased appetite
   C. no change in appetite
   D. unrelated to appetite
   E. none of the above

304. Obesity
   A. is not a risk factor associated with any disease
   B. is unimportant to the dentist
   C. may act as a risk factor associated with coronary heart disease
   D. is a disease in the strict sense of the term
   E. is none of the above

305. Obesity may occur in association with
   A. Cushing's syndrome only
   B hypothalamic brain tumor only
   C. insulinoma only
   D. Cushing's syndrome, hypothalamic brain tumor, and insulinoma
   E. none of the above

306. The symptoms of galactosemia are
   A. hepatosplenomegaly only
   B. cataracts only
   C. hepatosplenomegaly, cataracts, and mental retardation
   D. mental retardation only
   E. none of the above

307. The organic composition of bone is
   A. 10% collagen
   B. 23% collagen
   C. 5% collagen
   D. 60% collagen
   E. none of the above

308. The organic composition of dentin is
   A. 20% of its dry weight
   B. 10% of its dry weight
   C. 30% of its dry weight
   D. 3% of its dry weight
   E. none of the above

309. The chemical composition of cementum is obscure but is presumed to be similar to
   A. bone and dentin
   B. dentin only
   C. enamel
   D. secondary dentin only
   E. none of the above

310. Bone and enamel contain
   A. similar concentrations of magnesium
   B. lower concentrations of magnesium
   C. higher concentrations of magnesium
   D. no magnesium
   E. none of the above

311. Concretions removed from the salivary glands contain
   A. 40% mineral matter
   B. 80% mineral matter
   C. 60% mineral matter
   D. 95% mineral matter
   E. none of the above

312. The saliva is composed of
   A. mucin
   B. amino acids and vitamins
   C. minerals
   D. buffers
   E. all of the above

313. Fluoride
   A. definitely postpones the onset of carie'
   B. may only postpone the onset of caries
   C. does not postpone the onset of caries
   D. enhances the onset of caries
   E. is none of the above

314. In an initial carious lesion, fluoride
   A. fails to penetrate the partly demineralized enamel
   B. penetrates in a limited fashion into the carious lesion
   C. does penetrate the partly demineralized enamel
   D. does not react with the residual apatite crystals
   E. does none of the above

8. DENTAL ANATOMY

DIRECTIONS: Each of the questions or incomplete statements below is followed by five suggested answers or completions. Select the ONE that is best in each case.

---

315. The temporomandibular joint
    A. has a unilateral articulation with the cranium
    B. is a complex joint because an articular disc is interposed between the temporal bone and mandible
    C. has articular surfaces covered by hyaline cartilage
    D. is not influenced by the shape and position of the teeth
    E. is none of the above

316. The articulating surface of the temporal bone is situated
    A. anterior to the staphylion zygomaxillare
    B. anterior to the frontotemporale
    C. anterior to the tympanic bone on the squamous temporal comprising the articular fossa and articular tubercle
    D. posterior to the tympanic bone on the squamous temporal
    E. at none of the above

317. The articular disc is
    A. thinner at the periphery than at the center
    B. an oval, firm, fibrous plate thinner at the center than at the periphery
    C. thin at the posterior border
    D. full of blood vessels in the central area
    E. none of the above

318. The fibrous capsule of the mandibular joint
   A. unites with the temporomandibular ligament at the medial surface of the capsule
   B. is strengthened and united with the temporomandibular ligament at the lateral surface of the capsule
   C. is an oval plate of great firmness
   D. is located medially to the tympanic bone
   E. is none of the above

319. Which of the following ligaments are accessory ligaments of the temporomandibular articulation?
   A. Synovial capsule
   B. Mandibula lingula
   C. Intracapsular
   D. The sphenomandibular and stylomandibular ligaments
   E. None of the above

320. The opening movement of the mandible
   A. is a pure hinge movement
   B. is a pure sliding movement
   C. is neither a hinge or sliding movement
   D. is a combination of a hinge and sliding movement
   E. is none of the above

321. Centric position is
   A. when the mandibular musculature is at rest
   B. a pure hinge opening and closing of the mandible
   C. a position of total balance of the components of the masticatory organ
   D. all positions in which contact between some or all upper and lower teeth occur
   E. none of the above

322. The elevator muscles with retrusive power include which of the following?
   A. Masseter, medial pterygoid, and temporal muscles
   B. Geniohyoid muscle
   C. Digastric muscle
   D. Depressor muscles
   E. None of the above

323. Which of the following muscle pairs control mandibular movements and positions?
   A. Masseter and medial pterygoid muscles
   B. Temporal muscles
   C. Lateral pterygoid muscles
   D. Geniohyoid and digastric muscles
   E. All of the above

324. The depressor-retractor muscles of the mandible include the
   A. lateral pterygoid muscles
   B. masseter muscles
   C. temporal muscles
   D. geniohyoid and digastric muscles
   E. none of the above

325. The parotid duct opens into the oral vestibule
   A. opposite the first upper molar
   B. opposite the third upper molar
   C. at the level of the vestibule
   D. opposite the second upper molar
   E. at none of the above

326 The mucous membrane which covers the alveolar process to the necks of the teeth
   A. may be divided into the epimysium and fornix
   B. may be divided into the alveolar mucosa and gingiva
   C. is the tubercle of the oral mucosa
   D. is the transitional zone of the oral mucosa
   E. is none of the above

327. The soft palate is covered
   A. by a thick fold of mucosa containing an intricately arranged musculature
   B. by a thin layer of soft tissue
   C. by the vestibular gingiva
   D. by the narrow isthmus faucium
   E. by none of the above

328. The primary muscles of mastication with their actions are
   A. masseters (closure and some protrusion)
   B. temporals (closure and retraction) and digastrics (opening and retraction)
   C. lateral pterygoids (opening, protrusion, side to side movement)
   D. medial pterygoids (closure, protrusion, side to side movement)
   E. all of the above

329. The palatine bone
   A. determines the bony prominence of cheek
   B. consists of a horizontal plate (hard palate) and a vertical plate forming part of nasal cavity
   C. forms the lateral portion of the lower orbit
   D. lies between the orbital and nasal cavities
   E. does none of the above

330. Bilateral mental foramina are located
   A. below the premolar teeth
   B. below the lateral incisors
   C. below the cuspids
   D. distal to the first molar
   E. none of the above

331. Which of the following muscles are attached to the inner surface of the basal region of the mandible?
   A. Mylohyoid (mylohyoid ridge and line)
   B. Genioglossus (genial tubercle)
   C. Geniohyoid (genial tubercle)
   D. Digastric (lower border in chin region)
   E. All of the above

332. The mylohyoid muscle
   A. arises from the mylohyoid ridge on outer surface of mandible
   B. arises from the mylohyoid ridge on inner surface of mandible
   C. elevates the larynx
   D. fixes the lower jaw
   E. does none of the above

DIRECTIONS: Each group of questions below consists of lettered headings followed by a list of numbered words or statements. For EACH numbered word or statement, select the ONE heading that it is most closely associated with. Each lettered heading may be selected once, more than once, or not at all.

A. Parotid
B. Buccal glands
C. Sublingual gland
D. Incisive glands
E. Palatine glands
F. Submandibular gland
G. Lingual glands
H. Labial glands

333. A small group of glands found on the floor of the oral cavity close to the insertion of the lingual frenum

334. Small isolated mucous or mixed glands situated in the submucosa of the upper and lower lips

335. A round, biconvex body which occupies much of the digastric triangle

336. More numerous in the posterior part than in the anterior part of the cheek

337. Reaches medially to the styloid process and the muscles arising from it and upward to the external acoustic meatus which is situated in a groove of the gland

338. A long, flattened body situated close to the medial surface of the mandible which contains a shallow depression

A. Trigeminal nerve
B. Lacrimal nerve
C. Ophthalmic nerve
D. Maxillary nerve
E. Pterygopalatine nerve
F. Nasociliary nerve
G. Infraorbital nerve
H. Frontal nerve

339. This nerve is the intermediate branch of the maxillary nerve of the second trigeminal division

340. This is the second division of the trigeminal nerve and leaves the skull through a short horizontal canal

341. This nerve, the intermediate branch, is the strongest branch of the ophthalmic nerve

342. Arises with a larger sensory and a smaller motor root from the ventral surface of the cerebral pons at the boundary between its body and arm

343. The first division of the trigeminal nerve splits, immediately after reaching the orbit, into its three main branches

344. This is the external branch of the ophthalmic nerve

DIRECTIONS: Each of the following questions consists of a statement and a reason. Select

A if both the statement and the reason are correct and are related cause and effect
B if both the statement and the reason are correct but are not related cause and effect
C if the statement is correct but the reason is incorrect
D if the statement is incorrect but the reason is correct
E if both the statement and the reason are incorrect

---

345. It is a general rule that some of the lymph vessels which take their origin close to the midline cross to the other side because the median parts of the lips, tongue, and palate are drained to both sides.

346. The controversy as to the existence of lymph vessels in the dental pulp has been decided in a negative way because the lymph vessels draining the pulp and periodontal ligament have a common outlet.

347. The trigeminal nerve arises with a larger sensory and a smaller motor root from the ventral surface of the cerebral pons at the boundary between its body and arm because the origin is closer to the anterior or superior than to the posterior or inferior border of the pons.

348. The first trigeminal division, the ophthalmic nerve, courses anteriorly in the lateral wall of the cavernous sinus to the medial part of the superior orbital fissure, through which it enters the orbit because the second division, the maxillary nerve, is directed downward and forward.

349. A study of the complicated ramification of the sensory branches of the trigeminal nerve can be facilitated by subdividing each division into three sets of branches because each division sends fibers to the mucous membrane of the nasal or oral cavity.

350. The ophthalmic nerve, the first division of the trigeminal nerve, splits immediately after reaching the orbit into three main branches because the external branch of the lacrimal nerve runs anteriorly and laterally along the lateral border of the roof of the orbit toward the lacrimal gland and to the skin at the outer corner of the eye.

351. The maxillary nerve, the second division of the trigeminal nerve, leaves the skull through a short canal, the round foramen, because the anterior opening of the canal leads the first division into the pterygopalatine fossa.

352. The infraorbital nerve, the intermediate branch of the maxillary nerve, the first trigeminal division, continues the course of the main trunk anteriorly and slightly laterally because the infraorbital groove is roofed over to form the infraorbital canal which leads the infraorbital nerve through the infraorbital foramen to the superficial structures of the face.

353. The mandibular nerve, the first trigeminal division, is a mixed nerve which contains the entire motor portion because the mandibular nerve leaves the skull through the oval foramen and enters the infratemporal fossa.

354. The buccal nerve leaves the trunk of the mandibular nerve at its posterolateral circumference because in its first part it is combined with motor fibers which will constitute the anterior temporal and the lateral pterygoid nerves.

355. The inferior alveolar nerve, the intermediate branch of the mandibular nerve, the second trigeminal division, descends behind and slightly lateral to the lingual nerve between the two pterygoid muscles because it winds around the lower border of the medial pterygoid muscle, which separates the alveolar nerve from the mandibular ramus.

PART II

CLINICAL DENTAL SCIENCES

9. ORAL DIAGNOSIS AND TREATMENT PLANNING

DIRECTIONS: Each of the questions or incomplete statements below is followed by five suggested answers or completions. Select the ONE that is best in each case.

---

356. Oral diagnosis is
 A. executing proper and clear radiographs
 B. finding a tumor in the oral cavity
 C. the ability and skill of a clinician to detect, recognize, and know the nature of an abnormality
 D. examination of the areas surrounding the oral cavity
 E. none of the above

357. A successful clinician
 A. utilizes only clinical data
 B. utilizes only laboratory tests and procedures
 C. bases a diagnosis only on physical features
 D. must obtain data from clinical sources and laboratory tests and procedures and histopathology
 E. does none of the above

358. Laboratory diagnoses
 A. are necessary in order to resolve many diagnostic problems
 B. are unnecessary if clinical data is obtained
 C. are unnecessary when roentgenologic data are available
 D. are unnecessary when historical data are present
 E. are none of the above

359. Paget's disease of the maxilla and mandible can be diagnosed by
   A. means of clinical signs and symptoms
   B. means of a radiographic examination
   C. means of historical data
   D. means of clinical signs, radiographs, and laboratory findings
   E. none of the above

360. A differential diagnosis
   A. is based on the terminology of disease
   B. is based on the medical history
   C. is based on an understanding of many disturbances of development and growth of the oral and paraoral structures
   D. employs extensive and all-inclusive diagnostic procedures, i. e., the accumulation and study of all significant data
   E. does none of the above

361. Etiology is
   A. the treatment of disease
   B. the cause or causes of a disease
   C. how the disease develops, step by step
   D. the clinical sign of a disease
   E. none of the above

362. Pathogenesis is
   A. the histopathology of a disease
   B. the etiology of a disease
   C. how the disease begins, its step-by-step development, variances and behavior pattern, and final outcome
   D. the radiographic features, i. e., osteoblastic features of a disease
   E. none of the above

363. The medical history
   A. is not vitally important
   B. is essential in the evaluation of patients and is one of the most important aids in establishing a diagnosis
   C. is not affected by the competence of the interviewer
   D. is not affected by the ability of the patient to communicate
   E. is none of the above

364. The neck may be distorted due to
A. goiter, lymph node enlargement, and aneurysm
B. hemoptysis (coughing up blood)
C. orthopnea (shortness of breath)
D. bronchospasm (wheezing)
E. none of the above

365. Angina pectoris is characterized by
A. absence of pain following exercise
B. absence of pain following meals
C. absence of pain due to sudden change in environmental temperature
D. a dull, pressing pain in the retrosternal area lasting a few minutes
E. all of the above

366. Protrusion of the eyeballs (exophthalmos) is seen with
A. Horner's syndrome
B. ptosis (drooping of upper eyelid)
C. hyperthyroidism
D. miosis (narrow pupils)
E. none of the above

367. An abnormal protein of low molecular weight (Bence-Jones protein) is sometimes present in patients with
A. Horner's syndrome
B. multiple myeloma
C. hyperthyroidism
D. Parkinson's disease
E. none of the above

368. Glucose in the urine
A. indicates porphyria
B. indicates hypercalcemia
C. indicates polycythemia
D. reflects elevation of the blood glucose concentration
E. is none of the above

369. The white blood cell count is elevated in
A. infection
B. primary polycythemia
C. leukemia
D. tissue necrosis
E. all of the above

370. In blood typing the main groups include
   A. A, B, AB, and O
   B. A, B, O
   C. B, AB, and O
   D. AB and O
   E. none of the above

371. The dry socket (alveolar osteitis)
   A. produces severe pain which radiates widely
   B. produces dull pain
   C. produces a localized pain (transient)
   D. produces minimal or no pain
   E. does none of the above

372. Metabolic bone disease
   A. refers to those generalized skeletal disorders resulting from alterations in mineral metabolism or in production of bone matrix
   B. is due to deficiency of fat-soluble vitamins
   C. is due to deficiency of dihydrotachysterol
   D. is due to thyrocalcitonin
   E. is none of the above

373. Osteoporosis is accompanied by
   A. elevated serum calcium
   B. a decrease in serum phosphorus
   C. normal serum concentrations of calcium, phosphorus, and usually alkaline phosphatase
   D. elevated serum alkaline phosphatase
   E. none of the above

374. Hypoparathyroidism is accompanied by
   A. paresthesia and muscular cramps
   B. convulsions
   C. gastrointestinal disturbances, respiratory symptoms, and neurologic disturbances
   D. psychoneurosis and psychosis and trophic disturbances in skin, hair, and nails
   E. all of the above

375. Diabetes mellitus produces which of the following effects on the oral structure?
   A. Dry mouth
   B. Burning oral mucosae
   C. Recurrent gingival or periodontal abscesses
   D. Rapidly progressive periodontal breakdown in young adults
   E. All of the above

376. Pregnancy gingivitis occurs in
   A. 10-20% of all pregnant women
   B. 35-50% of all pregnant women
   C. 50-70% of all pregnant women
   D. 60-80% of all pregnant women
   E. none of the above

377. Which of the following varieties of histiocytoses are recognized?
   A. Hand-Schüller-Christian disease and eosinophilic granuloma
   B. Acute or subacute disseminated reticulosis (Letterer-Siwe disease), chronic disseminated reticulosis (Hand-Schüller-Christian disease), and localized reticulosis (eosinophilic granuloma)
   C. Letterer-Siwe disease and Hand-Schüller-Christian disease
   D. Eosinophilic granuloma and Letterer-Siwe disease
   E. None of the above

378. Letterer-Siwe disease has the following features
   A. An acute, severe, and widespread proliferation of cells of the reticuloendothelial system
   B. Disease occurs within the first two years of life
   C. Disease runs a rapid, fulminating course and terminates fatally in a short period of time
   D. Disease affects liver, spleen, lymph nodes, skin, lungs, and bone marrow
   E. All of the above

379. Hand-Schüller-Christian disease has which of the following clinical findings?
   A. Discrete oval or round radiolucencies in the jaws and skull
   B. Diabetes insipidus
   C. Exophthalmos
   D. Mucosal or skin lesions
   E. All of the above

380. Amelogenesis imperfecta has which of the following characteristics?
   A. A developmental disturbance of enamel formation
   B. Affects all teeth, both deciduous and permanent
   C. Involves enamel matrix formation and calcification
   D. Crown of teeth, may on occasion, be totally devoid of enamel
   E. All of the above

381. Dentinogenesis imperfecta has which of the following characteristics ?
   A. A developmental disturbance of dentin formation in deciduous and permanent teeth
   B. Disturbance affects mesodermal component of tooth only (enamel is sound)
   C. Disease is a dominant hereditary characteristic with no sex linkage
   D. Teeth have a translucent or opalescent appearance and a gray to bluish brown color
   E. All of the above

382. Periodontosis
   A. Is marginal gingivitis in young adults
   B. Occurs only in adolescent males
   C. Is operculitis (pericoronitis)
   D. Is demonstrated by a peculiar and extensive destruction of the attachment apparatus in adolescents or young adults, mostly females
   E. Is none of the above

383. The clinical features of osteomyelitis are
   A. of an acute or sudden onset
   B. intense pain with enlargement of the affected bone
   C. pus draining spontaneously from around the necks of many teeth
   D. generalized systemic toxic symptoms
   E. all of the above

384. The theory of focal infection
   A. is not tenable in cases of subacute bacterial endocarditis
   B. is tenable in all dental infections
   C. is tenable in cases of subacute bacterial endocarditis
   D. says elimination of any dental infection will cure a systemic disease
   E. is all of the above

385. Mandibular fractures show which of the following characteristics?
   A. Mandible is more frequently fractured than any facial bone
   B. Bilateral fractures may result from a single blow
   C. Pain is elicited by palpating the fracture site and upon chewing
   D. Masticatory force is markedly reduced in cases of complete fracture
   E. All of the above

386. The dentist must be alert to the presence of which of the following cardiovascular diseases in his patients?
   A. Rheumatic fever
   B. Subacute bacterial endocarditis
   C. Arteriosclerotic heart disease
   D. Hypertension and congestive heart failure
   E. All of the above

387. Which of the following dermal lesions are accompanied by oral manifestations?
   A. Lichen planus, pemphigus vulgaris
   B. Erythema multiforme, Behcet's disease, and Reiter's syndrome
   C. Benign mucous membrane pemphigoid, nevi (nonpigmented and pigmented nevi)
   D. Lupus erythematosus and scleroderma
   E. All of the above

388. The reversible oral keratotic lesions include
   A. pachyderma oralis, leukoedema, and mild leukoplakia
   B. "mild" leukoplakia
   C. speckled leukoplakia
   D. erythroplakia
   E. none of the above

389. The dentist may have to deal with which of the following allergic reactions?
   A. Contact allergies (delayed hypersensitivity)
   B. Angioneurotic edema
   C. Serum sickness
   D. Anaphylaxis
   E. All of the above

390. The role radiology plays in oral diagnosis is
  A. exploring the radiographic features of the lesions
  B. determining the size and shape of the lesion
  C. determining the margins of the lesion and the reaction of the surrounding bone tissue
  D. determining the radiopacity of the lesion (radiolucent or radiopaque)
  E. all of the above

391. Criteria for successful interpretation of radiographs include
  A. radiographic technique must be precise
  B. radiographic apparatus must be of good quality
  C. film must be reliable and properly stored away from chemicals and irradiations
  D. care should be taken over processing to avoid faulty development and fixation
  E. all of the above

392. Jaw lesions are varied but may be classified under which of the following headings?
  A. Odontogenic lesions
  B. Inflammatory bone disease
  C. Noninflammatory bone disease
  D. Fibro-osseous lesions and nonodontogenic neoplasms
  E. All of the above

393. The inflammatory and cystic odontogenic lesions of the jaw include
  A. dental granuloma, radicular cyst
  B. residual cyst, apical scar
  C. dentigerous cyst, traumatic cyst
  D. lingual mandibular bone cavity (latent bone cyst)
  E. all of the above

394. The patient who has bruxism should wear which of the following at night?
  A. Hawley-type appliance only
  B. Full occlusal splint only
  C. Double full occlusal splint only
  D. Hawley type appliance, full occlusal splint, or double full occlusal splint
  E. None of the above

395. The only clinical criterion available to test the efficacy of occlusal equilibrations is
   A. pocket depth
   B. mucogingival line
   C. mobility
   D. the presence of calculus on tooth
   E. none of the above

396. Diagnostic casts for study are usually prepared for cases of
   A. extensive restorative work
   B. orthodontic treatment
   C. occlusal discrepancies
   D. assessment of growth and development patterns and abnormal mineralizations patterns
   E. all of the above

397. Treatment planning for patients with a full complement of teeth includes
   A. operative
   B. operative and orthodontics
   C. endodontics, operative, and periodontics
   D. surgery, endodontics, periodontics, operative, fixed partial prosthodontics, or removable partial prosthodontics
   E. all of the above

398. Treatment planning for patients with a partial complement of teeth includes
   A. surgery, endodontics, operative, fixed and removable prosthodontics
   B. surgery, endodontics, operative, fixed and removable prosthodontics where periodontics will occupy the major part of operator's time
   C. prosthodontics only
   D. edentulous patients (surgery and prosthodontics)
   E. all of the above

399. Balanced occlusion refers to
   A. canine protection
   B. bilateral balance seen in complete denture service and bilaterally free and partial denture
   C. unilateral balance seen in complete denture service
   D. group protection
   E. none of the above

400. Vertical dimension may be maintained by
   A. restoring all four molars first and wating for an appropriate period before undertaking a full mouth approach and placing restorations in alternate quadrants and wating until they feel "natural"
   B. removing malpositioned third molars
   C. group protection
   D. a progressive Bennett movement
   E. none of the above

401. Which of the following considerations should always precede the construction of a prosthesis?
   A. Will the patient accept the prosthesis and utilize it in the manner it was intended? What is the projected oral hygiene of the patient?
   B. Should it be a fixed prosthesis? How long is the span?
   C. What is the condition of the abutment teeth: caries, periodontal involvement, or extensive old restorations?
   D. What will be the design of the prosthesis? What are the psychological, dental education, and economical profiles of the patient?
   E. All of the above

402. One of the important aspects of diagnosis is
   A. palpation, a step often neglected
   B. radiography
   C. hyperocclusion
   D. laboratory studies
   E. none of the above

403. Percussion is a useful modality in determining the presence of
   A. abnormal occlusion
   B. inflammation in the periodontal space
   C. fistula
   D. hypocclusion
   E. none of the above

404. Innovative treatment (tooth-supported dentures and retentive clip bar) is specifically indicated for the dental patient who demonstrates
   A. excessive loss of supporting bone regardless of etiology
   B. a widely divergent maxillomandibular relationship
   C. unfavorable anatomical position of muscle attachments and a large tongue which reduces stability of a conventional prosthesis
   D. anticipated lack of psychological adaptation to the acceptance of conventional complete denture service, a history of poor tissue tolerance to normal occlusal forces, and a systemic condition in which extractions would present a risk to the patient
   E. all of the above

405. One advantage for dental patients when using tooth-supported dentures with telescopic crowns is
   A. the flexibility incorporated in the event that a supporting tooth is lost
   B. the absence of flexibility in the event that a supporting tooth is lost
   C. lack of retentive quality
   D. patient disapproval
   E. none of the above

406. The obvious problems in implantology include which of the following?
   A. The profession has turned its head away from the field far too long
   B. People who need implants have insufficient bone to support an implant
   C. The oral cavity is less than ideal for maintaining an area free of epithelial invagination
   D. Implantology has been performed and insufficient attention was given to the manner in which the superstructure was fabricated
   E. All of the above

407. The contraindications for implants are
   A. systemic disease (collagen disturbances)
   B. insufficient bone to support implants
   D. patients who lack education and economic resources; and psychologically unfit patients
   E. all of the above

408. Which of the following represents the types of implants employed today?
   A. Blade implants-intrabony, tripod pin-intrabony (Scialom)
   B. Screw pin-endosseous, mattress type-subperiosteal (Chercheue), polymer (Hobish)
   C. Intramucosal inserts, transosseous
   D. Endosseous endodontic stabilizer, ramus implant
   E. All of the above

409. The process of maintenance and continual reappraisal (diagnosis)
   A. should be perpetual
   B. should be periodic
   C. should be perpetual, periodic, and performed with purpose
   D. should be performed with purpose
   E. should be none of the above

410. Patient-related factors in any decision of diagnosis include which of the following?
   A. General systemic health (extraoral and intraoral soft and hard tissues)
   B. An estimation of the patient's degree of desire and knowledge of the value of saving teeth
   C. Psychological status of the patient
   D. Does the patient have adequate time to have the treatment completed? Does the patient have access to financial resources? Is there an assessment of the patient's acceptance of the dentist?
   E. All of the above

411. Extraction of any teeth within an area receiving radiation therapy
   A. increases the likelihood of osteoradionecrosis
   B. is not satisfactory as endodontic therapy for these teeth
   C. is not satisfactory as apicoectomy for these teeth
   D. is undertaken in order to lessen the likelihood of osteoradionecrosis and radiation necrosis caries
   E. is none of the above

412. The retention and stability of complete dentures
   A. is not related to bony spicules or projections
   B. cannot be obtained without proper preprosthetic surgery
   C. can be obtained without proper preprosthetic surgery
   D. is based on the fact that all undercuts which directly interfere with denture insertion and removal should be removed
   E. is none of the above

413. The ability of oral tissues to support dentures is greatly dependent on
   A. the health of the oral tissues, which is affected by the general health of the individual
   B. the mental attitude of the patient toward prosthetic treatment
   C. the size, shape, and relationship of the jaws
   D. the degree of irritation imposed by the artificial appliances
   E. all of the above

414. The oral tissues are constantly exposed to
   A. mechanical agents
   B. thermal agents
   C. mechanical, thermal, and bacterial agents
   D. bacterial agents
   E. none of the above

415. Case presentation
   A. is unnecessary because of the high intelligence of modern patients
   B. is useful in 50% of patients
   C. refers to the conference that takes place between the patient and the dentist concerning the number of appointments and cost of the treatment
   D. should be utilized in 10% of patients
   E. is none of the above

416. According to Wolff's pathophysiology of pain, which of the following are pain-sensitive structures of the head?
   A. Tissues covering the cranium and great venous sinuses from the surface of the brain, the dural and cerebral arteries, and the fifth, ninth, and tenth cranial nerves and upper three cervical nerves
   B. Fifth, ninth, and tenth cranial nerves
   C. Upper three cervical nerves
   D. Intracranial structures
   E. None of the above

17. When a patient with overt bruxism has minor occlusal interferences combined with severe psychic tension, then psychotherapy
    A. is usually necessary
    B. is usually unnecessary
    C. cannot reestablish occlusal compatibility
    D. cannot affect parafunctional masticatory muscle activity which is not the result of various combinations of stimuli from voluntary or involuntary tension-relieving habits
    E. does none of the above

418. The occlusal forces that are generated during physiologic mandibular functions are
    A. of high magnitude
    B. of long-term but low magnitude
    C. of short-term and of low magnitude
    D. of short-term and high magnitude
    E. none of the above

419. Occlusal disharmony may result from
    A. premature contacts occuring in the following mandibular positions (centric relation, centric occlusion, working and balancing sides, lateral protrusive, and protrusive)
    B. iatrogenic causes (restorations, orthodontic therapy, occlusal equilibration, and extractions)
    C. developmental disturbances (incongruous arch forms, incongruous tooth forms, anodontia, and supernumerary teeth)
    D. malpositions of individual teeth (mesioversion, distoversion, labioversion or buccoversion, linguoversion, supraversion, infraversion, transversion, axiversion, and torsiversion
    E. all of the above

420. A cardinal rule of thumb is to limit the increase in vertical opening between the anterior incisors to a maximum of
    A. 2 mm
    B. 1 mm
    C. $1\frac{1}{2}$ mm
    D. 3 mm
    E. none of the above

421. Any infringement on the free way space results
   A. in resorption of the residual ridge which is of a reversible nature
   B. in no irritation and trauma
   C. in irritation and trauma to the mucosal bearing surfaces while the long-term effect is irreversible resorption of the residual ridge
   D. in reversible irritation and resorption of the residual ridge
   E. in none of the above

422. Occasionally during treatment of acute cases of the masticatory muscle pain-dysfunction syndrome with a palatal bite plate
   A. an exacerbation of the presenting symptoms does not occur
   B. an exacerbation of the presenting symptom will occur
   C. the syndrome is resolved
   D. pain is completely eliminated
   E. none of the above happens

423. As a rule, balancing side occlusal contacts
   A. are very necessary for optimal masticatory function
   B. may or may not be necessary for optimal masticatory function
   C. is not indicated in partial dentures
   D. are not necessary for optimal or normal masticatory function
   E. is none of the above

424. Condylar positions and movements can be extremely variable and therefore difficult to register and reproduce
   A. as long as the opposing teeth are in occlusal contact
   B. since movements on one side do not affect movements on the other side
   C. as long as the opposing teeth are not in occlusal contact
   D. while a translatory movement is present
   E. for none of the above reasons

425. In the so-called terminal hinge position
   A. only feasible reproducible mandibular positions occur when translation is completely blocked and condylar rotation is permitted
   B. only one condyle is in its posterior and cranial position
   C. one condyle is stabilized by the ligaments and structures of the temporomandibular joint
   D. positional relationship is not bone-to-bone
   E. none of the above is true

426. In centric relation
   A. there is a fuzziness and a break in the lamina dura
   B. the positional relationship (mandible to maxilla) is intentionally independent of the guiding influence of the occlusal surfaces
   C. the positional relationship is not independent of the guiding influence of the occlusal surfaces
   D. masticatory musculature is not free of any asynergy or hypertonicity
   E. none of the above are true

427. Centric relations
   A. occur when one condyle is in the terminal hinge position
   B. are due to horizontal and vertical vectors
   C. occur when mandibular closure occurs with both condyles in the terminal hinge position
   D. are a neuromuscular response
   E. are none of the above

428. Interferences between centric relation and centric occlusion are usually removed
   A. by decreasing the width and depth of the involved fossae
   B. by increasing the width and decreasing the depth of the involved fossae
   C. by increasing the width and depth of the involved fossae
   D. by decreasing the width and increasing the depth of the involved fossae
   E. by none of the above

429. Protrusive movement
   A. is not a border movement
   B. is a border movement
   C. is not important if malposed molars are present
   D. is related to interior group function
   E. is none of the above

430. A rule of thumb concerning irreversible selective grinding is
   A. maximize all grinding procedures
   B. if in doubt go ahead and grind cautiously
   C. grinding procedures are fully compensated for, although they are irreversible
   D. minimize all grinding procedures and when in doubt do not grind
   E. none of the above

431. The most common primary prematurity is
   A. the mesiolingual aspect of the buccal cusp of the maxillary first bicuspid
   B. on the maxillary first molar
   C. on the lower anterior teeth
   D. the mesiolingual aspect of the lingual cusp of the maxillary first bicuspid
   E. none of the above

432. The second most common prematurity is
   A. the mesiolingual aspect of the lingual cusp of the maxillary first bicuspid
   B. the maxillary first molar
   C. the mesiolingual aspect of the buccal cusp of the maxillary first bicuspid
   D. the mandibular anterior teeth
   E. none of the above

433. Radical alveolectomy means
   A. removal of alveolar bone
   B. removal of buccal plate
   C. that a major portion of the alveolus is removed
   D. removal of interradicular septa
   E. none of the above

434. Radical alveolectomy
   A. does not lead to excessive ridge resorption
   B. reduces postextraction healing time in half
   C. produces an excellent dental ridge
   D. leads to excessive ridge resorption
   E. is none of the above

435. Denture hyperplasia
   A. may occasionally be associated with chronic ulceration and frank malignancy
   B. is never associated with ulceration
   C. is never associated with malignancy
   D. should not be surgically removed
   E. is none of the above

436. Senescence is
   A. the result of some malignant regressive aging changes
   B. not the result of progressive aging changes
   C. the result of some benign regressive aging changes
   D. the development of hardy perenials who live to 100 years of age
   E. none of the above

437. Senescence is accompanied by
   A. use of bifocal glasses to counteract presbyopia
   B. hearing loss (presbycusis)
   C. slower gait (fibrosis of muscles)
   D. loss of moisture, fat, and elasticity from soft tissues and reduction of skeletal bone mass
   E. all of the above

438. Psychologically many geriatric patients
   A. notice an increase of immediate memory
   B. remember no remote incidents
   C. notice a loss of immediate memory
   D. never fabricate occurrences to make a story acceptable
   E. are none of the above

439. Geriatric patients are vulnerable to
   A. heart disease, diabetes, and arthritis
   B. cerebrovascular accidents
   C. cancer and hypertension
   D. atherosclerosis and respiratory disorders
   E. all of the above

440. In geriatric dentistry it is important for the dentist to observe
 A. the patient's constitution
 B. posture
 C. gait
 D. complexion and many other signs that might have some implications in dentistry
 E. all of the above

441. Aging changes are to be seen in
 A. perioral structures
 B. occlusion
 C. individual teeth
 D. oral soft tissues, jawbones, and saliva
 E. all of the above

442. Failure of the salivary flow in geriatric patients
 A. may be due to hypertrophy of the salivary glands
 B. may be due to xerostomia
 C. may be due to atrophy of the salivary glands
 D. may be due to the new phenomenon in dental caries in the advanced ages
 E. is none of the above

443. Oral diagnosis
 A. is the art of using scientific knowledge to identify oral disease processes and to distinguish one disease from another
 B. is the use of subjective symptoms
 C. is the use of signs
 D. is the use of objective findings
 E. is none of the above

444. Radiation injuries to the oral tissues include
 A. postradiation dermatitis and stomatitis
 B. pigmentation changes
 C. loss of skin appendages and salivary gland function
 D. radiation caries, incomplete tooth development, and osteoradionecrosis and/or carcinoma
 E. all of the above

445. The temporomandibular joint pain dysfunction syndrome (myofascial pain-dysfunction syndrome) has which of the following characteristics?
   A. Discomfort in the region of TMJ; pain of a chronic nature; discomfort is most intense upon arising and diminishes during the day
   B. Rarely does the syndrome occur in edentulous patients; many patients are females, 30-50 years of age; both sexes are involved; apprehension and emotional tension afflict women during the fifth and later decades of life; hysteria sometimes is present
   C. A person who is predisposed to suffer the pressures of day-to-day living in a stressful period of life may develop the syndrome; clicking in TMJ and trismus causes fears to heighten
   D. The oral region is exceptionally sensitive; emotional tension is common in subjects; excessive occlusal attrition may be observed, and there may be clenching or grinding of the teeth; bruxism may be present; etiology of discomfort appears to be related to prolonged involuntary overcontraction of the muscles of mastication and gives rise to pain within the muscles; minor abnormalities of the occlusion of the teeth are only contributing factors
   E. All of the above are true

446. Which of the following neuralgias are of importance to the dental practitioner?
   A. Neuritis, neuralgia
   B. Trigeminal neuralgia (tic douloureux)
   C. Sphenopalatine ganglion neuralgia (Sluder's headache)
   D. Glossopharyngeal neuralgia
   E. All of the above

447. Which of the following represent keratotic lesions of the skin?
   A. Psoriasis
   B. Pachyonychia congenita
   C. Keratoacanthoma, verruca vulgaris (wart)
   D. Seborrheic keratosis, molluscum contagiosum
   E. All of the above

448. The collagen diseases which affect the face and skin include
A. periarteritis nodosa (polyarteritis)
B. Wegener's granulomatosis
C. scleroderma
D. lupus erythematosus, dermatomyositis
E. all of the above

449. Which of the following represent malignant salivary gland neoplasms?
A. Malignant pleomorphic adenoma (malignant mixed tumor)
B. Adenocystic carcinoma (cylindroma, basaloid mixed tumor)
C. Mucoepidermoid carcinoma, epidermoid carcinoma
D. Adenocarcinoma, acinic cell adenocarcinoma, malignant stromal tumors of salivary glands
E. All of the above

450. Causes of xerostomia (dry mouth) include
A. aplasia of salivary glands
B. x-ray irradiation
C. sialadenitis
D. Mikulicz's syndrome; sjögren's syndrome (benign lymphoepithelial lesion)
E. all of the above

451. Macroglossia is a frequent finding during
A. cretinism or infantile myxedema
B. mongolism, acromegaly
C. gargoylism
D. glycogen storage disease
E. all of the above

452. Multiple myeloma has which of the following characteristics?
A. A malignant neoplasm arises primarily in bone and reveals the classic "punched-out" radiolucency without a distinct cortical border
B. It occurs predominantly in males in their fourth decade of life or later
C. The chief symptom is bone pain and occasionally pathologic fracture
D. Multiple lesions in various bones of the body (skull, spine, ribs, long bones, and mandible)
E. All of the above

453. The most serious emergencies in the dental office fall into which one of the following groups?
   A. Respiratory
   B. Cardiovascular (circulatory)
   C. Hemorrhagic diseases
   D. Respiratory, cardiovascular (circulatory), and hemorrhagic
   E. None of the above

454. Treatment planning in comprehensive care in dentistry is based upon the concept
   A. of partial treatment responsibility
   B. of a list of dental procedures commonly performed
   C. of whole treatment responsibility
   D. of changes in the list of dental procedures
   E. of none of the above

455. The responsibility of the dentist in providing comprehensive care can be divided into
   A legal
   B ethical
   C. moral
   D. legal, ethical, and moral
   E. none of the above

456. Which of the following represent the basic sources of requirements for administration in dental practice?
   A. Federal and state governments require that the type and source of income be recorded for income tax purposes
   B. Records of interactions with patients and treatment provided must be kept as a hedge against malpractice
   C. Records are maintained for the sake of simplifying and analyzing the management of a dental practice
   D. Dental records should include accounts payable, accounts receivable, patient records, recall system, billing system, and appointment system
   E. All of the above

457. Attitudes in dentists and dental students appear to
   A. become less tolerant with age
   B. become more tolerant with age
   C. be impossible to change through behavior modification techniques
   D. not become altered by role models
   E. be none of the above

458. Patients may be classified into which of the following groups according to their view of their dentist-patient relationship?
   A. Friend, savior, parent, servant, provider, or adversary
   B. Savior
   C. Parent
   D. Servant, provider, or adversary
   E. None of the above

459. Comprehensive care in group practice involves which of the following?
   A. The size and composition of a dental group has little effect on its commitment to comprehensive care
   B. Groups are frequently composed entirely of general practitioners
   C. Groups may be composed primarily of dental specialists
   D. Some group practices are built around certain dental specialists
   E. All of the above

460. Dental students under a comprehensive care system of teaching have an opportunity to
   A. apply management techniques learned in didactic dental courses
   B. undertake management of auxiliaries
   C. manage patient flow
   D. manage other parameters required on the part of the student, depending on the system in which he or she works
   E. do all of the above

461. Records are kept in dental practice for which of the following reasons?
   A. Requirement of the Internal Revenue Service
   B. Protection against malpractice
   C. Legal considerations
   D. Efficient and comprehensive practice management
   E. All of the above

462. Which of the following records are required by the Internal Revenue Service?
   A. Identification of sources of income
   B. Deductible income
   C. Social Security earnings
   D. Additional federal requirements and other government requirements
   E. For all of the above reasons

463. The patient's dental records should be
   A. easy to use
   B. consistent
   C. systematic
   D. logical, efficient, follow a natural order, be easy to update, and contain appropriate data
   E. all of the above

464. The information required in the patient's dental record includes
   A. medical and dental history
   B. psychological and attitudinal evaluation
   C. dental disease and conditions
   D. chronological list of services, diagnostic aids (radiographs, study casts, and photographs), and supplemental information
   E. all of the above

465. A well-constructed dental record will provide answers to which of the following questions?
   A. What information was collected from the patient?
   B. What was wrong or right with the patient?
   C. What plans were made to resolve the patient's problems, at what price, and how long will it take?
   D. Have the treatment plans been followed?
   E. All of the above

466. The ideal dental record should
   A. be simple to utilize
   B. contain a broad data base
   C. contain an easily located list of patient problems
   D. be clearly written and organized according to the natural order of activities and be easily read and understood
   E. all of the above

467. In a problem-oriented dental practice which of the following data bases should be utilized?
   A. Demographic, personal, and financial information
   B. Extensive interview data
   C. Self-completion or review of systems Health History Questionnaire
   D. A reasonable physical assessment; a complete oral hygiene appraisal; a thorough dental examination, periodontal assessment, and occlusal analysis; and appropriate radiographic surveys with a panographic radiograph
   E. All of the above

468. In the development of an on-line computer system for managing comprehensive care which of the following questions should be answered?
   A. What are the information needs?
   B. How are those needs being met now?
   C. What needs could be satisfied with a new system?
   D. What is the cost of the new system
   E. All of the above

10. OPERATIVE DENTISTRY

DIRECTIONS: Each of the questions or incomplete statements below is followed by five suggested answers or completions. Select the ONE that is best in each case.

469. The future oral health of a patient depends upon
   A. oral examination
   B. nature of dental disease
   C. diagnosis and treatment planning
   D. nature of systemic disease
   E. none of the above

470. A chalky appearance of the marginal ridge suggests
   A. no need for radiographic examination
   B. underlying dental caries
   C. no need for visual examination
   D. loss of translucency
   E. none of the above

471. Radiographic examination reveals
   A. caries and indicates depth of caries to a degree
   B. the extent of periodontal and periapical bone loss to a degree
   C. unerupted and impacted teeth
   D. the number, size, and shape of roots and root canals
   E. all of the above

472. Diagnosis and treatment planning requires
   A. clinical examination
   B. radiography
   C. study casts
   D. laboratory examinations and consultations with other dentists and physicians
   E. all of the above

473. Operative dentistry is
   A. purely mechanical
   B. treating a tooth
   C. devoid of physiologic and psychologic aspects
   D. treating the person
   E. none of the above

474. The types of caries evident in clinical examinations are
   A. pit caries and fissure caries
   B. pit and fissure and smooth surface caries
   C. smooth surface caries
   D. fissure caries
   E. none of the above

475. Extension for prevention in smooth surface caries is
   A. extension to dentinoenamel junction
   B. extension of cavity preparation to areas that are self-cleansing
   C. not related to removal of enamel defects
   D. not related to removal of pits and fissures on premolars and molars
   E. none of the above

476. Objectives of cavity preparation are
   A. to remove all decay
   B. to give protection to the pulp
   C. to locate margins of restorations in immune areas of the tooth
   D. that tooth or restoration will not fracture
   E. all of the above

477. Class IV cavities include
   A. cavities on proximal surfaces of incisors and canines that do not involve the incisal edge
   B. cavities on proximal surfaces of incisors and canines that do involve the incisal edge
   C. cavities on the incisal edge of anterior teeth
   D. cavities on the incisal edge of anterior teeth or on the occlusal cusp heights of posterior teeth
   E. none of the above

478. Extend the cavity margin
   A. as much as the individual dentist desires
   B. until solid tooth structure is obtained with no unsupported enamel
   C. to meet the lateral spread of caries
   D. to solid tooth structure (but unsupported enamel may be present)
   E. to none of the above

479. Factors to be considered in pit and fissure cavities in posterior teeth are
   A. the position of free margin of interproximal tissue
   B. the estimation of facial embrasure areas least susceptible to caries
   C. the estimation of lingual embrasure areas least susceptible to caries
   D. the location of contact point
   E. all of the above

480. Resistance form
   A. is that shape and placement of cavity walls that enables the tooth to withstand stress
   B. does not utilize the box shape and flat floor
   C. does not take into consideration resistance of the tooth to fracture
   D. utilizes a rounded pulpal floor
   E. is none of the above

481. Basic retention form in class II cavity preparations for amalgam include
   A. parallel proximal and occlusal walls
   B. reduced cusps
   C. a rounded pulpal floor
   D. proximal and occlusal walls converging occlusally
   E. none of the above

482. Considerations to be undertaken in the finishing of enamel walls and margins include
   A. the direction of enamel rods
   B. support of enamel rods
   C. the type of restorative material to be placed in preparation
   D. the location of margin and the degree of smoothness desired
   E. all of the above

483. The advent of ultra high speed requires consideration of which of the following factors in finishing enamel walls?
   A. Marginal seal
   B. Sealing gingival margin
   C. Lessening of tactile sense and rapid removal of tooth structure
   D. Marginal metal that is easily burnished
   E. None of the above

484. The basic consideration in performing cavity sterilization is
   A. the effectiveness of the agent
   B. the production of sterile field
   C. the harm to odontoblasts
   D. the harm to pulpal cells
   E. is all of the above

485. Hand cutting instruments are composed of
   A. a handle and blade
   B. a handle, shank, and blade
   C. a shank and blade
   D. a handle and shank
   E. none of the above

486. The effective use of any instrument is dictated by
   A. the ability and preference of the operator
   B. the metals used in manufacture
   C. the heat treatment and tempering
   D. the instrument design
   E. none of the above

487. A dry operative field affords
   A. better vision
   B. clean cavity walls
   C. adequate detection of caries
   D. development of full properties of dental materials used
   E. all of the above

488. An advantage of the rubber dam is
   A. a dry, clean, visible field
   B. protection of the patient and operator
   C. the economic factor (time more productive)
   D. improved properties of dental materials and retraction of soft tissues
   E. all of the above

489. A disadvantage of the rubber dam is
   A. time consumption
   B. patient objection
   C. it cannot be used in teeth that have not erupted sufficiently to clamp
   D. it cannot be used on malpositioned teeth
   E. all of the above

490. Amalgam restorations of proximal tooth surfaces are successful if they are placed
   A. in the proper cavity preparation
   B. with the proper matrix
   C. under the rubber dam
   D. with well-established principles in the handling of amalgam
   E. all of the above

491. The three-surface cavity preparation for amalgam includes
   A. an occlusal step
   B. isolation of proximal enamel
   C. proximal boxing and enamel walls
   D. a rubber dam
   E. all of the above

492. When caries are extensive,
   A. two cusps on the affected tooth must be capped
   B. buccal cusps should be capped
   C. lingual cusps should be capped
   D. all cusps on the affected tooth must be capped
   E. none of the above is true

493. The selection of a restorative material for the class III cavity preparation includes which of the following?
   A. Tooth in question
   B. Size and position of carious lesion
   C. Service and age of patient
   D. Esthetics and economics
   E. All of the above

494. In determining whether a class I cavity should be restored by a gold inlay, which of the following should be taken into consideration?
   A. Incidence and rate of proximal surface caries on other teeth
   B. Age of patient
   C. Extent of pit and fissure caries on the tooth
   D. Cost to patient and mouth rehabilitation by multiple tooth impression technique
   E. All of the above

495. Which of the following considerations are appropriate in determining whether the class II cavity should be prepared for a gold inlay?
   A. The rate and extent of caries on facial and lingual surfaces on all teeth
   B. The extent of proximal surface caries on the tooth in question
   C. Root canal therapy
   D. Dental rehabilitation with gold, economic factor, and splinting
   E. All of the above

496 Before operative dentistry is started it should be determined if
   A. the patient has adequate finances
   B. the patient requires splinting
   C. occlusal relationships are adequate and merit perpetuation in restorations
   D. patient appreciation is present
   E. none of the above

497. If a marginal ridge is severely weakened due to excessive extension into it
   A. the cavity outline should include the proximal surface
   B. the cavity outline should include the buccal surface
   C. the cavity outline should not include the proximal surface
   D. the outline form should remain unaltered
   E. none of the above should occur

498. Teeth that have had root canal therapy
   A. require no special restorations or design
   B. are strong and not subject to fracture
   C. decay rapidly
   D. are weak and subject to fracture due to occlusal forces
   E. are none of the above

499. The proper restoration for the tooth that has undergone root canal treatment is
   A. class II amalgam
   B. class II inlay
   C. class III inlay
   D. post-full crown or cusp capping post inlay
   E. none of the above

500. In splinting anterior teeth,
   A. three-fourths of the lingual surface should be included in outline form
   B. one-half of the lingual surface should be included in outline form
   C. none of the lingual surface should be included in outline form
   D. the entire lingual surface should be included in the outline form
   E. none of the above should be done

501. Forms and types of gold foil available include
   A. sheet foil in book form
   B. gold foil ropes
   C. gold foil pellets or cylinders
   D. mat gold
   E. all of the above

502. The advantage of goldent, a new type of cohesive gold, is
   A. it manipulates easily and can be placed in a short period of time
   B. it is semiplastic when annealed
   C. it has greater density than gold foil
   D. it can be used easily to restore incipient Class II cavities
   E. all of the above

503. Silicate cement, by virtue of its fluoride content,
   A. is not superior to acrylic resin in protecting teeth from recurrent caries
   B. is excellent in teeth of mouth breathers
   C. is indicated for patients with a high caries index
   D. is unaffected by dryness
   E. is none of the above

504. An advantage of silicate cement restorations is
   A. a conservative cavity preparation due to the anti-caries factor
   B. a natural initial appearance
   C. ease of manipulation, little time required for operation
   D. good insulation, coefficient of thermal expansion similar to that of tooth structure
   E. all of the above

505. An advantage of restoring (silicate) the proximal cavity from the lingual aspect is
   A. discoloration or dissolution of the filling material is not likely to be visible
   B. some unsupported enamel can be left on the facial wall since it is not a stress area
   C. facial enamel is preserved
   D. color matching is not critical and the lingual area is more apt to stay wet
   E. all of the above

506. Cavity outline forms for silicate cements are determined by
   A. the extent of preparation
   B. the size of caries
   C. the location and shape of caries
   D. enlargements necessary to provide access for vision and instrumentation
   E. all of the above

507. An advantage of desirable qualities of acrylic resin restorations is
   A. excellent tooth-matching ability and color stability
   B. ease of manipulation
   C. minimum time during placement
   D. only mildly irritating to pulp
   E. all of the above

508. Retention for acrylic resins
   A. has more effective retention by sharp angles
   B. has more effective retention and protection to pulp is obtained with round undercuts
   C. does not require special emphasis
   D. is similar to retention for gold inlays
   E. is none of the above

509. Dental caries
   A. were very common in early humans
   B. were comparatively rare in early humans
   C. never occurred in early humans
   D. never occurred in Bronz Age skulls
   E. were none of the above

510. The initial changes in dental caries are caused by
   A. a mineral phase phenomenon
   B. products of bacterial metabolism excreted at the surface of the tooth
   C. an organic phase phenomenon
   D. saliva
   E. none of the above

511. Theoretically, the presence of acid
   A. is essential for dissolution of tooth mineral
   B. is chelation
   C. is a nonionic complex
   D. is not essential for dissolution of tooth mineral
   E. is none of the above

512. Materials attached to the surface of enamel (dental plaque) are
   A. aggregations of salivary microorganisms
   B. deposits of mucin
   C. epithelial cells
   D. food debris
   E. all of the above

513. A low viscosity of the saliva is associated with
   A. a low caries experience
   B. a high caries experience
   C. an extremely high caries experience
   D. no caries at all
   E. none of the above

514. The dental plaque begins as
   A. particles of food on enamel
   B. deposits of fungi on enamel
   C. deposits of salivary mucoid on enamel
   D. deposition of acid on enamel
   E. none of the above

515. Preventive dentistry includes
A. oral hygiene
B. dietary measures
C. topical fluoride applications
D. ingestion of fluoride in tablets, milk, and salt
E. all of the above

516. There is no finer restoration in dentistry than
A. amalgam
B. silicate
C. a well-made gold inlay and nothing worse than a poor one
D. acrylic
E. none of the above

517. The direct inlay technic (method) is
A. less accurate than the indirect method
B. of the same accuracy as the indirect method
C. not an accurate method
D. more accurate than indirect because fewer steps are involved
E. none of the above

518. An inlay made with pins
A. should be sufficiently far away from the pulp
B. is dislodged readily
C. should not be far away from the pulp
D. causes serious pulp irritation
E. is none of the above

519. Wax patterns for full crowns may be made by which of the following?
A. All-wax method
B. Wax-and-gold matrix method
C. Semi-indirect-direct method
D. Direct-indirect method
E. All of the above

520. Every wax pattern
A. may be invested whenever desired
B. should be invested after 12 hours
C. may be held indefinitely in water
D. should be invested as soon as possible
E. is none of the above

521. With impression materials used today,
   A. all are entirely accurate
   B. some are entirely accurate
   C. reversive hydrocolloids are entirely accurate
   D. no impression is entirely accurate
   E. none of the above is true

522. Cavity preparation for silver amalgam
   A. should not minimize its weak points
   B. is the same as for the gold inlay
   C. must be designed to supplement the good properties of this material
   D. has strength not derived from bulk
   E. is none of the above

523. Retention for the silver-amalgam restoration
   A. should have only one retention area
   B. should provide separate retention for the occlusal and proximal portions
   C. should have only occlusal retention
   D. should have only proximal retention
   E. should do none of the above

524. The majority of fractures occurring with silver amalgam seem to concentrate
   A. at the gingival margin
   B. at the contact area
   C. in the area of the occlusal isthmus
   D. at dovetail area
   E. at none of the above

525. Moisture in an amalgam causes
   A. an increase in strength
   B. shrinkage of filling
   C. no marginal breakdown
   D. excessive delayed expansion with protrusion of the filling
   E. none of the above

526. A polished amalgam restoration
   A. will corrode
   B. will not retain its appearance
   C. will resist tarnish and corrosion
   D. will tarnish
   E. will do none of the above

527. Instruments for use in operative dentistry are made of which of the following stainless metals?
A. Stainless steel
B. Monel metal
C. Nichrome
D. Stellite and tarno
E. All of the above

528. Instruments for operative destistry may be classified as
A. cutting
B. miscellaneous
C. cutting, condensing, and miscellaneous
D. condensing
E. none of the above

529. Which of the following aid in determining the proper location for the cavity margins?
A. Extend margins until solid tooth structure, free from caries, is reached
B. Leave overhanging enamel margins
C. Do not extend the margins to include all the fissures and angular grooves
D. Do not unite two cavities close to each other
E. None of the above

530. Resistance form is
A. the shaping of the walls of the cavity so that they withstand stress
B. dependent upon the flare of the embrasures
C. dependent on mouth hygiene
D. related to the estimate of caries susceptibility
E. none of the above

531. Convenience form is
A. a restoration that resists displacement
B. a cavity that withstands stresses
C. a cavity shaped in such a manner that it may be most conveniently restored
D. a cavity of sufficient depth
E. none of the above

532. The characteristic feature of caries in pits and fissures is usually
   A. a small opening or orifice
   B. spreading in cone shape in the enamel, the base of the cone being in the deepest part
   C. rapid burrowing along the dentinoenamel junction
   D. spreading in the dentin in conical form, the base being at the surface of dentin and the apex pointing toward the pulp
   E. all of the above

533. The essential clinical feature of gingival third caries is
   A. carious area usually begins as a white line in the center of the gingival third of the labial and buccal surfaces
   B. marked sensitivity
   C. a process which generally spreads mesially and distally near the axial line angles
   D. often the least frequent of the usual types of caries
   E. all of the above

534. Which of the following major physical factors is involved in the use of cutting instruments for tooth tissue?
   A. Heat generated during the cutting operation
   B. Vibration developed during cutting operation
   C. Relative effectiveness of efficiency of various cutting instruments
   D. Effective operating life of a rotating instrument
   E. All of the above

535. Matrix bands should possess which of the following essential qualities?
   A. Easy adaptability and fixedness to the teeth
   B. Provision for proper contouring
   C. Resistance against the pressure necessary for insertion of restoration
   D. Capability of easy introduction and removal
   E. All of the above

536. The main objective to be attained in the restoration of teeth is
   A. arrest of the loss of tooth substance
   B. prevention of recurrence of caries
   C. restoration or maintenance of interproximal spaces and contact points
   D. establishment of proper occlusion and esthetic overall effect
   E. all of the above

537. Dental cements may be classified into
A. class I (zinc oxychloride, zinc oxide eugenol)
B. class II (copper phosphate, zinc phosphate)
C. class III (classes I and II, silver, copper, or mercury salts)
D. class IV (silicate, zinc phosphate-silicate)
E. all of the above

538. The characteristics of gold as a restorative material are
A. cohesiveness and weldability
B. softness during manipulation
C. ductility and tensile strength
D. malleability and hardness
E. all of the above

539. Cohesive gold foil is produced in which of the following types?
A. Soft type
B. Dead-soft type
C. Extra or special soft
D. Platinized soft gold
E. All of the above

540. The disadvantage of cohesive gold foil as a restorative material is
A. none; there is no disadvantage
B. low conductivity
C. inharmonious color, high conductivity, and difficulty in manipulation
D. ease of manipulation
E. none of the above

541. Indications for the use of gold are
A. all class I cavities
B. class V cavities
C. a majority of class II cavities of small and medium size
D. large class III cavities
E. all of the above

542. The inlay investments have been classified into
A. low plaster content only
B. low plaster content, high plaster content, and high-expansion investments
C. high plaster content only
D. high expansion investments only
E. none of the above

543. The size of the sprue former used
  A. should always be 8 gauge
  B. varies according to the technique of casting
  C. should be 5 gauge
  D. should be 12 gauge
  E. none of the above

544. Elastic impression materials for operative dentistry include
  A. hydrocolloids
  B. alginates
  C. Dr. Dietrich's elastic impression material
  D. Mizzy's trulastic sticks
  E. all of the above

545. Securing an impression for class II inlay cavities presents which of the following undercuts which may perplex the dentist?
  A. Unrelated undercuts, unintentional undercuts, and undercuts produced by normal constriction of tooth at cervix
  B. Only related undercuts
  C. Only unintentional undercuts
  D. Only undercuts produced by normal constriction of the tooth at the cervix
  E. None of the above

546. Fractured or destroyed angles (class IV) on the anterior teeth
  A. are readily restored
  B. require no special effort
  C. has an esthetic appeal of no importance
  D. may present the most intricate and perplexing of all the problems of operative dentistry
  E. are none of the above

547. The steps in porcelain inlay construction are
  A. preparation of the cavity for reception of the inlay
  B. making a platinum matrix which perfectly fits the cavity
  C. fusing porcelain into the matrix
  D. glazing and removal of the matrix from the porcelain and cementing inlay
  E. all of the above

548. For accurately fitting pins which of the following is necessary?
A. Production of a hole with a tapered orifice
B. Production of a clean-cut hole without a tapered or flared orifice
C. Production of a hole with a flared orifice
D. Production of a sloped and beveled hole
E. None of the above

549. It is axiomatic that pins
A. should not be parallel with each other
B. may be divergent
C. must be parallel with each other
D. may be convergent
E. be none of the above

550. Which of the following represent common uses for the cemented retentive pin?
A. Large amalgam restorations
B. Coping for crown and bridge abutment
C. Replacement of fractured incisal angles
D. Repair of bridge and crown facings
E. All of the above

551. Which of the following represent specifications for a suitable pin support?
A. Pins should be placed adjacent to an axial wall
B. Pins weaken composite dental materials
C. Perforation with the drill should be avoided, and pins should be spaced well apart and not adjacent to an axial wall
D. Perforations with the drill should be avoided
E. None of the above

552. The "pin-ledge" is a type of tooth preparation which consists of
A. incisal and axial reduction, proximal grooves, and ledges into which the pinholes are placed
B. incisal and axial reduction for bite clearance
C. axial reduction for bite clearance
D. incisal reduction into which the pinholes are placed
E. none of the above

553. Pin-ledge
   A. retainers are used as abutment retainers for small span bridges, and castings are difficult to prepare
   B. castings are easy to prepare
   C. cannot be used as abutment retainers for small span bridges
   D. consists of incisal and axial reduction for bite clearance
   E. is none of the above

554. The pinlay
   A. is perfectly acceptable for abutment retainers
   B. is not accepted for abutment retainers
   C. can resist heavy masticatory forces without angular bracing and is devoid of internal detail
   D. resists torquing forces
   E. is none of the above

555. The principle of "extension for prevention"
   A. is practical in the pinlay restoration
   B. is not practical in the pinlay restoration
   C. requires loss of labial enamel
   D. requires loss of proximal enamel
   E. is none of the above

556. A tooth suffering from abrasion
   A. requires that special provisions be made to hedge against it
   B. has extensive carious lesions
   C. has moderate carious lesions
   D. is not a likely candidate for the carious process
   E. is none of the above

557. If the incisal edge has not worn sufficiently to receive the placement of four pinholes for a cast pin restoration, the number of pinholes that should be used are
   A. only one pinhole
   B. three pinholes
   C. no pinholes
   D. only two pinholes
   D. none of the above

558. The twist drill for preparing pinholes
A. is a router
B. cuts only on the end as it penetrates dentin
C. can be used if dull
D. as a dull router can be used satisfactorily
E. is none of the above

559. An operator must observe which of the following biologic principles when preparing pinholes for retention of gold castings?
A. Interim dressings are vitally important
B. Pinholes must be sealed against the ingress of saliva or oral debris while the casting is made
C. Thermal conductivity is not influenced by pin depth
D. Pulp exposure must be recognized and treated as such
E. All of the above

560. Ordinarily the depth of a pinhole should be
A. under 2.5 mm
B. 2.5-3.0 mm
C. 3.0-3.5 mm
D. 2.0-2.4 mm
E. none of the above

561. For an acceptable impression
A. impression tray must be rigid
B. trays should have short flanges
C. gingival embrasures should be occluded, rubber or hydrocolloid material may be used, bristles must be accurately sized
D. bristles should not fall out of the pinholes, bristles should not engage the impression tray, impression bristles for Divestment Technic are smaller than pulled pattern technic, injection technics differ with knobbed and unknobbed bristles, and impression removal must be carefully controlled
E. all of the above are required

562. The operative dentist must consider which of the following questions, which should be answered in order to arrive at a logical conclusion?
   A. How long can the restoration be expected to remain intact?
   B. Is the patient willing to have the procedure repeated as needed? What is the biologic response to the acid-etch technique? What is the patient's age?
   C. Will the proposed treatment conserve tooth structure? Will it produce an acceptable esthetic result?
   D. Is it economically feasible for both the patient and the dentist? To what masticatory stress, if any, will the restoration be subjected? Can the patient be properly educated as to limitations of the service being contemplated?
   E. All of the above

563. Which of the following conditions are involved in the treatment of the young fractured incisor?
   A. Small pulp
   B. Incompletely formed root
   C. Cooperative patient
   D. A large pulp, partially erupted tooth, and young uncooperative patient
   E. None of the above

564. Fractures of the young incisor have been classified into which of the following categories?
   A. Class I fracture: minor chips of enamel from incisal edges
   B. Class II fracture: involving enamel plus dentin
   C. Class III fracture: one which exposes the pulp
   D. Class IV fracture: one involving the root of the tooth
   E. All of the above

565. The class III fracture presenting a pulp problem
   A. requires pulp capping
   B. automatically consigns the tooth to endodontic therapy
   C. requires pulpotomy
   D. requires a period of watching
   E. is none of the above

566. Which of the following factors make a restoration of the young fractured incisor difficult?
   A. An uncooperative patient
   B. Parent who demands ultimate cosmetic result, child with translucent enamel
   C. Demanding patient
   D. Tooth with translucent enamel
   E. None of the above

567. Notwithstanding occlusal interferences, a poorly shaped amalgam on an occlusal surface causes
   A. a great deal of irritation to the gingival tissues
   B. a common situation for all general practitioners
   C. no irritation to the gingival tissues
   D. a common situation for all prosthodontists
   E. none of the above

568. Carving of the amalgam is best facilitated by adhering to which of the following sequences?
   A. Wedge removed with serrated amalgam condenser
   B. Matrix band removed, proximal surfaces and embrasures carved
   C. Rubber dam removed, and occlusal height established while amalgam is still relatively soft
   D. Occlusal pits, grooves, and other carving completed
   E. All of the above

569. The proximal carver
   A. is a delicate knife-like instrument fabricated from spring steel
   B. for maxillary teeth has the blade at right angles to the handle
   C. is somewhat flexible and must be razor sharp
   D. has the ability to carve the external roll of the marginal ridge
   E. is all of the above

570. Cohesive gold foil
   A. fails to stand unopposed as the material of choice where it is indicated
   B. for the realistic practitioner uses all gold foil restorations
   C. for the pragmatic practitioner uses all gold foil restorations
   D. currently stands unopposed as the material of choice
   E. is none of the above

571. Gold foil
   A. has its place in the office of every "concerned" operative dentist
   B. fails to have a place in the office of every "concerned" operative dentist
   C. should be used only by state board examinations to fail aspiring applicants for licensure
   D. has no geographic boundaries bearing on distributions of its users
   E. is none of the above

572. Which of the following armamentarium is all that is requried for gold foil operators?
   A. Alcohol lamp and alcohol for annealing the gold
   B. Powdered cohesive gold (Goldent)
   C. Annealing broach used for annealing the gold over the alcohol flame
   D. Condensing instruments (Nos. LLGF20, LLGF21, and LLGF25)
   E. All of the above

573. Cavities prepared for cohesive gold (powdered gold)
   A. should be given a box-like shape
   B. should have definite line and point angles
   C. should have their margins terminate in solid, sound enamel with extensions into areas where caries do not occur
   D. have walls which should meet the tooth surface at right angles
   E. are all of the above

574. Powdered gold encased in a foil cover, i.e., "goldent,"
   A. condenses and finishes more satisfactorily against a butt joint
   B. is selected as the material of choice because of its unique characteristics
   C. is peculiarly plastic
   D. is up to 10 times more dense than a pellet of the same size of gold foil
   E. is all of the above

575. Overannealing of gold foil
   A. is the preferred method
   B. produces better adhesion properties
   C. is equally to be avoided
   D. is preferable to underannealing
   E. is none of the above

576. Inability to recognize improperly condensed gold by the operator is
   A. of no consequence
   B. due to underannealing
   C. due to overannealing
   D. an invitation to certain failure
   E. none of the above

577. An acceptable method used by the beginner to train to ascertain whether a gold foil restoration is condensed or not is
   A. use of a magnifying glass
   B. subject the surface to the penetrating power of a scaler
   C. use of a binocular microscope, subject the surface to the heavy penetrating force of an explorer
   D. subject the surface to the penetrating power of a large amalgam plugger
   E. none of the above

578. Finishing powder gold restorations includes
   A. superburnishing
   B. trimming off excess gold
   C. contouring to form
   D. burnishing incident to trimming, contouring, and final finishing touches
   E. all of the above

579. Which of the following motivational guidelines may be employed in patient interaction during plaque control for the treatment of periodontitis?
   A. Adopt the method of motivation to fit the interests and needs of each patient
   B. The motivational level of a patient is influenced by the patient viewing the reward of dental health as being worth the effort
   C. Motivation is related to the need to solve a problem
   D. Motivation and initial learning are the keys to retention of behavior changes; communication of the dentist's concern for the patient's dental health is important; and instruction in plaque control techniques is not sufficient without motivation
   E. All of the above

580. Root planning and gingival curettage are therapeutic procedures
   A. for pocket reduction/elimination
   B. to reduce inflammation and prepare the tissue for restorative dentistry to follow
   C. to reduce inflammation prior to periodontal surgical procedures
   D. to evaluate tissue response, as compromise thera, and in acute periodontal disease (gingival and periodontal abscesses)
   E. all of the above

581. Root planning and subgingival curettage are
   A. still the cornerstones of all periodontal therapy
   B. neither therapy nor surgical procedures
   C. of no value prior to restorative dentistry
   D. not effective for pocket reduction
   E. none of the above

582. Indications for orthodontics include
   A. periodontal patients where the teeth are in labioversion
   B. uprighting teeth in periodontal patients
   C. rotating teeth in periodontal patients
   D. intruding or extruding teeth in periodontal patients
   E. all of the above

583. Pathologic occlusions exhibit
   A. mobility
   B. fremitus patterns
   C. severe retrograde wear
   D. temporomandibular joint dysfunction and radiographic changes associated with occlusal trauma
   E. all of the above

584. The applications of electrosurgery for periodontal patients include periodontal surgery for
   A. mucogingival problems
   B. gingival enlargements
   C. irregular gingival contour, reshaping edentulous ridges, and periodontal abscesses
   D. incisions for flap surgery and thinning and scalloping of the flap prior to apposition and closure
   E. all of the above

585. Restorations are placed in teeth following periodontal therapy to
   A. rebuild the occlusion
   B. to replace missing teeth
   C. restore carious lesions
   D. to aid in stabilizing teeth and to prevent additional periodontal destruction
   E. accomplish all of the above

586. Surgical management of mucogingival problems in association with restorative dentistry is indicated in which of the following situaticns?
   A. An inadequate width or thickness of keratinized and attached gingiva
   B. Pull on the free gingival margin by the freni or muscle attachments
   C. Inadequate vestibular depth
   D. Gingival clefts or recession and pockets that approach or traverse the mucogingival junction
   E. All of the above

587. The objective of osseous surgery is
   A. to eliminate infrabony osseous defects and their accompanying soft tissue pockets
   B. has an obscure relationship with restorative dentistry
   C. plaque control and elimination
   D. elimination of absorbed endotoxins
   E. none of the above

588. The objective of osseous surgery is to
   A. eliminate formation of plaque
   B. produce deep infrabony defects
   C. eliminate infrabony osseous defects and their accompanying soft tissue pockets and to restore physiologic bony architecture that will help maintain healthy gingival forms and contours
   D. reduce exostoses or ledging of bone that has caused pocket formation
   E. do none of the above

589. The allograft relative to periodontal osseous graft therapy is
   A. an autograft
   B. a bone tissue graft between individuals of the same species
   C. the attachment apparatus
   D. a xenograft
   E. none of the above

590. Management of pulpo-periodontal disease should be performed in conjunction with periodontal management for which of the following indications?
   A. Root amputation to improve anatomical design for the periodontal supporting tissues
   B. To treat pulpal diseases
   C. To treat caries
   D. To treat calcification of the pulp
   E. None of the above

591. Signs and symptoms of embrasure problems are
   A. a change in coral pink to red color
   B. loss of stippling
   C. swollen or edematous papillae
   D. blunted papillae and irregular festooning and radiographic evidence of crestal bone involvement
   E. all of the above

592. Root amputation is indicated to
   A. safely remove a dowel from a canal
   B. produce a satisfactory overlay
   C. salvage a multirooted tooth by removing an offending root
   D. eliminate a fistula found between the tooth and near the gingival margin
   E. do none of the above

593. The advantage of retaining teeth in a healthy supportive environment is
   A. to eliminate subgingival caries
   B. retention
   C. for anterior esthetic considerations
   D. to prevent plaque development
   E. none of the above

594. The indication for the use of an overdenture is
A. whenever opposing natural dentition exerts a destructive effect on the supporting structures
B. when there are congenitally missing teeth or surgically corrected arches
C. in mandibular arches with severely resorbed ridges and few remaining anterior teeth
D. in maxillary arches of class III prognathic occlusions or class II, division II, vertical overlap relations; in malformed dental arches or in cases of severely worn teeth; in conjunction with a removable partial denture, providing a vertical position stop; whenever full mouth extractions of questionable teeth are diagnosed; as a transitional denture phase with endodontic implants; and when the psychological advantage for the patient overweighs the other considerations
E. all of the above

11. ORAL PHARMACOLOGY

DIRECTIONS: Each of the questions or incomplete statements below is followed by five suggested answers or completions. Select the ONE that is best in each case.

---

595. Drugs are substances that
   A. fail to modify the activity of biologic systems
   B. initiate new functions of cells
   C. modify the activity of biologic systems
   D. neither speed up nor slow down functions inherent and natural to cells
   E. do none of the above

596. The prescription
   A. is a written communication from the dentist to the pharmacist directing him or her to prepare a certain medication and dispense it to the patient
   B. is a complicated procedure and order to the pharmacist
   C. is an intricate order to the pharmacist
   D. is too difficult for a dentist to write
   E. is none of the above

597. The classic parts of the prescription include
   A. the superscription
   B. the inscription
   C. the subscription
   D. the signature
   E. all of the above

598. By means of local anesthetic agents, pain impulses may be blocked at
A. the pain fiber termination only
B. any place along a nerve
C. the spinal cord only
D. the pain fiber termination, any place along a nerve and at the spinal cord
E. none of the above

599. General anesthetics
A. are specific and block pain
B. block pain without abolishing consciousness
C. obliterate pain
D. both obliterate pain and cause loss of consciousness
E. are none of the above

600. The analgesics
A. obliterate pain and cause loss of consciousness
B. are nonspecific and block pain
C. are specific and block pain without abolishing consciousness
D. do not block pain
E. are none of the above

601. Aspirin (acetylsalicylic acid) is
A. the most potent pain reliever available
B. the least potent pain reliever available
C. of average potency as a pain reliever
D. free of toxicity
E. none of the above

602. Narcotic analgesics
A. have high analgesic potency
B. have distressing side actions
C. are not needed for long periods in dentistry
D. as less powerful narcotic analgesics are quite effective in dentistry
E. are all of the above

603. Codeine has which of the following uses?
A. Analgesic action
B. Cough suppressant
C. Aborting a cold
D. Hangover remedy combined with aspirin
E. All of the above

604. Morphine
   A. is effective only if given subcutaneously
   B. is equally effective by any route of administration
   C. has a faster onset of effect when administered orally
   D. addiction does not occur with habituation
   E. is none of the above

605. Meperidine hydrochloride (demerol)
   A. is an analgesic
   B. has been regarded as a morphine substitute
   C. has analgesic potency not quite as great as that of morphine
   D. has analgesic potency greater than that of codeine
   E. is all of the above

606. Methadone hydrochloride (dolophine)
   A. has a low level of sedative-producing properties
   B. has a low level of euphoria-producing properties
   C. cannot be used to allay apprehension or relieve anxiety
   D. exhibits side effects, i.e., constipation, nausea, and vomiting
   E. is all of the above

607. Local anesthetics
   A. obliterate pain and sensation in a local area without loss of consciousness
   B. cause paralysis of the sensory or afferent nerve endings
   C. is accomplished by injecting a solution of the agent into the region surrounding a nerve trunk
   D. diffuse into the nerve trunk, paralyzing all the nerve fibers, whether afferent or efferent
   E. are all of the above

608. Para-aminobenzoic acid esters include
   A. Novocain (procaine)
   B. Pontocaine (tetracaine)
   C. Monocaine (butethamine)
   D. Ravocaine (propoxycaine), nesacaine (2-chloroprocaine), and duocaine (procaine and butethamine)
   E. all of the above

609. Vasoconstrictors with regional anesthetics
   A. produce their effect by acting on the postganglionic sympathetic nerve fiber terminations
   B. are responsible for the success of dental regional anesthesia
   C. should contain the lowest concentration of the vasoconstrictor as possible
   D. should not be injected into a blood vessel
   E. are all of the above

610. The most widely used vasoconstrictor is
   A. Cobefrin
   B. Epinephrine
   C. Neo-Synephrine
   D. Neo-Cobefrin
   E. none of the above

611. An anaphylactic reaction
   A. never accompanies the administration of a local anesthetic
   B. is not due to the synthetic chemical substances of local anesthetics
   C. is a possibility in a patient sensitive to a local anesthetic agent
   D. is due to the vasodilator in local anesthetics
   E. is none of the above

612. Topical anesthetic agents used in dentistry
   A. are supplied in the form of aqueous solutions
   B. do not remain sterile
   C. are somewhat hazardous due to possible evaporation from improperly closed bottles
   D. may be a hazard because of possible oxidation of the ingredients when exposed to air for a long period
   E. are all of the above

613. General anesthesia for use in dentistry
   A. requires the selection of an agent with a rapid onset of action
   B. requires an agent with a short duration of effect
   C. requires an agent which will allow rapid restoration of consciousness
   D. requires an agent which allows full recovery of mental faculties as soon as oral surgery or other dental procedure is completed
   E. is all of the above

614. The stages of general anesthesia include the
   A. first stage: induction
   B. second stage: excitement
   C. third stage: surgical anesthesia
   D. fourth stage: medullary paralysis
   E. all of the above

615. Inhalation anesthetics
   A. may be liquid at room temperature
   B. are liquids easily vaporized because of low boiling point
   C. may be gases at room temperature
   D. as gases must be stored in tanks and administered with special apparatus
   E. are all of the above

616. Nitrous oxide
   A. produces anesthesia only if the concentration is high (above 85%)
   B. is a nonflammable, nonexplosive, colorless gas with no taste or odor
   C. may be used in high concentrations up to 95%
   D. recovery is rapid and is the safest of all general anesthetic agents
   E. is all of the above

617. Ether
   A. is a volatile liquid
   B. is administered by the open method or by a vaporizer bottle attached to anesthetic machine in the semiclosed or closed method
   C. has a slow onset of action and slow recovery
   D. inhalation produces irritation of the oral mucosa, pharyngeal mucosa, and salivation
   E. is all of the above

618. Barbiturates
   A. are soporifics found readily acceptable in dental practice
   B. with 50 related chemical substances have been marketed
   C. are classified as long-acting
   D. are classified as intermediate-duration-of-action, short-acting, and ultra-short acting
   E. are all of the above

619. Tranquilizers
   A. are not curative
   B. only abolish symptomatology
   C. are antianxiety drugs
   D. do not stop the original symptom complex from returning upon stoppage of medication
   E. are all of the above

620. Antidepressants
   A. are called psychic energizers
   B. are psychotropic drugs
   C. raise the mental state out of lethargy and depression back to normal
   D. are opposite in action to that of the tranquilizers
   E. are all of the above

621. Antibiotics used in dentistry are usually administered
   A. parenterally
   B. by intramuscular injection
   C. orally in the form of capsules or tablets
   D. topically in the form of solutions applied locally
   E. in all of the above ways

622. Concerning penicillin G, USP,
   A. it is the current basic penicillin from which variations are derived
   B. there is no therapeutic difference between it and potassium penicillin G
   C. there is no therapeutic difference between sodium penicillin G and buffered crystalline penicillin G
   D. there is no therapeutic difference between potassium penicillin G and sodium penicillin G
   E. all of the above are true

623. The tetracyclines
   A. have dosages expressed in units
   B. are never followed by gastrointestinal upsets
   C. are not useful in penicillin-resistant strains of pathogenic bacteria
   D. are broad-spectrum antibiotics
   E. are none of the above

624. Chloramphenicol
- **A.** is a broad-spectrum antibiotic
- **B.** is rapidly absorbed after oral administration
- **C.** in oral dose must be repeated every 6-8 hours to maintain adequate blood levels
- **D.** when used, the white cell count and morphology should be followed closely because of blood dyscrasias developing
- **E.** involves all of the above

625. Treatment of allergic reactions in the skin and oral mucosa include
- A. epinephrine (adrenalin) should be used for immediate effects, 1/2 to 1 cc of a 1:1000 solution intramuscularly, it may be necessary to repeat the injection in 1-2 hours
- B. anaphylatoxin
- C. histamine
- D. precipitin
- E. none of the above

626. Emergencies in the dental office
- A. are very frequent
- B. may cause considerable consternation
- C. always produce effective treatment
- D. do not require an oxygen machine and an adequate emergency kit in the modern dental office
- E. do not involve any of the above

627. The principles involved in formulation of a plan of action include
- A. an adequate history
- B. an adequate clinical evaluation
- C. the use of premedication to prevent emergencies
- D. recognition of the early signs and symptoms of the emergency
- E. all of the above

628. An emergency anaphylactic kit for a dental office where injection of penicillin and other drugs takes place should include
   A. epinephrine (adrenalin), 0. 2-0. 5 cc dosage of 1:1000 via a tuberculin syringe
   B. oxygen, 10 liter flow administered by inhalation under pressure
   C. methoxamine hydrochloride, 15 mg IM or 5 mg IV to support circulation
   D. diphenhydramine, 20-50 mg IV if necessary to assist antihistaminic therapy
   E. all of the above

629. In patients on steroid therapy the problem in dentistry is
   A. to perform all extractions aseptically
   B. to avoid secondary infection
   C. to avoid any stress (operation) to the patient who has been on therapy and has recently stopped medication
   D. to avoid bacteremias (transient)
   E. none of the above is true

630. The primary aim of good emergency treatment is
   A. oxygenation of the patient
   B. adequate respiration
   C. maintenance of normal circulation of the blood
   D. to administer 20% oxygen via ambu bag and mask
   E. all of the above

631. An emergency kit for a dental office (separate from anaphylactic emergency kit) should contain
   A. pentobarbital, IV, 30-100 mg, sedation, toxicity, and convulsions
   B. diphenhydramine, IV, 10-50 mg, allergic reactions
   C. epinephrine IV 0. 1-0. 2 cc; SC 0. 2-0. 5 cc, anaphylactic shock, and other life-threatening allergic reactions only
   D. methoxamine HCl, IV, or IM, 15 mg IM or 5 mg IV, asthma and hypotension; meperidine HCl, IV, analgesic for coronary or other pain; aminophylline, IV, 3. 75-7. 5 gr, bronchodilator; nitroglycerin, sublingually, 1/200 gr, angina pectoris; hydrocortisone sodium succinate, IV, 100 mg, adrenal insufficiency and anaphylactic shock; dextrose 50%, IV, 50 cc 50%, insulin shock; ammonia ampule, inhalation, syncope; and gelfoam, thrombin, for hemorrhage
   E. all of the above

632. Antagonism implies
   A. that two drugs are helping one another
   B. potentiation of actions
   C. exaggeration of actions
   D. that there is a reduction of the effect of one drug in the presence of another
   E. none of the above

633. The stages of general anesthesia include the
   A. stage of induction
   B. stage of excitement or delirium
   C. stage of surgical anesthesia
   D. stage of medullary paralysis or impending death
   E. all of the above

634. Halothane
   A. has no depressant effect on the heart
   B. is inflammable
   C. is a potent anesthetic used in concentrations of 1-3%. delivered from a special apparatus
   D. is explosive
   E. is none of the above

635. The advantages of intravenous thiopental sodium anesthesia include
   A. rapid and pleasant induction
   B. little salivation
   C. no fire or explosion hazard
   D. rapid recovery and minimal aftereffects
   E. all of the above

636. Vinyl ether has which of the following properties?
   A. Toxic to liver and kidney, irritant, and relaxation moderate
   B. Rapid action, no cardiac toxicity
   C. Moderate anesthetic potency
   D. Inflammable liquid
   E. All of the above

12. COMPLETE DENTURE PROSTHODONTICS

DIRECTIONS: Each of the questions or incomplete statements below is followed by five suggested answers or completions. Select the ONE that is best in each case.

---

637. Failure of full dentures can often be traced to
   A. poor patient instructions and information
   B. immediate insertion of denture
   C. the first five minutes of evaluation of the patient
   D. learning time
   E. none of the above

638. Evaluation of the full denture patient should include
   A. ridge shape
   B. the position of remaining teeth to be extracted
   C. maxillomandibular space
   D. health, tolerance, and adaptability
   E. none of the above

639. Important diagnostic factors for complete dentures include
   A. geriatric nutrition
   B. border extension
   C. muscles of the pharynx
   D. age, social position, position of remaining teeth, ridge size and shape, and saliva
   E. none of the above

640. The torus mandibularis
  A. should never be removed surgically
  B. has a known etiology
  C. may be irritated by movements of the denture
  D. is always larger than a hazelnut
  E. is none of the above

641. The denture-bearing area covering the incisive foramen
  A. should be relieved routinely to prevent impingement of nasopalatine nerves and blood vessels
  B. should not be relieved routinely
  C. should be relieved routinely to prevent impingement on the mental nerve
  D. is surrounded by a sharp narrow annular ridge
  E. is none of the above

642. The temporomandibular joint is
  A. a sliding hinge capable of hinge, lateral, bilateral and protrusive movements, and combinations of the latter
  B. capable of only lateral and protrusive movements
  C. capable only of opening and closing the jaws
  D. not a sliding hinge joint
  E. none of the above

643. The Bennett movement is
  A. caused by contraction of one external pterygoid muscle
  B. caused by the sphenomandibular ligament
  C. caused by the articular disk (meniscus)
  D. a direct lateral slide occurring simultaneously with a lateral mandibular movement
  E. none of the above

644. Malposition of the mandible due to occlusal disharmony
  A. may result in muscular imbalance, trismus, and pain
  B. causes drifting of teeth
  C. causes sleeping habits
  D. results in neoplasms of the TMJ
  E. does none of the above

645. Occlusal errors are
  A. always easily recognized
  B. detected by roentgenogram of TMJ
  C. due to maximum relaxation of jaws
  D. not always easy to recognize
  E. none of the above

646. A patient whose occlusal abnormalities have been corrected once
   A. becomes less sensitive to slight changes in occlusion than before correction
   B. becomes more sensitive to slight changes in occlusion than before correction
   C. shows no change in sensitivity to slight changes in occlusion
   D. is caused pain by wet heat to the jaws
   E. is none of the above

647. Rugae
   A. may be distorted in an impression to provide comfort to patient
   B. are areas of hard tissue
   C. should not be distorted in an impression to provide comfort to the patient
   D. are located in the posterior part of the palate
   E. are none of the above

648. A well-made impression
   A. may overcome the difficulties resulting from malocclusion
   B. may in specific instances overcome the difficulties resulting from malocclusion
   C. does not require our best efforts
   D. can never overcome the difficulties resulting from malocclusion
   E. is none of the above

649. The external oblique ridge
   A. does not govern the extension of the buccal flange
   B. does govern the extension of the buccal flange
   C. does not help to determine the relative amount of resistance or lack of resistance of border tissues
   D. is not a valuable landmark in prosthetic dentistry
   E. is none of the above

650. The lingual extension on impressions
   A. has been abused and misunderstood
   B. is limited by the ramus of the mandible
   C. is limited by the retromolar fossa
   D. is limited by the buccinator muscle
   E. is none of the above

651. Hypertrophied tissue ridges
   A. are caused by trauma under an old denture
   B. take very great biting stress
   C. with pressure placed on them will not lead to more irritation
   D. should be treated similar to normal tissue during impression making
   E. are none of the above

652. Registration of centric relation
   A. is exact and can be proved
   B. is not exact
   C. cannot be proved
   D. with correct vertical dimension cannot be arrived at without question
   E. is none of the above

653. Errors in the arrangement of teeth for complete dentures include
   A. setting mandibular anterior teeth too far forward to meet maxillary teeth
   B. failure to make cuspids the turning point of the arch
   C. setting mandibular first bicuspids to the buccal side of the cuspids
   D. failure to establish the occlusal plane at the proper level and inclination
   E. all of the above

654. Anterior artificial teeth should be placed
   A. in exactly the same positions as the previous natural teeth
   B. in a labial position to the previous natural teeth
   C. in a lingual position to the previous natural teeth
   D. in infraocclusion compared to previous natural teeth
   E. in none of the above

655. Setting teeth with their long axes parallel to each other
   A. produces very natural looking teeth
   B. causes people to be happy with their dentures
   C. never causes patients to be irritated by the appearance of their dentures
   D. produces an artificial appearance to the dentures
   E. does none of the above

656. The plane of occlusion which results in enhanced stability is one with
   A. end-to-end relations
   B. reduced incisal inclination
   C. increased incisal inclination
   D. horizontal overlap
   E. none of the above

657. Balanced occlusion refers to
   A. the balancing side
   B. occlusion with simultaneous contacts of the occlusal surfaces of teeth of both sides of the arch, regardless of mandibular position
   C. the working side
   D. centric occlusion
   E. none of the above

658. Centric occlusion and centric relation with tooth contact
   A. always coincide
   B. may not coincide
   C. coincide only in the adult
   D. never coincide in a child
   E. do none of the above

659. Occlusion of all complete dentures should be
   A. perfected after the patient wears them
   B. partially perfected before and partially after the patient wears them
   C. perfected before the patient is permitted to wear them
   D. delayed until the patient discovers errors in occlusion
   E. none of the above

660. Errors in occlusion may result from
   A. unavoidable changes in the denture base material
   B. making the impression
   C. making the waxed dentures
   D. a difference in incisal guidance
   E. none of the above

661. Factors important in the retention of dentures are
   A. the basal surface
   B. the impression surface
   C. the leverage position and occlusal surface of the teeth
   D. the shape of the polished surfaces of the dentures
   E. all of the above

662. Types of occlusal error in centric occlusion are
   A. any pair of opposing teeth can be too long and hold teeth out of contact
   B. upper and lower teeth can be too nearly end-to-end
   C. upper teeth can be too far bucally in relation to lower teeth
   D. A, B, and C can be corrected by specific grinding for each error
   E. all of the above

663. Important factors in diagnosis and treatment planning for complete dentures include
   A. mental attitude
   B. systemic status
   C. local factors
   D. diagnostic procedures
   E. all of the above

664. Anatomic landmarks in the maxillary arch of importance in complete denture impressions are
   A. the labial frenum which may be single or multiple
   B. the labial vestibule or labial flange area
   C. the buccal frenum
   D. the buccal vestibule area, hamular notch
   E. all of the above

665. Inflammatory reaction of the basal mucosa is the result of
   A. removing dentures to allow tissue to rest
   B. absence of hyperemia
   C. endocrine disturbances
   D. good oral hygiene
   E. none of the above

666. Dislodgement of complete dentures during function is the result of
   A. overextension in the masseter groove area
   B. lateral extension beyond the external oblique line
   C. overextension of lingual flanges
   D. placing occlusal plane too high
   E. all of the above

667. The temporomandibular joint
A. is not a sliding hinge joint
B. is a monarthrodial ginglymous joint
C. has only one joint acting as a hinge of rotation
D. is unique and set apart from all other joints of the skeleton
E. is none of the above

668. Denture stability is enhanced
A. by placing the occlusal areas distant from their support
B. by placing the occlusal areas close to their support
C. when the patient does not chew vertically
D. by not centralizing the occlusal areas
E. by none of the above

669. Vertical dimension
A. is the face height at physiologic rest position
B. is occlusal contact
C. of rest position is the vertical separation of the jaws when tonic contraction of maxillofacial musculature exists
D. is the interocclusal gap
E. is none of the above

670. The arrangement of teeth on an articulator
A. gives a full indication of the way the teeth will look in the oral cavity
B. gives only a partial indication of the way the teeth will look in the oral cavity
C. is the final functional form
D. will always be in harmony for muscle action
E. is none of the above

671. Synthetic resin teeth
A. are more easily individualized than porcelain ones
B. are less easily individualized than porcelain ones
C. cannot appear individualized
D. cannot be made as thin as necessary
E. are none of the above

672. In selecting porcelain teeth, it is well to judge their suitability not only according to their labiolingual thickness but also according to
   A. bite
   B. the three divisions of the lingual side (bite, pin-seal, and ridge-lap)
   C. pin-seat
   D. ridge-lap
   E. none of the above

673. Some of the most common errors in arrangement are that
   A. all incisors are too even
   B. upper lateral incisors are too low
   C. upper lateral incisors are rotated away from central incisors
   D. lower incisors are tipped too much lingually at incisal ends
   E. all of the above are true

674. A simple and accurate way of producing both protrusive and lateral balance is by
   A. means of individually made lower second molars
   B. means of individually made upper bicuspids
   C. placing balancing occlusal unit labially to upper working occlusal unit
   D. placing balancing occlusal unit mesial to the upper working occlusal unit
   E. none of the above

675. Rehabilitation of persons with maxillofacial defects or problems requires a team effort and which of the following in a comprehensive approach to the problem?
   A. Pertinent questionnaires
   B. Discussions providing medical, psychological, and socioeconomic information to influence the treatment planning
   C. The patient should be examined comprehensively, i. e., objectively and subjectively
   D. Accurate and adequate study casts (intraoral and extraoral) should be obtained
   E. All of the above

676. Technical indications for a provisional prosthesis are
   A. postsurgical sequelae (trismus, need for irradiation therapy, changes in dimensions of defect, interim or transitional prosthesis)
   B. existing intraoral conditions (pathology, occlusion, retention factors, undesirable anatomic structures)
   C. unsatisfactory opposing prosthesis
   D. broken clasps and/or rests, incorrect occlusal plane, inadequate retention and stabilization factors of opposing prosthesis
   E. all of the above

677. The causes of maxillofacial defects requiring maxillofacial prosthetics are
   A. oral and paraoral defects as a consequence of surgery
   B. abnormal morphologic conditions with or without altered physiologic function
   C. conditions precipitated by trauma or any surgical intervention required to debride or close wounds or stabilize or replace lost parts
   D. injuries to the head and neck produced by a weapon (such as in war) or vehicular or other accidents
   E. all of the above

678. Patients with maxillofacial defects
   A. require treatment of the patient's personality
   B. do not require an interview of their attitudes
   C. do not require a psychosocial assessment
   D. fail to have any negative assessments of the effect of the deformity on personality
   E. need none of the above

679. The clinical examination of any patient for a maxillofacial prosthesis
   A. need not have panaoramic, occlusal, and periapical dental radiographs
   B. should not have cephalometric films produced
   C. must be supplemented by radiographic and diagnostic cast examination
   D. should not have diagnostic casts made for observation of total occlusal relationships
   E. needs none of the above

680. A guide-flange prosthesis
   A. is used for correction of speech deficiencies
   B. is a mandibular prosthesis designed for the patient who is able to achieve an appropriate mediolateral position of the mandible but is unable to repeat this position consistently
   C. represents the adjunctive phase of treatment for the congenital defect
   D. is the pharyngeal section of a speech-aid prosthesis
   E. is none of the above

681. Which of the following represent acquired maxillary defects?
   A. Fixed prosthodontic needs
   B. Alveolar ridge defect
   C. Hard palate defect, soft palate defect
   D. Partial maxillary resection
   E. All of the above

682. The common errors observed in the clinical management of congenital defects revolve around
   A. vertical dimension of occlusion
   B. prosthesis contours
   C. velar extension design
   D. obturator placement and design, oral hygiene
   E. all of the above

683. Which of the following structures may be altered as the result of the effects of radiation on the structures of the head and neck?
   A. Oral mucosa
   B. Salivary glands
   C. Taste
   D. Neuromuscular function, teeth, bone
   E. All of the above

684. The prevention of osteoradionocrosis lies with an understanding of which of the following predisposing factors?
A. Inadequate healing of previous surgery prior to the initiation of therapy
B. Proximity of irradiated lesions to bone
C. High radiation dosage, combination of external and interstitial radiation sources
D. Poor oral hygiene and tissue abuse, unnecessary surgery involving irradiated tissues, indiscriminate use of prostheses following radiotherapy without resolution of primary problems, bony trauma in irradiated areas, disregard for physical health and nutrition problems
E. All of the above

685. Splints are appliances for the fixation of displaced or movable parts. Which of the following splint may be utilized in maxillofacial prostheses?
A. Gunning splint in the edentulous patient
B. Labiolingual splint
C. Fenestrated splint
D. Kingsley splint, occlusal wafer, palatal-occlusal splint, cast-metal splints
E. All of the above

686. The most common problem confronting the dentist in constructing maxillofacial prostheses is
A. anterior end guidance
B. management of teeth, both natural and artificial, at the stump or surgical resection line
C. wax wafers for interocclusal registrations
D. speech
E. none of the above

687. Materials currently utilized for extraoral prostheses include
A. methyl methacrylate resin
B. latexes
C. vinyl plastisol, silicone rubber
D. room-temperature vulcanizing silicones, heat-vulcanizing silicones, polyurethane polymers
E. all of the above

688. Adhesives that have been used successfully with facial prostheses include
   A. biface adhesive tape works with polyvinyl chloride resin
   B. davol works with polyvinyl chloride and polyurethane
   C. medico adhesive works with polyvinyl chloride, silicone, and acrylic
   D. epithane-3 adhesive works with polyvinyl chloride and silicone, Prosad adhesive is effective with silicone
   E. all of the above

13. PARTIAL DENTURE PROSTHODONTICS

DIRECTIONS: Each of the questions or incomplete statements below is followed by five suggested answers or completions. Select the ONE that is best in each case.

---

689. On the basis of how support is achieved or how occlusal work loads are transferred to the supporting bone, the types of prostheses used for the replacement of teeth include
   A. tooth-borne partial denture
   B. tooth-borne partial denture, tissue-borne complete denture, and tooth-tissue-borne extension-base prosthesis
   C. tissue-borne complete denture
   D. tooth-tissue-borne extension-base prosthesis
   E. none of the above

690. The removable partial denture has
   A. an extension base
   B. tooth-tissue supported appliances
   C. at least one free-end base
   D. removable and tooth-borne
   E. none of the above

691. The extension-base partial denture has which of the following features?
   A. Removable and tooth-borne
   B. Stress is tensile
   C. An accurate elastic impression is required
   D. Major support is from structures underlying its base, and it has at least one free-end base
   E. None of the above

692. Methods of classification of removable partial denture prosthesis have been developed by
   A. Cummer only
   B. Cummer, Friedman, and Kennedy
   C. Friedman only
   D. Kennedy only
   E. none of the above

693. The Kennedy classification includes
   A. class I (bilateral edentulous areas located posterior to the remaining teeth)
   B. class II (a unilateral edentulous area located posterior to the remaining teeth)
   C class III (a unilateral edentulous area bounded anteriorly and posteriorly by remaining teeth)
   D. class IV (an edentulous area located anterior to the remaining teeth)
   E. all of the above

694. In the Applegate-Kennedy classification
   A. two groups have been removed from the Kennedy classification
   B. three more groups have been added to the Kennedy classification
   C. one more group has been added to the Kennedy classification for clarification
   D. two more groups have been added to the previous four of the Kennedy classification for clarification
   E. none of the above is true

695. The most important part of a partial denture is the
   A. connectors
   B. replaced teeth
   C. base
   D. reciprocal arm
   E. none of the above

696. In major connectors, the principle of counterleverage may be utilized to
   A. increase lateral stresses on abutments
   B. increase twisting stresses on abutments
   C. stimulate tissue tone
   D. decrease lateral, twisting (torque) stresses on abutments
   E. do none of the above

697. The occlusal rest
 A. prevents occlusal movement of the appliance on the abutment
 B. prevents cervical movement of the appliance on the abutment
 C. fails to assist in limiting lateral appliance movement
 D. fails to assist in maintaining occlusal efficiency
 E. does none of the above

698. The first requirement of an impression for partial prosthesis is the
 A. static relationship
 B. registration of perfect anatomic form
 C. contour of abutment teeth
 D. extension-base
 E. none of the above

699. A requisite of the impression for a removable extension-base prosthesis is
 A. the function of supporting occlusal loads
 B. a static relationship
 C. registration of the functional or supporting form of the subjacent foundation area
 D. the minute contour of abutment teeth
 E. none of the above

700. An advantage of hydrocolloid materials for partial dentures is
 A. it will remove from undercut areas without permanently deforming or tearing
 B. it is a one-piece impression
 C. no separating medium is required
 D. it can be used very quickly
 E. all of the above

701. The majority of surveyors have which of the following parts?
 A. Level platform
 B. Vertical upright
 C. Horizontal arm
 D. Table, base, mandrel and paralleling tool, analyzing rod, or guideline marker
 E. All of the above

702. The path of insertion is
   A. from rest position to last contact of its rigid parts with supporting teeth
   B. vertical right
   C. the movement of an appliance from the points of initial contact to the place of final rest position
   D. vertical posterior
   E. none of the above

703. The path of removal is
   A. movement of the appliance from the points of initial contact to the place of final rest position
   B. the appliance movement from rest position to the last contact of its rigid parts with the supporting teeth
   C. vertical position
   D. vertical-right
   E. none of the above

704. The path of insertion may be influenced by
   A. interference to insertion and removal
   B. retention of appliance against dislodging forces
   C. esthetics
   D. guiding planes
   E. all of the above

705. The uses of the surveyor include
   A. indicating where a retentive clasp could be located with greatest esthetics
   B. improving the esthetic result by lessening the need for mutilating the anatomic form of anterior tooth substitutes
   C. promoting more positive clasp retention and lessen clasp strain by indicating positive guiding planes in abutment preparations
   D. indicating the areas of critical importance in the final impression
   E. all of the above

706. The preliminary examination should be adequate to supply reliable data on
   A. any disease process in any of the oral structures
   B. the existence of a physical abnormality which would contraindicate the rendering of dental rehabilitation
   C. the patient's age, sex, occupational activity, and economic status
   D. any oral and/or systemic evidence of reduced tissue tolerance
   E. all of the above

707. The oral examination should be adequate to supply reliable data on the teeth regarding
   A. the nonvital status of any pulp
   B. the existence of a degenerative change in any pulp which might lead to a later condition of nonvitality
   C. the presence of new or recurrent caries or areas of demineralized enamel
   D. the number and location of teeth remaining in a dental arch which can be restored to a healthy condition
   E. all of the above

708. Conditions of prosthetic significance include
   A. oral health
   B. systemic health
   C. caries susceptibility
   D. bone of the jaw
   E. all of the above

709. Which of the following are serious defects inherent in a radiographic method of determining the balance of the patient's supporting bone?
   A. Favorable appliance support may be found in patients having less dense bone as well as those having bone which is dense
   B. There is a lack of agreement whether dense or less dense bone assumes extra work loads with least tendency to atrophic change
   C. The apparent density of the alveolar bone varies in the same specimen when there is a change in the angulation of film or in exposure or processing
   D. There is a wide difference of opinion as to what is really meant by "dense"
   E. All of the above are true

710. Mouth preparation for partial dentures is a term
   A. indicating operative dentistry
   B. indicating crown and bridge work
   C. indicating prophylaxis
   D. covering all types of changes affected in the teeth, ridges, or other oral structures
   E. meaning none of the above

711. To have occlusal imbalance means
   A. the teeth will receive forces tending to tilt them
   B. that the induced work loads will be magnified
   C. that areas of the periodontium will be subjected to stress
   D. overload very often exceeds the tolerance of the host's supporting structures
   E. all of the above

712. One very important advantage of the use of an abutment crown is that
   A. the lingual as well as the proximal surface may be made parallel to the path of insertion and removal
   B. the crown can be replaced as desired
   C. the crown can carry the occlusal rest
   D. the crown can have a lingual surface made parallel to path of insertion and removal
   E. none of the above

713. Multiple abutments will be increasingly utilized because
   A. of tilted teeth
   B. of new partial denture designs
   C. of stimulation of the gingiva
   D. many teeth are now being restored to health through periodontic therapy
   E. of none of the above

714. During multiple splinting the use of the inlay is avoided for anchorage of a splint because
   A. it may fracture
   B. it may cause fracture of the tooth
   C. of the danger of its becoming partially loosened
   D. it weakens the splint
   E. of none of the above

715. An excellent objective in partial denture prosthesis is
   A. to produce a highly complex design
   B. to devise an intriguing new design
   C. to utilize a new material
   D. to keep appliance design as simple as possible
   E. none of the above

716. Which of the following represent tooth-supported functional units of a removable partial denture?
   A. Major connectors and base
   B. Minor connectors
   C. Direct retainer
   D. Indirect retainers
   E. All of the above

717. A critical requisite of the free-end base is
   A. that its relationship to the ridge structures be such that the work load is distributed uniformly
   B. that it does not require an occlusal rest
   C. that it requires no major connector
   D. that it requires no direct retainer
   E. none of the above

718. The second auxiliary function of the extension base is
   A. to reduce maintenance
   B. to eliminate the occlusal rest
   C. to eliminate the minor connector
   D. to provide effectual resistance to torque stresses
   E. none of the above

719. The occlusal rests
   A. provide unification
   B. provide counterleverage
   C. are linguoplate connectors
   D. resist movement of the partial denture in a cervical direction
   E. none of the above

720. Rigidity of the major connector may be made more certain by employing one or more of which of the following?
   A. Use a cast rather than a wrought iron connector
   B. Avoid a flat or ribbon-shaped connector
   C. Increase the bulk of a major connector
   D. Utilize the linguoplate type of connector
   E. All of the above

721. The most frequently used direct retainer is
   A. the vertical upright
   B. the upright lug
   C. the trussarm
   D. the intracoronal and extracoronal retainer
   E. none of the above

722. Which of the following factors aid in determining clasp retentiveness?
   A. The angle of cervical convergence of the infrabulge abutment surface in the area where the clasp is to be placed
   B. The distance that the retentive arm is placed cervical to the height of the contour
   C. How well the retentive terminal contact is maintained
   D. The flexibility of the retentive clasp
   E. All of the above

723. Regarding the routine use of hinges or other types of stress-breakers for distal extension partial dentures,
   A. it is acceptable
   B. it causes no misuse
   C. it is not acceptable
   D. it is adequate support for the partial denture base
   E. none of the above is true

724. Which of the following represent phases of partial denture service?
   A. Patient education
   B. Treatment planning and design
   C. Adequate support for distal extension denture bases
   D. Establishment of occlusal relations
   E. All of the above

725. The oral examination for partial dentures should encompass
   A. thorough and complete oral prophylaxis
   B. placement of individual temporary restorations
   C. a complete intraoral roentgenographic survey
   D. vitality tests, exploration of teeth and investing structures, and impressions for casts
   E. all of the above

726. The final treatment plan for partial denture prosthesis should represent the best possible course for the patient after considering
   A. physical and mental factors
   B. mechanical factors
   C. esthetics
   D. economic factors
   E. all of the above

727. The effectiveness of tissue support is dependent upon
   A. quality of the residual ridge
   B. accuracy of the denture bases
   C. accuracy of impression registration
   D. total occlusal load applied
   E. all of the above

728. Which of the following factors influence the design of the removable partial denture?
   A. Which arch is to be restored
   B. Whether or not the denture will be entirely tooth-borne
   C. Type of replacement teeth to be used
   D. Materials to be used for framework and bases
   E. All of the above

729. When one or more distal extension bases are involved, which of the following factors must be considered?
   A. Need for indirect retention
   B. Clasp designs which minimize the forces applied to the abutment during function
   C. Need for later rebasing
   D. Secondary impression method to be used
   E. All of the above

730. The typical removable partial denture contains
   A. major and minor connectors
   B. rests and direct retainers
   C. reciprocal or bracing components
   D. indirect retainers and one or more bases
   E. all of the above

731. Indications for the use of a linguoplate in partial denture construction include
   A. stabilizing periodontally weakened lower teeth
   B. in the class I situations with residual ridges undergoing excessive vertical resorption
   C. when lingual frenum is high or the space available for a lingual bar is slight
   D. when the patient has found a past lingual bar objectionable
   E. all of the above

732. Maxillary major connectors include
   A. single palatal bar
   B. u-shaped palatal connector
   C. combination anterior and posterior palatal bar-type connectors
   D. palatal plate-type connectors
   E. all of the above

733. The function of the minor connector is
   A. not to transfer the effect of the retainers to the rest of denture
   B. to transfer functional stress to the abutment teeth
   C. to provide an internal clip attachment
   D. to provide a splint bar for the partial denture
   E. none of the above

734. A rest should be designed so that transmitted forces are directed
   A. horizontally
   B. along the long axis of the supporting tooth
   C. mesially
   D. distally
   E. in none of the above ways

735. The most satisfactory lingual rest, from the standpoint of support is
   A. one placed on a prepared rest seat cast restoration
   B. one placed on enamel
   C. one placed on acrylic
   D. one placed on silicate
   E. none of the above

736. Which of the following points are important in multiple spruing for partial denture construction?
   A. Use a few sprues of larger diameter rather than several smaller sprues
   B. Keep all sprues as short and direct as possible
   C. Avoid abrupt changes in direction and T-shaped junctions
   D. Reinforce all junctions with additional wax to avoid constrictions in sprue channel
   E. All of the above

737. The spruing of the cast for partial dentures should include which of the following considerations?
   A. The sprues should be large enough so molten metal in them will not solidify before the casting proper has frozen
   B. The sprues should lead into the mold cavity as directly as possible
   C. The sprues should leave a crucible from a common point
   D. The sprues should be attached to the pattern at its bulkier sections
   E. All of the above are true

738. Excellent dental castings are dependent upon
   A. the size of the sprues
   B. the length of the sprues
   C. the configuration of sprues
   D. the points of attachment and the manner of attachment of the sprues to the cast
   E. all of the above

739. Dental castings are dependent upon
   A. the restraint offered to the expansion of the investment, due to the investment ring
   B. setting time, burn-out temperature, and burn-out time
   C. the method of casting, gases (adhered, entraped, and absorbed), and force used in throwing the metal into the mold
   D. shrinkage on cooling, removal from the investment after casting, pickling, polishing, and heat handling
   E. all of the above

740. When finishing a dental casting, which of the following should be taken into consideration?
   A. High speeds are preferable to low speeds
   B. There is less danger of the casting being thrown out of the hands due to high speed
   C. The wheels or points and the speed of thier rotation should do the cutting
   D. A definite sequence for finishing should be adopted and followed in every case
   E. All of the above

741. Dental gold castings, which are subject to heat hardening, may be effectively hardened by which of the following?
   A. Quench the casting in the investment by shaking it vigorously in an ample volume of water as soon as the sprue bottom has lost its heat
   B. Remove the casting from the investment
   C. Thoroughly clean and do all the finishing necessary
   D. Heat harden the casting
   E. Do all of the above

742. Which of the following are types of anterior teeth used on partial dentures?
   A. Porcelain or resin denture teeth
   B. Ready-made resin denture teeth
   C. Resin teeth processed to a metal framework
   D. Porcelain or resin facings cemented to denture framework and anterior teeth hollowed out to receive resin veneers
   E. All of the above

743. Rules for forming the interdental papilla state that
   A. the papilla must extend to the point of tooth contact for cleanliness
   B. the papillae must be of various lengths
   C. interdental papilla must be convex in all directions
   D. the papillae must be shaped according to the age of the patient
   E. all of the above

14. CROWN AND BRIDGE PROSTHODONTICS

DIRECTIONS: Each of the questions or incomplete statements below is followed by five suggested answers or completions. Select the ONE that is best in each case.

---

744. The purpose of replacing a lost member is
   A. functional
   B. aesthetic and functional
   C. aesthetic
   D. to remove caries
   E. none of the above

745. A removable partial denture replacing one tooth
   A. is an acceptable permanent method
   B. is not an acceptable method unless it is temporary treatment until a fixed partial denture is placed
   C. does not result in caries under the clasps
   D. has no danger of aspiration of prosthesis
   E. is none of the above

746. A fixed splint
   A. is a gold inlay
   B. is a type of fixed prosthesis used to stabilize two or more teeth
   C. is an abutment
   D. is a connector
   E. is none of the above

747. Failures in fixed partial dentures can be minimized by compliance with
   A. physiologic requirements
   B. mechanical requirements
   C. hygienic requirements
   D. aesthetic requirements
   E. all of the above

748. Considerations in fixed partial denture treatment are
   A. the age of the patient
   B. the teeth involved
   C. the pathologic condition of the teeth
   D. the position of teeth
   E. all of the above

749. An abutment tooth tilted beyond 25° is
   A. usually ruled out as an abutment
   B. occasionally used as an abutment
   C. never ruled out as an abutment
   D. suitable for an abutment
   E. none of the above

750. A disadvantage of the direct method for constructing fixed partial dentures is
   A. it cannot be readily used for all types of retainers
   B. it requires more appointments than the indirect method
   C. marginal adaptation of retainers is difficult to obtain
   D. it is more difficult to master
   E. all of the above

751. An advantage of the direct method for constructing fixed partial dentures is
   A. it requires more chair time
   B. an accurate adaptation of marginal lines can be obtained and it requires less chair time
   C. accurate adaptation is impossible
   D. it is easier to master the direct method
   E. none of the above

752. From study casts, each tooth can be studied to determine
   A. the crown length
   B. the crown contour
   C. the position of the tooth in the arch
   D. the relation of the arches to each other
   E. all of the above

753. The objectives of correcting centric occlusion are
   A. to achieve harmony of centric relation and centric occlusion by repositioning the mandible
   B. to bring cuspid teeth in contact
   C. to secure uniform contact of all teeth
   D. to provide a balanced stop
   E. all of the above

754. Reduce a cusp tip
   A. when the mesial incline on upper is reduced
   B. only when it is an interfering contact in centric, working, and balance positions
   C. when the distal incline of the lower is reduced
   D. when the fossa is deepened
   E. when none of the above occurs.

755. A fixed partial denture provides
   A. stability
   B. an excellent appearance
   C. improved function
   D. patient comfort
   E. all of the above

756. The choice of method of tooth replacement should be considered in which of the following orders?
   A. Fixed partial denture, complete denture, removable partial denture
   B. Complete denture, fixed and removable partial denture
   C. Removable partial, complete denture, fixed partial denture
   D. Fixed partial denture, removable partial denture, complete denture
   E. None of the above

757. An indication for occlusal equilibration is
   A. excessive occlusal wear
   B. periodontal problems
   C. temporomandibular disturbances attributed to occlusion
   D. extensive restorative procedures involving two or more quadrants
   E. all of the above

758. An indication for inlay abutments is
   A. tooth replacement should not exceed a single tooth
   B. abutment teeth should be bulky and well-supported with crown length above average
   C. biting stresses should be minimal
   D. abutments should be in good alignment and distal retainer should be a MOD inlay
   E. all of the above

759. A contraindication for the inlay abutment is
   A. long span
   B. weak, short, and broken-down teeth
   C. abutments in poor alignment
   D. heavy biting stresses and dentition with low caries resistance
   E. all of the above

760. The partial veneer retainer is indicated on maxillary and mandibular anteriors and bicuspids and maxillary molars when
   A. the facial surface is in good condition
   B. sufficient sound dentin remains to permit replacement of adequate retention
   C. the crowns are of good length
   D. there is adequate alignment
   E. all of the above are true

761. Contraindications to the partial veneer crown are
   A. maxillary or mandibular incisors, triangular in shape or with minimal faciolingual thickness
   B. mandibular molars with shape not adaptable to this type of retainer
   C. maxillary second molar with low and poorly developed distal marginal ridge and short distal surface
   D. any badly broken-down tooth with insufficient sound dentin for retention
   E. all of the above

762. Indications for the complete veneer crown as a retainer on anterior teeth are
   A. teeth which have eroded or carious surfaces
   B. teeth which have proximal surfaces involved with large interproximal caries and restorations
   C. teeth which require alterations in length
   D. teeth which require alterations in alignment for cosmetic reasons
   E. all of the above

763. Indications for the complete veneer crown as a retainer on posterior teeth are
A. teeth which have high caries suceptibility
B. teeth which have no ability, due to caries, to support other types of retainers
C. teeth which have mandibular molars shaped for adequate retention
D. maxillary second molars with low and poorly developed distal marginal ridge and contour
E. all of the above

764. Fixed splints
A. are used when periodontal tissues have been exposed to the traumatic influence of excessive tooth movement
B. may not involve a single loose tooth
C. depend upon span length and cosmetic qualities
D. should be the size and shape of the coronal portion of the tooth
E. are none of the above

765. The choice of retainers used for a splint is governed by
A. the retention needed
B. the length of span involved
C. the health of coronal portion of teeth
D. the caries and existing restorations in the teeth
E. all of the above

766. Broken-down vital teeth may be used as an abutment for a full crown retainer
A. never
B. when iridioplatinum wire in the form of a staple is used for reinforcement
C. after placing silver alloy filling
D. after placing oxyphosphate of zinc cement
E. when none of the above are true

767. An advantage of the knife-edge gingival margin is
A. it provides a definite marginal finish line with minimal removal of tooth structure
B. it can be established more rapidly and with fewer instruments
C. it provides sufficient bulk for the wax pattern and gold for good marginal adaptation
D. its strength is adequate when the correct type of gold is used
E. all of the above

768. The gingival marginal finish must be extended below the gingiva
    A. when existing restorations or caries are subgingival on surfaces involved in preparation
    B. in teeth requiring restorations in mouths exhibiting rampant caries
    C. in uncontrolled sensitivity of exposed supragingival cementum and erosion
    D. in interproximal areas without periodontal pockets
    E. in all of the above

769. Because of stresses received by the fixed partial denture, the inlay abutment preparation should provide
    A. parallelism of cavity walls
    B. no undercuts
    C. flat, deep, pulpal wall to provide strength
    D. sufficient proximal surface width to accommodate an adequate connector
    E. all of the above

770. The retentive aspect of the partial veneer crown is in
    A. the amount of gold adapted to facial surface
    B. the amount of reduction of axial walls
    C. its length and depth of grooves and bulk of cingulum
    D. the undercuts produced
    E. none of the above

771. An advantage of ultrahigh-speed hand pieces is
    A. less annoyance because vibration is minimized
    B. less time spent in the chair for the patient
    C. less operating force required on the tooth
    D. less bone-conducted noise and less physical and mental trauma
    E. all of the above

772. An advantage of ultrahigh-speed hand pieces to the operator is
    A. increased efficiency makes quadrant restorative methods easy to accomplish
    B. less patient resistance to tooth preparation
    C. the possibility to make better tooth preparations through increased operator control
    D. less physical and mental trauma with greater efficiency
    E. all of the above

773. The plane of occlusion is
   A. the anatomic curvature of the occlusal alignment
   B. an imaginary surface related anatomically to the cranium
   C. a fixed factor in all prosthetic procedures
   D. the opposing functional occlusion
   E. none of the above

774. In the past few years, procelain has been widely accepted because
   A. of the advent of the diamond and carbide tooth-reducing instruments and high-speed handpieces
   B. of the ease in accomplishing tooth preparation
   C. method was developed for preparing gold with porcelain
   D. acrylic materials available today are inadequate
   E. of all of the above

775. An advantage of the complete porcelain veneer crown is
   A. it has withstood the test of time by satisfying cosmetic demands
   B. it is more readily tolerated by soft tissues than any other material used if properly fused and contoured
   C. it is excellent for maintaining a normal, healthy, and vital pulp on properly prepared teeth
   D. it is an excellent insulating material for protecting the pulp from thermal shock
   E. all of the above

776. Porcelain should be the material of choice
   A. when a facing is demanded for cosmetic reasons
   B. when the material is to be used without the support of metal
   C. for other than for veneer purposes
   D. since extensive inflammatory changes occur in adjacent soft tissue
   E. for none of the above situations

777. Acrylic facings are used in
   A. pin or interchangeable flat-back facings
   B. fabricated to gold facing
   C. long pointed pin facing
   D. pin pontic facing
   E. none of the above

778. Color has
   A. hue
   B. saturation
   C. hue, brilliance, and saturation
   D. brilliance
   E. none of the above

779. The method of designing the anterior facing for a facing with a porcelain ridge portion is
   A. to reduce size (mesiodistally and incisocervically)
   B. to adapt the ridge
   C. to perfect contour and form
   D. to accomplish arch alignment and tooth inclination
   E. to do all of the above

780. Restoring a finish to a ground facing can be accomplished
   A. by polishing only
   B. by polishing by fusing dry porcelain to surface and applying an overglaze
   C. only by fusing dry porcelain to surface
   D. only by applying an overglaze
   E. by none of the above

781. The requirement of the connector is
   A. to supply mechanical strength to fixed partial denture
   B. to provide proper occlusal, buccal, lingual, and interproximal embrasures
   C. to provide correct occlusal function without interference
   D. not to impinge on any marginal finish line of a retainer
   E. to do all of the above

782. A semirigid connector is used
   A. because of difficulty in soldering
   B. if a rigid connector interferes with the physiologic movement of abutment teeth and does not transmit torsional stresses
   C. where parallelism exists in the abutment teeth
   D. where long spans are present
   E. for none of the above

183. The semirigid connector
A. is always located in the distal surface of the anterior retainer
B. is in the mesial surface of the anterior retainer
C. is in the strongest abutment tooth
D. is in long spans
E. is none of the above

784. The complete seating of a fixed partial denture requires evaluation of
A. contact areas
B. marginal finish lines
C. centric occlusion
D. functional occlusion and stability
E. all of the above

785. Which of the following is used to provide space for cement between the internal axial walls of the metal crown and the tooth preparation?
A. Occlusal stone index
B. Aqua regia or electrolytic stripping of gold
C. Hinge bow record
D. Interocclusal records
E. None of the above

786. Patients with fixed partial dentures are instructed on
A. using dental floss under the pontics
B. the use of pipe cleaners to clean interproximal embrasures
C. the use of the toe of the toothbrush to clean under lingual pontic areas
D. additional home-care methods
E. all of the above

787. Failures of fixed partial dentures may be classified into failures due to
A. one or more of the retainers
B. one or more of the connectors
C. inadequate functional occlusion
D. one or more of the pontics
E. all of the above

788. When making abutment tooth preparations
   A. it is not necessary to have the abutments parallel to each other
   B. sufficient tooth structure must be removed to permit paralleling the attachments
   C. there must be gold between the female attachment and the tooth
   D. attachments should be within the contour of the coronal portion of the tooth
   E. all of the above must be considered

789. A bridge
   A. is a nonremovable prosthesis
   B. reproduces a portion of the surface anatomy of the clinical crown
   C. reproduces the entire surface anatomy of the clinical crown
   D. is a removable prosthesis
   E. is none of the above

790. Requirements (intangibles) of bridge construction include
   A. forces developed by the oral mechanism and by the resistance of the tooth and supporting tissues to them
   B. modifications of normal tooth form that reduce forces or increase resistance to them
   C. establishing normal tissue tone
   D. maintaining normal tissue tone
   E. all of the above

791. Requirements (technical proficiency and concern) in bridge construction include
   A. removal of caries from abutment or associated tooth
   B. sterilization or cleansing of the tooth surface
   C. protection of the pulp during tooth preparation and construction of bridge
   D. restoration of tooth surface for normal function
   E. all of the above

792. Indications for bridges are
   A. whenever any teeth are present
   B. when any length space can be replaced by bridge
   C. whenever there are properly distributed teeth to serve as abutments
   D. where there is space existing opposite natural teeth only on one end of bridge
   E. none of the above

793. Contraindications to bridges are
   A. when space is of such length that additional load will impair tissue health around abutments
   B. when the space length requires a beam of such dimension that embrasures will be greatly reduced and underlying tissue overprotected
   C. when previous prosthesis produced an unfavorable reaction in mucous membrane
   D. when, in the anterior, there has been a loss of alveolar bone making excessively long pontics
   E. all of the above occur

794. Diagnostic casts are
   A. positive reproductions of the maxillary and mandibular arches mounted in accurate relationship on an articulator
   B. reproductions of the arches
   C. not to be mounted on articulators
   D. not necessary in the diagnosis and planning of treatment for bridges
   E. none of the above

795. The ideal clinical crown for an abutment is
   A. a short tooth
   B. a frail tooth
   C. a tapered tooth
   D. one of average length, of square form and of average bulk
   E. none of the above

796. When possible, the gingival margin of fixed partial prostheses should be located
   A. at least 2 mm above the gingival crest
   B. at least 1 mm above the gingival crest
   C. at least 4 mm above the gingival crest
   D. exactly at the gingival crest
   E. at none of the above

797. Concerning the full veneer crown preparation,
   A. it secures the greatest amount of retention possible with the use of parallel walls
   B. in addition to the mesial and distal walls, the gingival third of the facial and lingual walls are virtually parallel and offer good retention
   C. on posterior teeth additional length may be secured by surgical intervention
   D. if much of the coronal portion of the tooth is destroyed, a pin or post buildup may be necessary to obtain sufficient retention
   E. all of the above are true

798. Investing encompasses which of the following features?
   A. Investment begins by cleansing the wax pattern surface
   B. As soon as the vacuum investing instrument has been assembled, proceed to select, mix, and pour the investment material itself
   C. Use a hygroscopic investment
   D. Investment should secure much of its expansion from prolonged setting in a water bath
   E. all of the above

799. The casting may be heat treated to harden it by simply letting the ring cool slowly after casting and quenching it
   A. below 1000°F
   B. below 500°F
   C. above 1000°F
   D. above 250°F
   E. none of the above

800. Removing the fixed prosthesis may be accomplished by
   A. passing a double strand of dental floss through the embrasure of the pontic and retainer and while holding the occlusal surfaces with the thumb, exerting intermittent tension on the dental floss to free the prosthesis
   B. passing a brass wire ligature through the embrasure between the pontics and the retainer, attaching the wire to the handle of a hand instrument, and gently tapping the handle with a mallet
   C. cutting a conservative groove on the lingual or buccal surface of the retainer with a No. 699 cross-cut fissure bur and then cautiously prying the casting loose from the cement bond
   D. using the Jack screw method as a more certain approach for removing a prosthesis and to preserve the margins of the retainer (a radical technique is to use a Clevedent crown and bridge remover)
   E. all of the above

801. Chewing involves which of the following factors?
   A. There is a definite pattern to chewing; it involves wide lateral closing movements, tooth gliding, and a period of high force during the occlusal phase
   B. In some malocclusions the neuromuscular system shows control during chewing to avoid occlusal interferences
   C. Restorative procedures based on lateral retruded border registrations are applicable to functional chewing movements
   D. The looseness of the TMJ seen in the sagittal view of the working-side condyle plots is important for prosthetic dentistry; the working-side first molar has an anterior component of final closing movement; forces during the occlusal phase of chewing and swallowing are 36.2 and 41.0%, about 40% of the patient's maximum biting force; the force-time contact in chewing is one-half that of nocturnal bruxing; and steep anterior guidance does not appear to expose the teeth to extreme lateral forces
   E. All of the above are true

802. The patient's response to occlusal therapy is related to which of the following factors?
   A. Alteration of the occlusion by splint therapy and occlusal rehabilitation clearly reduce muscle soreness and nocturnal EMG activity
   B. Increasing the vertical dimension of occlusion is based upon the favorable results of the occlusal splint test
   C. Rehabilitation of the occlusion and reduction in muscle soreness are affected by the chewing pattern
   D. Jaw movements are more affected by chewing hard foods than soft foods following occlusal changes; the natural chewing motions may have diagnostic value in patients with dysfunction
   E. All of the above are true

803. Occlusion refers to
   A. the static intercuspal relationship of the teeth plus the act of closing the teeth together
   B. proprioception
   C. border positions
   D. occlusal forces during swallowing
   E. none of the above

804. Centric location is the
   A. unilateral chewing position
   B. ending location of good chewing strokes and is a comfortable physiologic position for all patients who have healthy TMJ and good mandibular muscle control
   C. efferent stimuli to the muscles of mastication
   D. movement of the mandible during chewing
   E. none of the above

805. Eccentric molar contacts on the nonworking side results from
   A. flexion of the mandible
   B. compressibility of the meniscus and periodontal ligament
   C. powerful masseter and temporalis muscles
   D. tough food on the working side acting as a fulcrum to tip the mandible and make molar contacts on the working side; wearing and shortening of the anterior teeth; flat condylar paths; large amounts of sideshifts; and improper posterior tooth inclinations
   E. all of the above

806. The causes for bruxism are
- A. myofacial pain syndrome
- B. rehabilitative restorative dentistry
- C. minimal muscle activities of jaw muscles
- D. those of psychogenic origin and those of occlusal disharmonies
- E. none of the above

807. When planning the therapy for patients with poor relationships of the anterior teeth, primary consideration should be given to
- A. prosthetics
- B. orthodontics
- C. endodontics
- D. periodontics
- E. none of the above

808. In the practice of occlusal equilibration, which of the following is undertaken?
- A. Anterior splint therapy
- B. Maxillary training
- C. Posterior eccentric interferences are removed, resulting in less muscle stress
- D. The production of an overlap of the anterior teeth
- E. None of the above

809. The functions of an articulator are
- A. diagnosis
- B. treatment planning
- C. communication of as much static and dynamic information as possible; diagnosis and treatment planning
- D. diagnosis and treatment planning
- E. none of the above

810. The aim of occlusal therapy is
- A. to restore function to the stomatognathic system
- B. to encourage the physiological reshaping of the bony structures of the TMJ
- C. the treatment of choice for any degenerative change of the TMJ due to occlusal disharmonies
- D. to restore the function of the stomatognathic system and to encourage physiological reshaping of the bony structures of the TMJ
- E. none of the above

811. The subjective signs and symptoms of jaw dysfunction include
   A. headache as the most common symptom
   B. occlusion difficulty
   C. jaw noise
   D. facial pain, earache, and pain upon biting or chewing
   E. all of the above

812. The treatment of jaw pain and dysfunction should be based upon
   A. a correct differential diagnosis
   B. reason and purpose
   C. the relative urgency of the presenting symptoms
   D. being directed toward eliminating or neutralizing the cause of the symptoms
   E. all of the above

813. Conservative treatment of the facial pain patient with myofascial pain and TM joint dysfunction includes
   A. ASA
   B. heat
   C. soft diet
   D. rest, Valium (5 mg HS)
   E. all of the above

814. Conservative therapy alternatives for myofascial pain include
   A. spray and stretch
   B. heat
   C. ultrasound
   D. triggerpoint injection
   E. all of the above

815. Stress control treatment alternatives for myofascial pain include
   A. nerve blocks
   B. counseling, biofeedback, and self-hypnosis
   C. acupuncture
   D. psychiatric evaluation
   E. none of the above

816. An examination of occlusal function in a patient with pain should include
   A. uneven centric stops
   B. lateral deviation in the slide from retruded contract to maximum intercuspation
   C. balancing interferences
   D. protrusive guidance by posterior teeth, lateral guidance by posterior teeth, crossover interferences, and incorrect occlusal vertical dimension
   E. all of the above

817. The myofacial pain-dysfunction patient demonstrating noxious clenching or bruxism should be treated with
   A. stress control alternatives
   B. a bite stent worn at night
   C. acupuncture
   D. therapeutic nerve block
   E. none of the above

818. Occlusal traumatism is
   A. marginal periodontitis
   B. a form of periodontal pathology induced by occlusal trauma
   C. jiggling forces on a tooth
   D. temporal arteritis
   E. none of the above

819. The sequelae of partial edentulism are
   A. undermined esthetic appearance
   B. modification in areas of support
   C. loss of masticatory efficiency
   D. migration of teeth, extrusion of teeth, depression and attrition of teeth, deviation of the mandible and a distorted occlusal position, loss of vertical dimension, TMJ disorders, and loss of alveolar bone
   E. all of the above

820. A characteristic of a satisfactory occlusion is
   A. the need for simultaneous bilateral contacts between premolars and molars in the intercuspal position for a free, undisturbed and relaxed closing from postural position and after a passive hinge movement into a retruded contact position
   B. the elmination of occlusal disharmonies eliciting untoward alterations in the masticatory system
   C. the establishment of an adequate number of bilateral tooth contacts
   D. a stable tooth-to-tooth contact relation of the cusp-fossa relationships on premolars and molars in the intercuspal position that directs forces axially
   E. all of the above

821. The choice of an articulator should be based upon which of the following considerations?
   A. The articulator should accept and maintain an accurate hinge-axis relationship and be adaptable for a face bow
   B. The articulator should maintain a definite interarch relationship
   C. The articulator should accept interocclusal records or positional relation records for mounting casts
   D. The articulator should provide for variation in the side-shift and condyle guidance angle; it also should have an incisal guide table to establish and maintain incisal guidance control
   E. All of the above

822. Vertical dimension is
   A. symmetrical bilateral displacement
   B. maximum intercuspation
   C. the facial height between any two selected points
   D. a symmetrical displacement
   E. none of the above

823. Extraoral devices for the measurement and study of vertical jaw position are
   A. massive headgear for long-term studies with calibration
   B. continuous recordings providing control for lateral and protrusive movements
   C. massive headgear for long-term studies with calibration, and continuous recordings providing control for lateral and protrusive movements
   D. telemetry
   E. none of the above

824. Which of the following factors affect wear (time-dependent removal of tooth surfaces that are in motion relative to each other)?
   A. Increasing the occlusal force
   B. Decreasing the contact area
   C. Increasing the sliding distance and increasing the surface roughness
   D. Increasing the contact frequency and increasing the chemical activity
   E. All of the above

825. One of the contributing factors to periodontal disease is
   A. tooth malposition and early loss of primary teeth with loss of space
   B. abnormal tongue habits
   C. anterior proprioceptive guidance
   D. splint therapy
   E. none of the above

826. Pathologic occlusion produces
   A. excessive wear of teeth
   B. temporomandibular joint disturbances
   C. pulpal involvement (hyperemia, pulpitis, and necrosis)
   D. periodontal alterations
   E. all of the above

827. A pathologic occlusion can be modified to a therapeutic occlusion by correcting
   A. alignment
   B. esthetics
   C. interarch relationships
   D. vertical positioning and transverse positioning
   E. all of the above

828. Requirements of an effective biteguard include
   A. esthetics
   B. vertical positioning
   C. transverse positioning
   D. it must fit the maxillary teeth accurately to provide stability and retention; during centric relation closure all mandibular teeth should contact the biteguard simultaneously; in any position (except centric relation contact position) the working-side mandibular canine should be the only tooth contacting the biteguard
   E. none of the above

829. The advantage oi fabrication of a biteguard include which of the following?
   A. The biteguard can be fabricated from a maxillary cast only (no mandibular cast necessary)
   B. The biteguard can be adjusted intraorally, and casts are not required to be mounted on an articulator
   C. Treatment is started immediately
   D. There is no additional laboratory expense
   E. All of the above

15. ORAL SURGERY

DIRECTIONS: Each of the questions or incomplete statements below is followed by five suggested answers or completions. Select the ONE that is best in each case.

---

830. Treatment of mixed tumors of the salivary glands consists of
   A. irradiation
   B. surgery or electrosurgery removing adequate uninvolved tissue when no capsule is present
   C. excision of adjacent teeth and bone
   D. injection of sclerosing solution into tumor
   E. none of the above

831. In osteomyelitis of the body of the mandible, an alveolar process of the maxilla drainage
   A. may be accomplished by extraction of offending teeth
   B. may be undertaken by incision into the oral mucosa
   C. results from application of heat
   D. results following the Caldwell-Luc operation
   E. does none of the above

832. Treatment of the odontoma consists of
   A. enucleation from extraoral approach
   B. enucleation from intraoral approach, extraoral approach only in very extensive lesions
   C. hemimandibulectomy
   D. resection
   E. none of the above

833. Treatment of the average ameloblastoma should consist of
   A. radium implantation into neoplasm
   B. curettage for all channels and niches harboring neoplastic cells
   C. intraoral block, excision, peripheral osteotomy, and resection of the complete segment containing neoplasm
   D. irradiation
   E. none of the above

834. Oral visibility requires
   A. any type of light to illuminate the oral cavity
   B. that the patient must be positioned so that the dentist can clearly see without stooping, crouching, bending, or twisting
   C. overhead lights
   D. that the patient is allowed to move without it affecting the amount of light in the oral cavity
   E. none of the above

835. Indications for the extraction of teeth include which of the following?
   A. Teeth that are hopelessly carious
   B. Teeth with nonvital pulps, acute or chronic pulpitis when root canal therapy is contraindicated
   C. In cases of severe periodontal disease
   D. Teeth in which apicoectomy is contraindicated
   E. All of the above

836. Contraindications to extraction of teeth or to other oral surgical operations (unless patient's physician approves) include which of the following
   A. Cardiac disease
   B. Rheumatic heart disease
   C. Subacute bacterial endocarditis
   D. Blood dyscrasias
   E. All of the above

837. Oral surgery for the pregnant woman should include
   A. emergency treatment for pain and nonemergency but necessary treatment (periapical chronic abscess)
   B. only emergency dental treatment
   C. only elective dental treatment
   D. emergency, nonemergency, and elective dental treatment
   E. none of the above

838. Complications arising from retained impacted teeth include
A. infection
B. pain
C. fractures
D. ringing in the ear, otitis, and affections of tne eye
E. all of the above

839. Methods of oral radiographic localization include
A. stereoscopic
B. shift-sketch
C. occlusal (topographical, cross section)
D. extraoral (lateral head, posterior-anterior) and use of contrast media
E. all of the above

840. Vital points to remember in the extraction of teeth include
A. never refering to an extraction as a simple extraction
B. forewarning the patient of the possibility of breakage or fracture with alarm
C. never covering up breakage of roots
D. always removing root fragments from the socket
E. all of the above

841. Root breakage during exodontia include
A. peculiar root formation
B. excessive density of surrounding bone
C. incorrect application of force during extraction of teeth
D. beaks of forceps not parallel to long axis of tooth
E. all of the above

842. Components of a detailed examination for oral surgery should include
A. the tooth or teeth to be extracted
B. dental radiographs
C. examination of supporting hard tissues
D. the age of the patient and previous extractions
E. all of the above

843. A reason for root breakage during extractions is
A. improper application of beaks of forceps
B. the wrong type of forceps
C. extensive caries
D. brittleness due to age or nonvitality
E. all of the above

844. Complications during or after the removal of impacted teeth include
A. disruption of the blood supply due to injury to the inferior alveolar artery and vein
B. traumatization or dislodgement of adjacent teeth
C. discoloration of soft tissues overlying and below the mandible, below the eye, and in the cheek or lip
D. injury to the lips, cheeks, or mucous membrane
E. all of the above

845. The treatment of pericoronitis includes
A. conservative treatment with irrigation
B. extraction of the third molar
C. surgical removal of overlying flap
D. electrosurgical removal of overlying flap
E. all of the above

846. Complications accompanying the removal of impacted teeth include
A. exposure of the inferior alveolar canal
B severance of the inferior alveolar nerve or injury resulting in paresthesia of lip
C. acute trismus
D. fracture of roots or fracture of a large section of the alveolar process
E. all of the above

847. A factor complicating the removal of impacted maxillary cuspids includes
A. pronounced curvature at the apical third
B. danger of injury to adjacent teeth and vital structures in the area of surgery
C. openings of various sizes may be created in the maxillary sinus
D. the possibility of forcing the cuspid root into the maxillary sinus
E. all of the above

848. The most important factor in the removal of impacted teeth is
A. a radiograph of the tooth
B. adequate exposure with removal of overlying and surrounding bone
C. soft tissue flap
D. Miller elevators
E. none of the above

849. A history for an oral surgery patient should include which of the following?
   A. Chief complaint and history of present illness
   B. Past medical history and family history
   C. Systemic review and social habits
   D. Summary and clinical impression
   E. All of the above

850. Therapeutic clinical antibiotic usage may be used for localization of which of the following acute infections prior to oral surgery?
   A. Acute cellulitis
   B. Ludwig's infection
   C. Parapharyngeal infections
   D. Osteomyelitis and acute suppurative infections of major salivary glands
   E. All of the above

851 Therapeutic clinical antibiotic usage may be used in the treatment of which of the following acute infections preparatory to oral surgery?
   A. Acute gingivitis and stomatitis
   B. Pericoronitis
   C. Treatment of a sinusitis prior to closure of an oral-antral fistula
   D. Infection of oral mucosa during agranulocytosis and aplastic anemia
   E. All of the above

852. Alveoplasty is
   A. cutting into the alveolar process
   B. surgical contouring of the alveolar process
   C. surgical excision of the alveolar process
   D. surgical contouring of the gingival tissues
   E. none of the above

853. Vestibuloplasty
   A. corrects ankyloglossia
   B. results in deepening of the mandibular sulcus
   C. corrects a hypertrophied labial frenum
   D. corrects a diastema
   E. does none of the above

854. Oral surgical procedures for dental prosthesis include
   A. surgery necessary for the insertion of immediate dentures
   C. the transplantation of developing teeth
   D. excision of tissue which prevents the normal eruption or position of the teeth
   E. all of the above

855. Pain may accompany which of the following situations even though local anesthesia is present?
   A. When pressure is created by the roots or instruments on the inferior alveolar nerve in spite of local anesthesia
   B. When pulps are exposed as a result of the splitting or sectional technique
   C. Following compression of the inferior alveolar nerve
   D. Following compression of an exposed pulp
   E. All of the above

856. Infections of the face and neck are located in which of the following anatomical locations?
   A. Periapical area and pericemental pocket
   B. Upper lips, palate, and canine fossa
   C. Subperiosteal maxilla and mandible, sublingual, mental areas
   D. Buccal space, submandibular or submaxillary areas, and pterygomandibular and zygomaticotemporal spaces
   E. All of the above

857. Postoperative orders should include
   A. removal of tongue suture and sponges when patient reacts
   B. 10 grains ASA with 1/2 grain codeine orally for pain, every 3 hours
   C. ice packs to face for first 24 hours, 30 minutes each hour, followed by heat on second day
   D. soft diet (nonchewing), forced fluids, and multivitamins
   E. all of the above

858. The oral examination prior to oral surgery should include
   A. teeth, mucosa, and gingiva
   B. palate, pharynx, lips, cheeks, floor of mouth, and sublingual tissues
   C. tongue, breath and oral hygiene
   D. lymph nodes, TMJ, and face
   E. all of the above

DIRECTIONS: Each group of questions below consists of lettered headings followed by a list of numbered words or statements. For EACH numbered word or statement, select the ONE heading that is most closely associated with. Each lettered heading may be selected once, more than once, or not at all.

A. Immediate complications associated with oral surgery
B. Syncope
C. Cardiac infarction in dental practice
D. Closed-chest cardiac massage
E. Angioneurotic edema
F. Cardiac arrest
G. Shock
H. Delayed complications associated with oral surgery

859. A circulatory deficiency, which is either cardiac or vasomotor in origin and characterized by decreased cardiac output and hemoconcentration

860. Acute cerebral anemia, the earliest form of shock, and generally transient

861. A rare complication of oral surgery but may follow the administration of any anesthetic, local or general

862. A symptom complex frequently recognized as having a varied mechanism of underlying hereditary and psychophysiologic factors

863. Midsternal thoracic pain, impending suffocation, shortness of breath, sudden and profuse perspiration, vomiting hypotension, tachycardia, and leukocytosis

864. Include syncope, cardiac arrest, myocardial infarction, and acute allergic reactions to antibiotics and anesthetic solutions

DIRECTIONS: Each of the questions or incomplete statements below is followed by five suggested answers or completions. Select the ONE that is best in each case.

865. In a preoperative evaluation of the oral surgery patient, which of the following useful questions should be asked?
A. "Do you suffer from shortness of breath (dyspnea)?"
B. "Have you ever suddenly awakened at night with difficulty in breathing?"
C. "Do you suffer from chest pains?"
D. "Can you sleep flat at night, or do you have to be propped up on pillows? Do you suffer from ankle swelling?"
E. All of the above

866. Examples of other clinical highlights which are suggestive of disease entities include
A. hirsutism and "moonface" (Cushing's disease or excessive steroid therapy); exophthalmos (hyperthyroidism)
B. jugular vein distention (right-sided cardiac failure); lymphadenopathy of submental, submandibular, and deep cervical nodes (Hodgkin's disease or underlying malignant disease)
C. thyroid gland enlargement (goiter or thyroid disease); tremor of hands (Parkinsonism, cerebrovascular disease, hyperthyroidism)
D. clubbing of fingers (chronic diseases of the heart, lung and alimentary system); erythema of palms of hands and increased whiteness at the bases of the nails (cirrhosis of the liver); swelling and pitting edema of ankles (cardiac failure, kidney disease, thrombophlebitis); shuffling gait (Parkinson's disease, hemiplegia after stroke)
E. all of the above

867. Oral surgery in the controlled diabetic is
A. 50% more hazardous than in the nondiabetic patient
B. 10% more hazardous than in the nondiabetic patient
C. no more hazardous than in the nondiabetic patient
D. contraindicated
E. none of the above

868. Which of the following blood dyscrasias affect oral surgery procedures?
  A. Anemia
  B. Leukemia
  C. Agranulocytosis
  D. Bleeding disorders (abnormalities in the coagulation factor system)
  E. All of the above

869. Some of the important and common drug interactions to avoid for the oral surgery patient are
  A. central nervous system depressants (sedatives, hypnotics, tranquilizers, narcotic analgesics), which are potentiated by barbiturates, antihistamines, and alcohol
  B. penicillin, which is antagonized by any of the tetracycline group of broad spectrum antibiotics
  C. the sulfonureas (Tolbutamide, Chlorpropamide, Tolazamide), which are released from binding sites in serum by aspirin and phenylbutazone
  D. monoamine oxidase inhibitors which are antidepressant drugs and are greatly potentiated by vasopressor amines and narcotic analgesics; anticoagulants are potentiated (prothrombin time increased) by aspirin, acetaminophen, tetracycline, and chloral hydrate; prothrombin time is decreased by vitamin C, barbiturates, meprobamate, and most nonbarbiturate sedatives
  E. all of the above

870. Which of the following are general objectives guiding oral surgery responsibilities?
  A. To use a standard methodical pattern for clinical examination
  B. To use a foundation of professional knowledge which guides surgical skill
  C. To recognize and select those problems which lie within the range of the operator's ability and to refer other surgical problems wisely
  D. To develop a sense of confidence in basic surgical skills and improve clinical judgment which stimulates a desire for self-improvement in oral surgery
  E. All of the above

871. Oral-facial pain has been classified as
   A. superficial somatic pain
   B. deep pain, referred pain
   C. odontogenic pain, myogenic pain
   D. arthralgic pain, vascular pain, inflammatory pain, neurogenic pain
   E. all of the above

872. The diagnosis of oral-facial pain is based upon
   A. history, onset, character
   B. duration, localization, modifiers
   C. neurologic signs, response to previous therapy, psychological status
   D. previous injury or infection, concurrent medication
   E. all of the above

873. Diagnoses which often indicate the extraction of teeth are
   A. dental caries (pulp exposure, abscess, granuloma, cyst, residual roots)
   B. periodontitis with or without pericemental abscess
   C. fractured teeth with pulp exposure or pulp necrosis
   D. malposed teeth, impacted teeth, supernumerary teeth, odontogenic cysts
   E. all of the above

874. Which of the following represent diagnoses which modify routine oral surgical procedures?
   A. Acute inflammation (gingivitis, pericoronitis, stomatitis, oral sepsis)
   B. Presence of undiagnosed soft tissue or bone lesions, irradiated supporting bone
   C. Diseases caused by biologic agents, physical agents, chemical agents
   D. Congenital or rheumatic heart disease, congestive heart failure, advanced heart disease, liver disease, severe hypertension, severe malnutrition, blood dyscrasias, systemic diseases, medication with anti-coagulants and steroids
   E. All of the above

875. Which of the following are contraindications for tooth removal?
   A. Acute infections, gross oral sepsis, serious risk to adjacent structures when extraction is elective
   B. Prosthetic problems, undiagnosed malignancy in the area, irradiated bone support from prior treatment of malignancy
   C. Extremes in chronic degenerative diseases, severe malnutrition
   D. Bleeding tendency, first and third trimesters of pregnancy, no adequate antibiotic protection where there is need for subacute bacterial endocarditis prophylaxis
   E. All of the above

876. The significance of the patient with coronary artery occlusion to oral surgery is
   A. hemorrhage following oral surgery
   B. proneness to infection
   C. danger of myocardial infarction precipitated by stress; uncontrolled hemorrhage following oral surgery
   D. delayed healing
   E. none of the above

877. The significance of the patient with rheumatoid arthritis and allergic diseases is
   A. that long-term corticosteroid therapy can cause suppression of adrenocortical function and decreased resistance to stress and infection
   B. that stress precipitates seizure
   C. myocardial infarction
   D. uncontrolled hemorrhage
   E. none of the above

878. The significance of the patient with blood dyscrasias to oral surgery is
   A. it is frequently fatal, there is a possibility of uncontrolled hemorrhage, and the patient is vulnerable to infection
   B. decreased resistance to stress
   C. diabetic acidosis and coma
   D. stress can precipitate seizure
   E. none of the above

879. The significance of the patient with hypertensive heart disease to oral surgery is
   A. stress can precipitate seizure
   B. the danger of cerebral vascular accident from severe hypertension; postural hypotension potentiates drug depression
   C. myocardial infarction precipitated by stress
   D. uncontrollable hemorrhage
   E. none of the above

880. Which of the following are guidelines for the priority of teeth to be removed during multiple extractions?
   A. Any tooth producing pain or teeth with large associated pathology demand immediate attention
   B. In the choice between the two jaws for tooth removal, it is preferable to remove the mandibular teeth or tooth first
   C. In removal of the third molar, the lower third molars should be removed first
   D. A significant hazard is encountered in the removal of residual maxillary molars, i.e., fracture of the maxillary sinus wall; in removal of a single tooth where adjacent teeth are in contact, do not attempt mobilization with elevators placed in the interproximal space
   E. All of the above

881. Conditions that are of special significance in radiographic diagnosis before tooth removal are
   A. root morphology
   B. adjacent bone
   C. regional radiographic landmarks
   D. root morphology, adjacent bone, and regional radiographic landmarks
   E. none of the above

882. When anticipating the removal of multiple adjacent teeth
   A. it is advantageous to incise around the necks of teeth and reflect the mucoperiosteum
   B. it is not wise to incise around the necks of the teeth and reflect the mucoperiosteum
   C. elevators should be used
   D. elevator #1, #2, #303, or #77R should be used
   E. none of the above is true

883. Which of the following teeth can be removed without pre-operative radiographs?
   A. Dilaceration
   B. Hypercementosis
   C. Ankylosis
   D. Gigantism of maxillary central incisors
   E. None of the above

884. Closing of extraction sites by careful suturing requires
   A. suture over bone crest from labial to lingual
   B. suture from the more reflected to the more stabilized flap margin
   C. suture with equal depth and equal distance from margins; suture flaps that are mobile and displaced by controlling them by grasping with the beaks of a tooth beaked, tissue, thumb forceps
   D. suture with instrument tie technique; grasp only the end of the suture in tying the knot to avoid snarling of doubled or excess suture material
   E. all of the above

885. The third molar often is abnormally positioned because
   A. of loosening of adjacent teeth
   B. its formation can be irregular and delayed
   C. of fracture of adjacent teeth
   D. of fracture of the buccal plate; resistant soft tissue
   E. of none of the above

886. Malposed third molars often
   A. displace the second molars into either buccal or lingual malposition or into hypereruption
   B. cause radicular cysts
   D. cause dental caries
   D. cause hypercementosis
   E. do none of the above

887. Any unerupted tooth which lies impacted in the jaws has the potential for
   A. the development of hypercementosis
   B. periodontal disease
   C. the development of a cyst from the reduced enamel epithelium in the paracoronal crypt
   D. paracoronal infections
   E. none of the above

888. If the maxillary tuberosity does fracture during an extraction, which of the following suggestions should prove useful?
   A. If motion is slight and the segment is small, section the tooth and remove it, leaving bone segments attached to the periosteum
   B. If fracture of tuberosity is severe, with a large segment of bone involved, stop the extraction and equilibrate the tooth
   C. If the tooth is partially extracted and a fracture of the tuberosity occurs, section the crown and leave the roots in place; remove the roots after the tuberosity is no longer mobile, i. e., in 6 weeks
   D. If necessary, in a large fracture of the tuberosity, splint the teeth so that the fracture may heal
   E. All of the above

889. Excessive intraoperative hemorrhage
   A. is seldom a problem for the oral surgeon
   B. is rare to encounter (vascular bleeding disorder or clotting deficiency)
   C. with major arteries are quite easy to avoid when designing mucoperiosteal flaps for exodontia
   D. with arterial bleeding may be found in the retromolar area where one or two small arteries may emerge distal to the third molar
   E. involves all of the above

890. The most frequent reasons for extracting erupted permanent teeth are
   A. apical abscesses
   B. periapical granulomas
   C. arch length discrepancies and other orthodontic indications
   D. dental caries (advanced)
   E. none of the above

891. Which of the following factors should be considered in any omergency situation?
A. Observe and record the cardinal physical signs, maintain composure, and act deliberately and with sound judgment
B. Assure patent airway, support the blood pressure, and keep the patient flat unless he is dyspneic or complaining of heart pain
C. If the pulse is slow (less than 40) and the blood pressure is low (less than 90 systolic), give atropine 0.5 mg intravenously; if the pulse is rapid, do nothing; if the pulse is rapid and the blood pressure is low, support the blood pressure with a vasopressor
D. Treat obvious acute allergic emergencies with epinephrine (5 cc of a 1:10, 000 mixture), give the comatose diabetic intravenous glucose (50 g), and treat pain only if you are sure of the etiology
E. All of the above

892. Which of the following represent operative considerations in the prevention of hemorrhage?
A. Planning incisions
B. Handling tissues
C. Bleeding from intrabony vessels and capillary soft tissue bleeding
D. Use of absorbable hemostatic agents
E. All of the above

893. Bacterial factors related to infections of the maxillofacial region are
A. the number of bacteria
B. the species of bacteria
C. devitalized tissue and foreign bodies
D. bacterial enzymes, toxins, and spreading factors
E. all of the above

894. Which of the following represent deep space infection and the site of origin of the maxillofacial regions?
A. Mental abscess (from mandibular incisors)
B. sublingual abscess (from mandibular incisors, cuspids, bicuspids, and molars)
C. Submandibular abscess (from the mandibular bicuspids and molars), Ludwig's angina (from all mandibular teeth), buccal abscess (from the maxillary and mandibular bicuspids and molars), parapharyngeal abscess (from maxillary and mandibular molars, especially third molars)
D. Canine space abscess (from maxillary cuspids), masticator abscess (from lower molars, especially third molar, and needle infection), infratemporal abscess (secondary to other maxillofacial space infections)
E. All of the above

895. Antibiotic usage is indicated when oral surgery is performed in the presence of
A. rheumatic heart disease, congenital heart disease, and a valvular prosthesis
B. diabetes mellitus (uncontrolled or severe) uremia
C. leukemia, multiple myeloma, marrow depressing (anticancer) drugs; hypogammaglobulinemia
D. steroid therapy where infection threatens; disseminated cancer with depleted defenses
E. all of the above

896. Each case should be judged on its own merits. However, the indications for antibiotic therapy in oral surgery are
A. acute cellulitis of dental origin and acute pericoronitis with trismus
B. deep fascial space infections and osteomyelitis
C. open mandibular and maxillary fractures, deep oral lacerations, and oral surgery performed with diminished host defenses
D. prophylaxis (rheumatic and congenital heart disease, cardiac valvular prosthesis) and postoperative bacteremia
E. all of the above

897. Early detection of oral cancer requires that the dentist be alert to
   A. chronicity, bleeding, and friability
   B. hyperkeratosis and hyperplasia
   C. submucosal swelling, induration, and infiltration
   D. retarded healing, regional lymphadenopathy, and bone abnormality
   E. all of the above

898. Which of the following represent types of bone grafts?
   A. Autogenous or self-donor
   B. Homogenous or donor of same species
   C. Heterogenous or donor of different species
   D. Alloplastic bone substitutes
   E. All of the above

899. Bone grafts are responsible for which of the following?
   A. They promote osteogenesis and so may be used in cases showing delayed healing or nonunion to fill large bone cavities and to restore continuity defects
   B. They serve in the fixation of fractures and reconstruction of the jaws after osteotomy
   C. They restore contour and may be used following ridge loss to correct an asymmetry and in genioplasty
   D. They add strength when the risk of pathologic fracture is present
   E. All of the above

900. Which of the following represent bone grafting principles?
   A. The physical status of the patient should be good
   B. Appropriate and adequate antibiotic coverage should be provided
   C. The graft bed should be well prepared, be infection-free, have no scar, and be well vascularized
   D. The wound closure must be water-tight, and hematoma must be avoided; the graft must be adequately fixed and immobilized; there should be an adequate supply of cancellous bone tissue; and there should be adequately restored function

901. Orthognathic surgery refers to
   A. autotransplants
   B. the concept of surgical orthodontics
   C. replantation of teeth
   D. biologic replacements (replants and transplants)
   E. none of the above

903. Surgical management of mandibular retrognathism is accomplished by
A. C-osteotomy
B. vertical L-osteotomy
C. sagittal split osteotomy of the mandibular rami
D. C-osteotomy, vertical L-osteotomy, and sagittal split osteotomy of the mandibular rami
E. none of the above

904. The surgical procedure utilized to correct maxillary retrusion (maxillary retroposition) is
A. high level horizontal osteotomy of the maxilla corresponding to the Le Fort type I maxillary fracture
B. sagittal split osteotomy
C. vertical-oblique osteotomy
D. C-osteotomy
E. none of the above

16. ANESTHESIA

DIRECTIONS: Each of the questions or incomplete statements below is followed by five suggested answers or completions. Select the ONE that is best in each case.

---

905. The selection of an anesthetic for oral surgery during pregnancy includes the consideration that
    A. local anesthesia is the simplest and safest technique
    B. impairment of uterine blood flow can adversely affect the fetus
    C. most drugs cross the placenta and enter the circulation of the fetus
    D. teratogenic effects of drugs given the mother are most likely to occur during the first trimester
    E. all of the above must be considered

906. Premedication is given preceding a general anesthetic
    A. to allay apprehension and produce a degree of amnesia preceding the anesthetic
    B. to depress reflex irritability
    C. to lessen metabolic activity
    D. to raise the pain threshold when indicated
    E. for all of the above reasons

907. Complete local anesthesia of normal pulp tissue is
    A. more difficult to obtain if the pulp is inflamed
    B. less difficult to obtain if the pulp is inflamed
    C. only possible with special supplementary injections
    D. easy to obtain in patients with physical and mental fatigue
    E. none of the above

908. Pain perception
   A. is not dependent upon other anatomical structures
   B. is localized within the cortex of the brain
   C. is not dependent on afferent sensory fibers conducting impulses
   D. is not dependent upon a stimulus
   E. is none of the above

909. Psychogenic pain
   A. is that unpleasant sensation that has an organic basis
   B. is that unpleasant sensation that has no organic basis
   C. is the result of raising the pain threshold
   D. is due to failure to block the pathway of painful impulses
   E. is none of the above

910. Analgesia refers to
   A. raising the pain threshold
   B. pain perception
   C. the loss of pain sensation without a loss of consciousness
   D. psychosomatic methods for relief of pain
   E. none of the above

911. Nerve block
   A. is a field block
   B. applies to a method of securing regional anesthesia
   C. is local infiltration
   D. is topical analgesia
   E. is none of the above

912. In performing a paraperiosteal injection the needle is inserted
   A. in proximity to or contacts the periosteum and the solution is deposited so that it diffuses through the cancellous bony plate
   B. beneath the mucosal layers
   C. into the osseous tissue
   D. between the periosteum and bone
   E. in none of the above

913. Indications for regional analgesia include which of the following?
   A. No additional trained personnel are necessary
   B. Techniques not difficult to master
   C. Percentages of failures is small
   D. There is no additional expense to the patient
   E. All of the above

914. Indications for the mental nerve block are
   A. for surgery on the lower lip or mucous membrane in the mucolabial fold anterior to mental foramen
   B. surgery on the mandibular buccal mucosa
   C. procedures on mandibular teeth
   D. surgical procedures on teeth posterior to the second bicuspid
   E. none of the above

915. Areas anesthetized by the lingual nerve block include
   A. the floor of the mouth
   B. the anterior third of tongue
   C. the mucosa on lingual side of mandible
   D. the mucoperiosteum on lingual side of mandible
   E. all of the above

916. Areas anesthetized by the intraoral inferior alveolar nerve block include
   A. the body of the mandible
   B. the inferior portion of the ramus
   C. mandibular teeth
   D. the mucous membrane and underlying tissues anterior to the first mandibular molar
   E. all of the above

917. Areas anesthetized by the maxillary nerve block include
   A. the anterior temporal and zygomatic regions
   B. the lower eyelid and side of nose
   C. the anterior cheek and upper lip
   D. the maxillary teeth, maxillary alveolar bone, hard and soft palate, tonsil, pharynx, nasal septum and floor of nose, nasal mucosa, and turbinate bones
   E. all of the above

918. Indications for extraoral techniques for infraorbital nerve block include which of the following?
   A. When anesthesia of the entire distribution of maxillary nerve is required
   B. Diagnostic purposes
   C. When the anterior and middle superior alveolar nerves are to be anesthetized and intraoral approach is not possible due to infection and trauma
   D. Therapeutic purposes
   E. None of the above

919. Epinephrine
   A. has a synergistic action with the free base of local anesthetics
   B. prolongs the action and increases the intensity of the anesthetic but does not potentiate it by any synergistic action with the free base
   C. shortens the duration of action by acting upon the free base
   D. decreases the intensity of analgesia
   E. does none of the above

920. The ideal local anesthetic should
   A. have a rapid onset and sufficient duration to be advantageous
   B. have sufficient penetrating properties to be effective topically
   C. be free from allergic or idiosyncratic reactions
   D. be stable in solution and either be sterile or capable of being sterilized by heat
   E. have all of the above

921. Local anesthetics used in dentistry
   A. are drugs which have little or no irritating effects when injected into the tissues
   B. permanently interrupt nerve conduction
   C. are not synthetic compounds
   D. in wide use do not include cocaine
   E. are none of the above

922. The cause of toxicity (i.e., true overdose) is
   A. inadvertent intravenous injection
   B. too great a percentage strength
   C. injecting rapidly into vascular areas
   D. too large a volume
   D. all of the above

923. An anesthetic complication resulting from the absorption of the anesthetic solution is
   A. toxicity
   B. idiosyncrasy
   C. allergy and anaphylactoid
   D. an infection due to contaminated solutions
   E. all of the above

924. Mepivacaine
 A. does not produce anesthesia of moderately long range
 B. produces anesthesia with a duration of 1 hour
 C. is very similar to lidocaine in its action within the body
 D. of maximum dosage is approximately 600 mg
 E. is none of the above

925. Lidocaine
 A. when injected rapidly may have a slight local irritating effect on tissues
 B. first signs of toxicity are stimulation
 C. fails to potentiate the barbiturates
 D. fails to possess topical anesthetic properties
 E. does none of the above

926. Tetracaine is
 A. not a potent local anesthetic
 B. a potent, nontoxic, local anesthetic
 C. a potent, relatively toxic local anesthetic
 D. capable of potentiating procaine when in combination
 E. none of the above

927. Syncope
 A. is perhaps the most frequent complication associated with local anesthesia
 B. is the least frequent complication of local anesthesia
 C. is always associated with loss of consciousness
 D. is treated in late phases
 E. is none of the above

928. Muscle trismus is
 A. rare following regional analgesia or anesthesia
 B. not obvious to patient or dentist
 C. a fairly common complication of regional analgesia or anesthesia
 D. not treated by the dental practitioner
 E. none of the above

929. The physical evaluation should include
 A. inspection
 B. blood pressure and pulse
 C. breath-holding test
 D. laboratory tests
 E. all of the above

930. Anesthesia means
   A. regional anesthesia
   B. without sensation
   C. spinal, epidural, and paravertebral anesthesia
   D. depression
   E. none of the above

931. Which of the following factors influence the absorption and elimination of volatile anesthetics?
   A. Tension or concentration in the inspired mixture
   B. The tidal exchange
   C. The total minute volume exchange and the functional residual air volume
   D. The solubility coefficient of drug in blood, the diffusability through alveoli, blood flow through lungs, blood flow through tissues, penetration into brain, and solubility in the tissues
   E. All of the above

932. Cardiac arrest is used to denote ineffective propulsion of blood by the heart. It is due to
   A. stoppage of the heart
   B. stoppage of the heart, ventricular fibrillation, and ineffective propulsion due to a feeble myocardium
   C. ventricular fibrillation
   D. feeble myocardium
   E. none of the above

933. Most local anesthetics in present-day use are derived from
   A. aliphatic chains
   B. hydroxy compounds
   C. antihistamine compounds
   D. benzoic or para-aminobenzoic acid
   E. all of the above

934. The anaphylactoid-type reaction due to allergy to a local anesthetic
   A. is of common occurrence
   B. is severe, comes on immediately, and usually terminates fatally
   C. involves a large dose necessary to induce sudden syncope
   D. is not an antigen-antibody reaction
   E. is none of the above

935. Absorption of local anesthetics (topical) from the mucous membranes
   A. fails to produce detectable blood level
   B. produces blood levels that simulate those of rapid intravenous injection
   C. produces higher blood levels than those following rapid intravenous injection
   D. produces much lower blood levels than those following rapid intravenous injection
   E. does none of the above

936. The usefulness of a local anesthetic drug is determined by
   A. the pH of the tissue
   B. the buffering mechanism of the proteins
   C. its solubility, potency, and toxicity
   D. the amino portion of the molecule
   E. none of the above

937. A local anesthetic solution is
   A. more potent at low pH (higher C_m)
   B. less potent at high pH
   C. more potent (has a lower C_m) at high pH
   D. a potent topical anesthetic at a low pH
   E. none of the above

938. The duration of a nerve block depends upon
   A. the rate of removal of anesthetic drug
   B. the firmness of bond between drug and nerve membrane
   C. the firmness of the bond between the anesthetic and nerve membrane and the rate of drug removal
   D. the rapidity of injection of anesthetic drug
   E. none of the above

939. The higher the local anesthetic blood level and the longer it remains elevated
   A. the greater the chance of an adverse systemic reaction
   B. the less the chance of an adverse systemic reaction
   C. the less the chance of respiratory depression
   D. the less the chance of hypotension
   E. none of the above is true

940. The action of nitrous oxide on the central nervous system is
   A. irreversible
   B. reversible
   C. dependent on the circulation time of the blood
   D. dependent on the lipoid content of the blood
   E. none of the above

941. A good analgesic state may be induced in a dental patient with a mixture of
   A. 98% oxygen and 2% nitrous oxide
   B. 100% oxygen and 0% nitrous oxide
   C. 90% oxygen and 10% nitrous oxide
   D. 95% oxygen and 5% nitrous oxide
   E. none of the above

942. Pharmacologic properties of nitrous oxide include which of the following?
   A. Elimination of nitrous oxide takes place largely through the lungs
   B. There is no change in the composition or volume of the cerebrospinal fluid due to nitrous oxide
   C. Nitrous oxide causes the cough reflex to be suppressed only moderately when used as a general anesthetic
   D. Nitrous oxide does not cause any change in the heart rate or cardiac output or changes in arterial pressure or venous pressure
   E. All of the above

943. The stage of relative analgesia is comprised of
   A. plane 1, plane 2, and plane 3
   B. plane 1 and plane 2
   C. plane 2 and plane 3
   D. plane 1 and plane 3
   E. none of the above

944. With the use of relative analgesia
   A. the dentist can perform major surgery
   B. it is impossible to attain complete analgesia and amnesia all of the time
   C. it is possible to attain complete analgesia and amnesia all of the time
   D. inspiration is prolonged
   E. none of the above is true

945. Under relative analgesia, the muscles show which of the following signs?
   A. No movement, muscles relaxed
   B. Facial expression of a conscious individual
   C. Nausea extremely rare
   D. Purposeful but delayed resistance as result of the trauma
   E. None of the above

946. Which of the following represent vital factors during the performance of a venipuncture?
   A. Immobilizing the arm steadily with low cross-light
   B. The venipuncture site should be desensitized before puncture
   C. The skin should be stretched, with approach about 30°, then align; needle taped in position, syringe clipped nearby
   D. Visual and aspiration checks before any injection; if any pain or doubts, stop at once
   E. All of the above

947. The current success of conscious sedation is
   A. due to the concept of increasing the oxygen concentration administered rather than the nitrous oxide
   B. due to increasing the nitrous oxide concentration rather than the oxygen
   C. due to administration of diazepam
   D. due to administration of meperidine
   E. none of the above

948. Conscious sedation provides which of the following benefits?
   A. Apprehension and anticipatory apprehension are reduced
   B. Pain sensation is reduced from skin, mucous membrane, and periosteum (not tooth sensitivity)
   C. The time estimate for dental work is reduced, and appointments seem much shorter
   D. Absence of need to administer a premedication
   E. All of the above

949. A contraindication to conscious sedation is
   A. hypertension
   B. nasal obstruction
   C. a crying child with a blocked airway
   D. epilepsy, asthma, and early pregnancy
   E. all of the above

950. The concept of minimum anesthetic concentration is
   A. analgesia
   B. the concentration of an agent which produces a 50% obtundation and a 50% response in a group of patients to a skin incision and measures the quality of anesthesia
   C. one which produces focus of the eyes
   D. one which alters response to command
   E. none of the above

951. Concerning hypnoanalgesia or hypnosis for control of pain,
   A. hypnosis is not a placebo in itself
   B. highly hypnotizable patients derive much more relief from hypnosis than from a placebo alone
   C. hypnoanalgesia is not correlated with the amount of pain relief obtained from a placebo
   D. 90% of dental patients can be helped by hypnotic analgesia
   E. all of the above are true

952. Drugs frequently used to allay apprehension include
   A. barbiturates
   B. phenothiazines
   C. ataractic drugs (hydroxyzine)
   D. narcotics (potentiated by other drugs)
   E. all of the above

953. The use of premedication prior to general anesthesia is used
   A. to prevent cardiac arrhythmias and to allay the patient's anxiety
   B. to reduce the amount of general anesthetic required
   C. to increase the speed of recovery from the anesthesia
   D. because the premedication acts for long periods after the oral procedure
   E. for none of the above

954. Agents used for general anesthesia in dentistry are
   A. nitrous oxide plus oxygen
   B. halothane
   C. enflurane
   D. trichloroethylene and methoxyflurane
   E. all of the above

955. Endotracheal intubation
  A. guarantees the safety of the patient
  B. neither guarantees the safety of the patient and the protection of the airway nor absolves the dentist from extreme care in operating around the oropharynx
  C. protects the airway
  D. absolves the dentist/oral surgeon from extreme care in operating around the oropharynx
  E. does all of the above

956. Which of the following represent types of local anesthetics?
  A. Esters of para-aminobenzoic acid (procaine, 2-chloroprocaine, tetracaine, butethamine, propoxycaine)
  B. Esters of benzoic acid (piperocaine, isobucaine, meprylcaine)
  C. Esters of meta-aminobenzoic acid (metabutethamine, primacaine)
  D. Amide derivatives (lidocaine, mepivacaine, prilocaine, pyrrocaine, parethoxycaine, hexylcaine, bupivacaine, etidocaine)
  E. All of the above

957. The speed of injection of a local anesthetic
  A. causes injection into a vascular channel
  B. probably modifies the actual final blood level obtained from a local anesthetic
  C. reduces the actual peak blood level attained
  D. increases the vascularity of the local area
  E. does none of the above

958. The Gow-Gates injection
  A. is a new method of attaining local anesthesia of the mandibular division of the fifth cranial nerve
  B. is an inhalation method for general anesthesia
  C. is an intramuscular method for general anesthesia
  D. requires three or four needle inserts
  E. is none of the above

959. Regarding vasoconstrictors in the United States,
  A. they are all sympathomimetic amines and act similarly
  B. they do not produce any side effects
  C. no systemic changes occur to administration of epinephrine
  D. ischemic ulcers are common adverse effects
  E. none of the above is true

960. Which of the following drugs are capable of interacting with monoamine oxidase inhibitors?
   A. Barbiturates and phenothiazines
   B. Chloral, anti-Parkinsonism drugs, meperidine
   C. General anesthetics, succinylcholine, cocaine
   D. Thiazides, reserpine, insulin, food and drinks
   E. All of the above

961. Any checklist of anesthetic equipment should include
   A. evaluation of the pressure levels in the circuit, review of the oxygen safety features of the equipment
   B. availability of reserve gases, check of connections in the circuits, review of flow rates delivered when the machine is turned on
   C. check for leaks in the high-pressure and low-pressure sides of the circuit, evaluation of valves to ensure they are not sticking
   D. check of the masks for cleanliness and presence of pollutants and defects, review of the emergency equipment available (critically important point)
   E. all of the above

962. In conscious sedation
   A. each patient will require different quantities of sedation
   B. the response of the patient varies at different times of the day and changes by the type and length of the dental procedure
   C. no serious amount of depression is produced
   D. more precise guides are currently needed to determine the exact level of sedation
   E. all of the above are true

963. Conscious sedation in dentistry
   A. is not safe
   B. is not effective
   C. has proven safe and effective
   D. is accompanied by amnesia for 10 hours
   E. is none of the above

964. The types of patients suitable for conscious sedation are
   A. handicapped patients
   B. new patients
   C. teenagers
   D. emergency patients, elderly patients, children
   E. all of the above

965. Signs and symptoms of the common faint of vasodepressor syncope are
   A. pallor and diaphoresis
   B. mydriasis, hyperventilation, and hyperpnea
   C. weak slow pulse and severe decrease in blood pressure
   D. impairment or loss of consciousness, collapse with muscle flaccidity, and tonic and/or clonic seizure activity
   E. all of the above

966. Indications for general anesthesia are
   A. adverse reactions to local anesthesia
   B. cardiorespiratory disease
   C. hemorrhagic diathesis and congenital abnormalities
   D. infection and a major procedure
   E. all of the above

967. The complications of conscious sedation include
   A. overdosage (as with barbiturates), major
   B. regurgitation of stomach contents, major
   C. nausea and vomiting, minor
   D. headache, dizziness, and postoperative hypnosis
   E. all of the above

17. COMMUNITY DENTISTRY

DIRECTIONS: Each of the questions or incomplete statements below is followed by five suggested answers or completions. Select the ONE that is best in each case.

---

968. Topic areas in community dentistry are listed as
   A. ethics, jurisprudence, office management or administration
   B. manpower, biometry, hospital organization, hospital dental service
   C. systems for delivery of health care, systems for delivery of dental care
   D. methods of financing dental care, methods of financing health care, history of dentistry and public health, health legislation, dental health legislation
   E. all of the above

969. New methods of delivery of oral health care in the United States include
   A. group practice
   B. hospital dental practice, health departments
   C. nursing home dental practice, partnerships, corporations
   D. dental schools, dental clinics, credit and insurance groups
   E. all of the above

970. Preventive care seeks to prevent
 A. effects of abnormal changes in the tissues of the mouth and jaws through early recognition and therapeutic control
 B. potential aberrations in the normal growth and development of the mouth and jaws through preventive manipulation of dental tissues during eruption of the primary and secondary dentition
 C. dental caries
 D. periodontal disease
 E. all of the above

971. The oral hygiene section of the dental rehabilitation team has responsibility for
 A. development of the dental history and oral evaluation for all patients admitted to the hospital (out-patient and in-patient)
 B. evaluation of DMF status, oral hygiene index
 C. evaluation of periodontal index, classification of occlusion
 D. health status of the soft tissues of the oral cavity, indications of acute or chronic inflammation and infection of the oral cavity and other pertinent data related to the oral health of the individual patient
 E. all of the above

972. A survey of hospitals in the nine county New York region for information on the number of patients with oral, facial and speech defects revealed
 A. there are approximately 20, 000 persons per year in the New York Metropolitan Region who would benefit from oral rehabilitation consultations
 B. there is a distinct need for the development of an orofacial profile for these patients and system for retrieval of this information to support follow-up observation, rehabilitation and maintenance services, and clinical research
 C. a large majority of the hospitals recognize the desirability of a well-organized network of orofacial rehabilitation centers and would be willing to develop and utilize linkages with such centers
 D. there is some small but good evidence that where there is a dental service functioning in the hospital in the area of general dental care, there is more recognition for specialized teams for oral justification for the development of a regional plan on which to structure an economically sound network of oral, facial and speech rehabilitation centers
 E. all of the above

973. The present gap that exists between delivery and demand for dental care is dependent upon
A. distribution of resources and dental needs, and dental treatment
B. distribution of resources
C. dental needs and dental treatment
D. dental treatment
E. none of the above

974. Which of the following represent features of a dental group practice?
A. All personnel including dentists must be salaried
B. Payment for dental health care will be on a capitation or budgeted basis, rather than fee-for-service; the group will be multidisciplinary, involving specialists and dentists with areas of special interest
C. Auxiliary personnel will be used to the maximum extent possible; the group will operate in facilities owned by a nonprofit organization with consumer and provider representation
D. The group practice will be part of a regional network, with responsibility for a specific geographic area
E. All of the above

975. A group dental practice should be based on
A. salaries for all personnel
B. capitation payment for services
C. full utilization of expanded duty auxiliaries
D. multi-disciplinary abilities of the dental staff and community ownership of the facilities
E. all of the above

976. Which of the following represent the reasons why a fluoridation bill was signed into law in the state of Connecticut?
A. Legislators became convinced of the value of fluoridation through various committees' educational efforts
B. Legislators became convinced there were many individuals in favor of fluoridation with many large, organized and reputable groups behind them
C. The opposition was not able to come up with a backing of a reliable, authoritative organization
D. The offensive methods of the antifluoridationists lobbying daily in the state capitol completely annoyed many legislators
E. All of the above

977. Preventive dentistry programs should consist of
A. a lecture and discussion on oral health in the school classroom by the dentist with dental students, presentations before community organizations on the need for oral health and prevention
B. screening of school children by a dentist or dental student in school one to two months after the lecture
C. a preventive visit at the health center where the child would receive a 1/2-hour visit for dental health education, prophylaxis and fluoride treatment and inspection
D. the child being able to receive dental care on a regular basis at the health center after the preventive visit
E. all of the above

18. DENTAL PRACTICE ADMINISTRATION

DIRECTIONS: Each of the questions or incomplete statements below is followed by five suggested answers or completions. Select the ONE that is best in each case.

---

978. Work simplification in dentistry means
   A. a shorter and easier way to practice dentistry, the right tool placed in the right position at the right time
   B. the auxiliaries do all the dental work under supervision
   C. a group dental practice
   D. use of new equipment in a dental practice
   E. none of the above

979. Ergonomics is
   A. time and motion studies
   B. time lapse movie analysis
   C. the study of man in relation to his working environment
   D. arrangement for dental work
   E. none of the above

980. Motions of the operator have been classified into which of the following types, from the simplest to the more complex patterns?
   A. Class I motion is movement of fingers
   B. Class II motion is movement of the fingers and wrist
   C. Class III motion is the movement of the fingers, wrist and elbow
   D. Class IV motion is the movement of the entire arm from the shoulders; class V motion is movement of the arm and twisting of the body
   E. All of the above

981. The results of the Westchester-Fairfield work simplification studies revealed that
   A. seated operators worked no faster than standing operators having the same operating facilities
   B. standing operators made more tiring body movements
   C. seated operators tended to be more relaxed, but became tired of sitting down for long periods of time
   D. the chair assistant whose height was different from that of the operator found difficulty in accomodating the seated operator
   E. all of the above are true

982. Factors to be considered in operatory planning are
   A. mobility
   B. versatility
   C. uniformity, economy
   D. acceptance, standardization
   E. all of the above

983. Types of dental chairs available today are
   A. fixed full-body curve chairs
   B. fixed lower-body curve chairs
   C. full-power lounge chairs
   D. rest-curve adaptations
   E. all of the above

984. Which of the following represents a school of thought concerning coolants?
   A. One group feels that large amounts of water supplied in solid streams coming from the contra angle and supplemented by a water syringe stream is necessary
   B. One group favors the spray of water
   C. One group favors only a stream of air
   D. One group feels that large amounts of water supplied in solid streams coming from the contra angle and supplemented by a water syringe stream is necessary; another group favors the spray of water; another group favors only a stream of air
   E. None of the above

985. The main essentials for any arrangement of high output lights include which of the following?
   A. They should be of high intensity; 1000-1800 footcandles
   B. The light should be variable in intensitv; it should not be too hot
   C. It should be adjustable both vertically and horizontally and should rotate in 360° arc around both a horizontal and vertical axis; the beam should be able to be focused
   D. The physical dimensions should be small enough so that it can be located close to the field of operation without being interfered with by the heads of the operating team; the quality of light should not cause eye fatigue; it should be balanced with overall lighting in the proper ratio, 3 to 1 footcandles; the light bulb should be easily replaced; the light should move easily if hit by a head
   E. All of the above

986. One of the most effective ways to conserve time and motion is to
   A. avoid obsolete equipment
   B. use adjustable bracket tables and operating magnifiers
   C. use a pre-prepared tray system in which the more commonly used instruments and accessories are placed on one tray convenient to the operating area
   D. use audio machines
   E. do all of the above

987. Some of the benefits of the pre-prepared tray system are
   A. it allows you to serve the same number of patients in less time
   B. a minimum of two extra patients per day may be seen with less effort, increasing your income
   C. it permits you to have every instrument you need at your fingertips, eliminating the delay involved in searching for instruments
   D. the system is just as adaptable to a one-chair, one-girl office as it is to a multiple operatory; the clean up and make ready time is reduced regardless of the number of operatories; the system is inexpensive and is readily adaptable to any procedure
   E. all of the above

988. Which of the following represents general principles of simplified training of dental assistants?
   A. Before you can instruct, you must be sure you know the material
   B. Know what the duties of the new dental assistant are
   C. Have the necessary materials ready before beginning training; remember that dental assistants tend to do those things they think are important to you
   D. Be prepared to have patience; acquaint her with the vocabulary of dentistry; have a larger plan of instruction
   E. All of the above

989. When managing special patients
   A. call the child from the waiting room by his first name
   B. act calm and matter of fact; be firm but look pleasant
   C. make no reference to behavior, fear, pain or hurt
   D. if child refuses to enter the operating room, call doctor; do not reprimand child yourself; if there is any resistance, forget it, don't push
   E. all of the above

19. PEDODONTICS

DIRECTIONS: Each of the questions or incomplete statements below is followed by five suggested answers or completions. Select the ONE that is best in each case.

990. Preventive methods utilized in pedodontics include
   A. oral hygiene
   B. dietary factors
   C. fluoride prophylaxis
   D. prevention of malocclusion
   E. all of the above

991. Educational programs for the public may include
   A. talks before school groups, PTA, service organizations, etc.
   B. school projects
   C. poster, essay, perfect smile contests
   D. free X-rays or dental examinations
   E. all of the above

992. A child's behavior pattern is governed first by
   A. conditioning received from the environment
   B. the father
   C. the inherited physical and mental endowment
   D. the mother
   E. none of the above

993. Fear
   A. is one of the primary emotions acquired soon after birth
   B. is acquired in utero
   C. is not a primitive response
   D. is acquired several years after birth
   E. is none of the above

994. Techniques of reconditioning the child for dental treatment include
   A. reconditioning the child through guidance from the dentist
   B. determining if the child has undue fear of dentistry
   C. familiarizing the child with dental treatment
   D. gaining complete confidence of the child
   E. all of the above

995. A complete examination of the child dental patient includes
   A. the patient's chief complaint
   B. the prenatal, natal, postnatal and infancy history
   C. general appraisal of the patient
   D. a detailed oral examination and supplementary examination and special tests
   E. all of the above

996. The recorded history of a pedodontic patient includes
   A. vital statistics
   B. parental history
   C. prenatal and natal history
   D. postnatal and infancy history
   E. all of the above

997. Examination of the oral cavity of children in a diagnostic survey includes
   A. breath
   B. lips, labial and buccal mucosa
   C. saliva
   D. gingiva, tongue and sublingual space, palate, pharynx, tonsils and teeth
   E. all of the above

998. Special roentgenographic surveys for children are generally made
   A. routinely
   B. once annually
   C. very frequently
   D. to show structures not shown on the usual dental roentgenograms
   E. by none of the above

999. Radiation exposure during oral diagnostic pedodontic roentgenography can be reduced by
   A. use of a properly constructed X-ray machine
   B. use good chairside and darkroom techniques
   C. use open end cones and if possible a recessed filter
   D. use a shield for the gonads
   E. all of the above

1000. Hypnotic-sedative agents include
   A. barbiturates
   B. chloral hydrate
   C. bromides
   D. paraldehyde
   E. all of the above

1001. It is desirable to place a permanent restoration in any tooth which will remain in the arch for
   A. three months
   B. six months or more
   C. one year
   D. one month
   E. none of the above periods

1002. For physically handicapped or physically inadequate children
   A. full restorative care can be provided during one long operative period under local anesthesia
   B. restorative mouth care is impossible
   C. let the teeth decay and extract all teeth
   D. full mouth restorative care can be provided during one long operative session under general anesthesia
   E. do none of the above

1003. The rubber dam is one of the most valuable approaches a dentist can develop in rendering restorative dental care to a child because
- A. it gives the operator the key to successfully managing nearly all children
- B. it increases the quality and quantity of work produced in a unit of time
- C. it provides a dry field for bases, pulp capping or pulpotomy
- D. it allows the use of air-water spray on high speed burs and affords the operator greater total visibility and accessibility
- E. it does all of the above

1004. Some of the differences between deciduous and permanent teeth are
- A. thin (1 mm) enamel covering
- B. broad molar proximal contacts
- C. enlarged pulp chamber
- D. enhanced cervical bulge and pronounced constriction at the neck of the tooth
- E. all of the above

1005. Before amalgam is inserted into any cavity
- A. the area should not be clean
- B. the occlusal enamel wall should not be parallel to axis tooth
- C. the area should remain dry during the entire insertion and carving procedure
- D. the pulpal wall should not be flat or smooth
- E. none of the above should be done

1006. Crowns are indicated on deciduous teeth when
- A. rampant caries involves three or more surfaces of a tooth
- B. the primary molar has had pulp therapy
- C. a child has rampant caries
- D. malformed teeth are present, such as hypoplastic enamel and in a handicapped child with poor oral hygiene
- E. all of the above are true

1007. The steps in dealing with silver amalgam include
- A. proportioning
- B. trituration
- C. condensation
- D. carving and polishing
- E. all of the above

1008. Amalgam restorations
- A. should be placed in deep-seated cavities
- B. should never be placed in deep-seated cavities because of thermal changes and an excellent conductor
- C. are not good conductors of thermal changes
- D. are not good conductors of electrical impulses
- E. are none of the above

1009. Silicate cement restorations are not permanent; their life expectancy is
- A. one year
- B. four to five years
- C. seven years
- D. ten years
- E. none of the above

1010. Zinc oxide and eugenol is used in pedodontics
- A. as a protective base or sub-base
- B. as a temporary filling
- C. as an anodyne dressing for inflamed pulps
- D. as a temporary or permanent cement for crowns
- E. for all of the above

1011. Calcium hydroxide
- A. neutralizes free phosphoric acid in zinc phosphate cement
- B. increases the density and hardness of the dentin under the base of the cavity
- C. stimulates odontoblastic activity and formation of secondary dentin
- D. is only moderately irritating to pulpal tissue
- E. is all of the above

1012. In indirect pulp capping the medication of choice is
- A. zinc oxide and thymol
- B. zinc oxide and eugenol
- C. calcium hydroxide
- D. zinc oxide and eucalyptol
- E. none of the above

1013. The mandibular teeth are best anesthetized with
  A. a long buccal injection
  B. infraorbital injection
  C. an inferior alveolar and long buccal injection
  D. mental injection
  E. none of the above

1014. The simplest form of pulp therapy is
  A. pulpotomy
  B. pulpectomy
  C. apicoectomy
  D. pulp capping
  E. none of the above

1015. Pulpotomy is
  A. enlargement of carious exposure
  B. complete removal of the coronal portion of the dental pulp
  C. pulp capping
  D. sterilization of remaining carious dentin
  E. none of the above

1016. Formocresol pulpotomy is indicated for
  A. all carious exposures on primary molars and incisors
  B. all carious and accidental exposure on primary molars and incisors
  C. all accidental exposures on primary teeth
  D. all carious exposures on permanent molars
  E. none of the above

1017. Pulpectomy refers to
  A. removal of the coronal pulp
  B. removal of the radicular pulp
  C. removal of all pulpal material from the tooth (coronal and root portions)
  D. pulp capping
  E. none of the above

1018. Primary teeth
  A. have no ancillary canals
  B. have canals free of tortuosity
  C. have no multifaceted root canals
  D. are noted for their many ancillary canals
  E. are none of the above

1019. When performing endodontics on primary teeth, which of the following must be taken into consideration?
A. A resorbable compound should be used as the filling material
B. Silver points and gutta-percha should be avoided
C. Do not penetrate past the apical foramen when reaming canals
D. Apicoectomy should not be performed
E. All of the above

1020. There is a real relationship between the incidence of fractured anterior teeth and the
A. caries in those teeth
B. hardness of the enamel
C. hardness of the dentin
D. protrusion of those teeth
E. none of the above

1021. The incidence of fractures to teeth in the maxilla is
A. 25%
B. 75%
C. 95%
D. 50%
E. none of the above

1022. Clinical examination of injuries to the teeth of children should include
A. type of abnormality (fracture, displacement, loss, laceration)
B. reaction to percussion
C. transillumination examination for congestion
D. mobility, vitality, occlusion, and radiographic examination
E. all of the above

1023. Maternal attitudes affect the child patient in regard to
A. overprotection
B. overindulgence
C. underaffection
D. rejection, authoritarianism
E. all of the above

1024. Child dental patients may be classified as
A. cooperative children
B. tense-cooperative children
C. outwardly apprehensive children, fearful children
D. stubborn or defiant children, hypermotive children. and handicapped children
E. all of the above

1025. Which of the following techniques have been used to manage the disruptive child patient?
A. Voice control, physical restraint
B. Hand-over-mouth technique and its variations
C. Hypnosis, nitrous oxide oxygen analgesia
D. Premedication (sedative-hypnotics, antianxiety drugs, and antihistamines), general anesthesia
E. All of the above

1026. Which of the following represent intravenous methods of conscious sedation?
A. The Jorgensen technique
B. The Shane technique
C. Intermittent methohexital sodium sedation
D. Intravenous diazepam sedation
E. All of the above

1027. The advantage of intravenous conscious sedation is
A. rapid onset
B. controlled dose
C. minimum recovery period
D. rapid onset, controlled dose, and minimum recovery period
E. none of the above

1028. Which of the following problems may accompany the venipuncture technique?
A. Hematomas
B. Irritation
C. Venospasm; phlebitis
D. Intra-arterial injection
E. All of the above

1029. Diagnosis in pedodontics involves
A. obtaining a full written health questionnaire from the patient
B. interviewing parent and child to supplement the questionnaire
C. performing extra- and intraoral examination of the patient
D. taking additional x-rays, models, and tests
E. all of the above

1030. The main areas of concern in diagnosis and treatment planning for the child are
A. oral-medical problems
B. periodontal considerations over the long term
C. dental caries and restorative dentistry
D. occlusion and craniofacial growth and development
E. all of the above

1031 Children may exhibit which of the following toxic reactions to local anesthetic solutions?
A. Restlessness, apprehension, and tremors progressing to excitement and convulsions
B. Increased blood pressure and increased pulse rate
C. Increased rate of respiration
D. Respiratory and cardiovascular depression with loss of reflexes and consciousness
E. All of the above

1032. Problems associated with tooth eruption in the child patient are
A. ankylosed deciduous teeth
B. supernumerary teeth
C. maxillary labial frenectomy
D. lingual frenectomy, inadequate attached gingiva
E. all of the above

1033. Factors which influence the quality of radiographs for children are
A. density, contrast, sharpness, distortion
B. contrast
C. sharpness
D. distortion
E. none of the above

1034. Unnecessary radiation exposure to pedodontic patients may be reduced by
- A. high-speed film and high kVp techniques
- B. filtering the X-ray beam
- C. collimating the X-ray beam
- D. care in filming and processing
- E. all of the above

1035. The acid-etch technique has been used for
- A. fissure sealants
- B. restoring fractured incisors, cementing orthodontic appliances
- C. sealing of anterior restorations, remodeling miss-hapen teeth, restoring teeth with developmental defects
- D. splinting loose teeth, face-lifting discolored teeth, and temporary bridges or space maintainers
- E. all of the above

1036. The prognosis of traumatized teeth depends upon
- A. a careful history, complete clinical and radiographic examination, and correct emergency treatment
- B. history
- C. the radiographic examination
- D. the clinical examination
- E. none of the above

1037. Space maintenance is
- A. preservation of a space for a permanent tooth in a child's mouth
- B. preservation of the total arch length in the child's mouth or of all of the permanent teeth in the arch
- C. replacement of a lost tooth
- D. prevention of mesial drift after loss of a tooth
- E. none of the above

1038. Vertical problems encountered in orthodontics include
- A. digit sucking
- B. lip sucking
- C. tongue thrusting
- D. mouth breathing
- E. all of the above

1039. Treating a handicapped dental patient involves
- A. the ability to transfer patients from wheelchairs (slide-board transfer, one person transfer)
- B. some special office design
- C. special radiographic techniques when the following are present: macroglossia, limited oral access, hyperactive gag reflex, management problem, poor muscle control, inadequate muscle strength
- D. special head support for cerebral palsy patient; patient restraints; specialized equipment
- E. all of the above

1040. All preventive dentistry programs are based upon
- A. an accurate diagnosis and treatment plan plus reinforcement of the program at various steps
- B. flossing
- C. a behavior change program
- D. behavior goals and strategies for persuasive prevention
- E. none of the above

1041. Fluoride supplements used in preventive dentistry are
- A. prenatal fluoride
- B. infant fluoride supplementation
- C. chewable fluoride tablets for youths and adolescents
- D. topical fluorides (stannous fluoride, acidulated phosphate fluoride, thixotropic gels)
- E. are all of the above

1042. Bacterial invasion of the teeth of children can be prevented by
- A. scaling the teeth
- B. prophylaxis once a year
- C. the use of pit and fissure sealants applied to the occlusal surfaces, along with fluoride therapy
- D. persuasive strategies
- E. none of the above

1043. The preventive dentistry program should be made up of the
- A. establishment of regular professional care
- B. development of proper prevention care at home
- C. use of systemic and topical fluorides
- D. establishment of proper eating habits, with a reduction in the intake of refined carbohydrates
- E. all of the above

1044. Expected benefits from fluoridated water are
A. a sixfold increase in the number of caries-free children (50-70% reduction in dental caries)
B. a 75% decrease in first permanent molar loss
C. a decrease in the size and complexity of new carious lesions
D. better appearance of teeth, fewer malocclusions among children, continued dental benefits into adulthood, a lower rate of osteoporosis in elderly women, lower death rate from falls for elderly women, less otosclerotic hearing loss
E. all of the above

20. ORTHODONTICS

DIRECTIONS: Each of the questions or incomplete statements below is followed by five suggested answers or completions. Select the ONE that is best in each case.

1045. Calcification of all primary teeth has begun by
   A. the eighth month of intra-uterine life
   B. the tenth month of intra-uterine life
   C. the fourth to sixth month of intra-uterine life
   D. the second month of intra-uterine life
   E. none of the above

1046. Interdentation of the primary teeth occurs
   A. before age 3 in most instances
   B. before age 2-1/2 years
   C. before age 2 years
   D. before age 1 year
   E. at none of the above

1047. The width at any given diameter across the bony alveolar arch
   A. shows a very large increase with age
   B. shows a decrease with age
   C. shows no large increase with age
   D. shows no increase with age
   E. shows none of the above

1048. If an excessive overbite is seen immediately upon the eruption of the incisors,
  A. a problem in the vertical relationship of the facial skeleton should be suspected
  B. a problem in the vertical relationship of the facial skeleton should not be suspected
  C. a problem in width relations should be suspected
  D. a problem in formation of primary teeth should be suspected
  E. none of the above is true

1049. The space occupied by the primary cuspid and first and second primary molars is necessary in order to
  A. permit eruption of the permanent cuspid
  B. permit eruption of the first and second bicuspids
  C. relieve incisor crowding
  D. provide for a late mesial shift of the permanent molars
  E. do all of the above

1050. Correct tooth position is
  A. necessary for proper function
  B. an important factor for proper function, esthetics, and overall preservation or restoration of dental health
  C. required for proper esthetics
  D. not imperative for overall preservation of dental health
  E. none of the above

1051. Which of the following represent prerequisites for orthodontic treatment?
  A. Adequate space
  B. Elimination of interferences
  C. Allowable axial inclination
  D. Correctable etiologic factors, favorable periodontal and periapical prognosis, and absence of contra-indications
  E. All of the above

1052. The classification of malocclusions involves which of the following types of versions?
A. Labio- or buccoversion (tooth is misplaced to the labial or buccal side of the dental arch)
B. Linguo- or palatal version (tooth is misplaced to the lingual or palatal side of the dental arch)
C. Mesioversion (tooth is displaced mesially to its normal position)
D. Infraversion (tooth has insufficiently erupted), supraversion (tooth has erupted further than usual with reference to the occlusal plane), torsiversion (tooth is abnormally rotated either mesially or distally), and transversion (one tooth has displaced another)
E. All of the above

1053. Horizontal (excessive) overjet (overlap) occurs
A. when the upper anterior teeth are protracted
B. when upper anteriors are retracted
C. when upper anteriors are rotated
D. when upper anteriors are in torsiversion
E. when none of the above occurs

1054. Vertical overbite (overlap) occurs
A. when upper anterior teeth are protracted
B. when approximately 10% of the labial surface of the lower incisor is overlapped by the maxillary incisor
C. when upper anteriors are in torsiversion
D. when skeletal deformities are present
E. when none of the above is true

1055. A common malocclusion which requires orthodontic treatment is
A. class I malocclusion is a discrepancy between tooth and individual jaw size
B. class II, division 1, malocclusion (distocclusion) occurs when the mandibular first permanent molar is distal to its maxillary counterpart due to a retrognathic mandible, a protracted maxilla, or a combination of the latter
C. class II, division 2, malocclusion (distocclusion) is characterized by a deep anterior overbite, lingual inclination of maxillary central incisors, labial tipped upper lateral incisors and an exaggerated curve of Spee in the mandibular arch (no crowding)
D. class III malocclusion (skeletal) is due to an overgrowth of the mandible resulting in a mesiooclusion and anterior cross-bite
E. all of the above

1056. A removable orthodontic appliance is
A. not easily cleaned
B. not firmly attached to the supporting tissues
C. easily removed for cleaning, firmly attached to the supporting structures so controlled pressure is brought to bear on the teeth to be moved
D. used for major tooth movement
E. none of the above

1057. The action of the removable orthodontic appliance is dependent upon which of the following auxiliary springs?
A. Labial wire spring (Hawley wire used for palatal or lingual tipping of the incisor teeth)
B. Free-ended spring (used for labial movement of teeth in cross-bite)
C. Accessory spring (used to accomplish very minor tooth movement along with primary treatment procedures)
D. The labial wire spring (Hawley wire), the helical coil spring or free-ended spring, the accessory spring
E. None of the above

1058. In planning anchorage of orthodontic appliances, much depends upon
A. the physical properties of wire
B. vectors of force in minor tooth movement
C. the physical properties of wire and the vector of force in tooth movement
D. the soldered joints
E. none of the above

1059. Which of the following principles are important when using finger springs or removable orthodontic appliances for limited orthodontic treatment?
A. It is almost impossible to grasp a tooth with the arm of the spring
B. Movement of the arm of the spring will always be radial and movement on any point of it will be part of the curve with its center at the coil
C. It may be necessary in certain situations to incorporate more than one coil in the spring to increase the range of action
D. In certain conditions, a compensatory bend may have to be incorporated in the arm to avoid contact with the adjacent teeth during treatment
E. All of the above

1060. Instruments used in the construction of orthodontic appliances are
A. wire-bending pliers (bird beak pliers, Howe straight pliers, Howe curved pliers, Weingardt utility pliers)
B. banding instruments (band pusher, band biter, band-contouring pliers, band-removing pliers)
C. wire cutters (pin- or ligature-cutting pliers, hard wire cutter)
D. ligature-tying pliers
E. all of the above

1061. The Hawley appliance has which of the following features and characteristics?
A. It is an acrylic and wire device
B. It is utilized to actively move teeth or passively retain teeth following orthodontic therapy
C. Retention is mainly borne by the tissue but its appliance is stabilized by clasps
D. The circumferential clasp is the most widely used means of retention
E. All of the above

1062. The active portion of the Hawley appliance is
A. the baseplate
B. the retentive clasp
C. the circumferential clasp
D. the anterior labial wire
E. none of the above

1063. Concerning the compressed legs of the mattress spring
A. it should be positioned at the cingulum of the tooth
B. it exerts a labial force on an anterior tooth
C. acrylic covers the spring and concentrates the pressure at the cingulum area of the tooth
D. the action of the mattress spring is derived by compressing the coils prior to placement of the appliance
E. all of the above are true

1064. The acrylic biteplate is
A. used to remove occlusal irregularities
B. utilized to disocclude the posterior teeth
C. used to decrease the vertical dimension
D. used to occlude the posterior teeth
E. is none of the above

1065. A properly fitting (tight-fitting) orthodontic band
- A. fails to protect the tooth from caries
- B. is used to place various attachments for application of forces
- C. protects the tooth from caries and is used to place the various attachments for the application of forces
- D. must contain certain crimpings of the band for a better fit
- E. does none of the above

1066. Various types of band attachments are
- A. a single edgewise bracket
- B. a single edgewise bracket with a vertical slot
- C. a single edgewise bracket with vertical slot and narrow ligature slot
- D. a single edgewise bracket with vertical slot and wide ligature slot; twin edgewise bracket with vertical slot, a Lee-Fisher edgewise bracket, a modified Lee-Fisher edgewise bracket
- E. all of the above

1067. The orthodontist utilizes the chin cup to
- A. correct a cross-bite
- B. redirect growth of the mandible in Class III and skeletal open bite malocclusions
- C. move a tooth labially or bucally
- D. to prevent the growth at the cartilagenous areas of the condyle to correct a Class II malocclusion
- E. do none of the above

1068. The real danger from prolonged thumbsucking is
- A. none
- B. torsiversion of the teeth
- C. changes to the occlusion sufficient to allow the more potent deforming muscular forces to create full-fledged malocclusion
- D. a negative overjet
- E. none of the above

1069. Maxillary anterior diastema is due to
- A. a hyperactive tongue
- B. a hypotonic perioral musculature
- C. discrepancies between tooth size and arch length
- D. ectopic tooth eruption
- E. all of the above

1070. A rule of orthodontics states that before a frenectomy is performed to correct a diastema
A. never attempt to close the diastema before surgery
B. an effort should be made to close the diastema
C. the resistant fibrous tissue will never disappear
D. scar tissue never develops following surgery
E. do none of the above

1071. Individual anterior crossbites are
A. often amenable to therapy by removable orthodontic appliances or by fixed and removable appliances (acrylic guide-plane treatment, limited fixed appliances)
B. not amenable to treatment by acrylic and wire appliances with mattress spring
C. treated by rapid palatal expansion
D. treated by palatal jackscrew
E. none of the above

1072. Third molar considerations include which of the following?
A. Not all third molars need to be extracted
B. 50% of patients with third molars must have them removed for one reason or another
C. Cyst formation often occurs around impacted third molars or around any impacted tooth
D. Third molars cause destruction to the adjacent second molar, ameloblastomas may be associated with impacted third molars, dentists should make every effort to preserve third molars if there is room in the jaws for the molars to erupt, the relationship between third molars and anterior crowding is currently controversial but the possibility has not been discounted
E. All of the above

1073. Orthodontic considerations for the adult patient include which of the following?
A. Tooth movement in adults is neither warranted nor indicated for all circumstances of malposition
B. If patients are functioning in comfortable harmony, there is no reason to alter the balance
C. The dentist/orthodontist must evaluate each adult individually and determine if a malocclusion will become a pathologic problem if left untreated
D. Adult patients should be evaluated individually for limited tooth movement
E. All of the above

21. ORAL PATHOLOGY

DIRECTIONS: Each of the questions or incomplete statements below is followed by five suggested answers or completions. Select the ONE that is best in each case.

1074. Congenital syphilis and Hutchinson's triad does not include
- A. interstitial keratitis
- B. ghon complex
- C. notched incisors
- D. nerve deafness, rhagades, saddle nose
- E. mulberry molars

1075. The oral lesion of tuberculosis of the tongue does not usually include
- A. a tendency to early central caseation
- B. a zone of epitheloid cells
- D. central giant cells are common
- D. orchitis
- E. a cuff of lymphocytes at periphery

1076. Osteoporosis of the jaws is not related to
- A. hyperthyroidism
- B. hypoandrogenesis
- C. Cushing's syndrome
- D. adenocarcinoma of the stomach
- E. ovarian agenesis

1077. The tongue shows macroglossia. It is enlarged with a homogenous material in the mesenchymal tissue which stains with congo red. This disease process is
A. secondary amyloidosis
B. paramyloidosis
C. hyaline degeneration
D. primary amyloidosis
E. fibrosis of stroma

1078. Characteristics of malignant oral neoplasms do not include
A. having viral etiology
B. scarce mitotic figures
C. invasive tumor
D. a tumor which spreads by transplantation and metastases
E. undifferentiated histologic components

1079. Characteristics of Hodgkin's disease do not include
A. Reed-Sternberg cells or Dorothy Reed cells
B. increased ground substance in lymph nodes
C. enlargement and coalescence of lymphoid follicles
D. bones involved in 20% of cases
E. eosinophilic infiltrate

1080. Precancerous lesions of the oral mucosa include
A. hyperkeratosis
B. leukoplakia
C. Bowen's disease of oral mucosa
D. leukoedema
E. papillomatosis of palate

1081. Ankylosis of fusion between bone and teeth may occur
A. if an apical granuloma is present
B. during malocclusion
C. during elongation of tooth
D. in replanted teeth
E. in none of the above cases

1082. Lymphosarcoma of the oral region does not occur in which of the following forms?
A. Reticulum cell sarcoma
B. Lymphosarcoma
C. Brill Symmers disease
D. Mycosis fungoides
E. Lymphoblastic lymphoma

1083. A professional specialty which shows a high incidence of leukemia is
A. prosthodontist
B. orthodontist
C. radiologist
D. pedodontist
E. oral surgeon

1084. Infectious mononucleosis involving cervical lymph nodes causes
A. chronic granulomatous inflammation
B. chronic inflammation
C. acute inflammation
D. leukemoid
E. necrosis

1085. The enlarged mandible of adults who have an eosinophilic adenoma of the pituitary is due to
A. Simmond's disease
B. Frohlich's syndrome
C. Addison's disease
D. acromegaly
E. Cushing's syndrome

1086. Oral findings in erythroblastosis fetalis are
A. notched teeth
B. hypoplastic teeth
C. pigmented teeth
D. dentinal dysplasia
E. mulberry molars

1087. Xerostomia is
A. lack of tears
B. atrophic oral mucosa
C. hyperplasia of salivary glands
D. dryness of the mouth
E. lack of hydrochloric acid and pepsin

1088. Amelogenesis imperfecta is
A. agenesis or hypoplasia of enamel
B. agenesis or hypoplasia of dentin
C. hypoplasia of enamel due to congenital syphilis
D. hereditary opalescent dentin
E. excessive thickness of the enamel

1089. Cleft palate results
- A. from complete formation of palate
- B. in a short skull and thick frontal bones
- C. from failure in fusion of the facial processes
- D. from fissural cysts
- E. from hyperplasia of palatal mucosa

1090. Torus palatinus and mandibularis
- A. are exostoses of bone of obscure etiology
- B. are rapidly growing
- C. are due to secondary infection
- D. never present oral surgical problems
- E. do not interfere with denture construction

1091. Paget's disease of the bone
- A is a local disturbance
- B. has a known etiology
- C. occurs below 30 years of age
- D. shows oral manifestations of enlargement of the maxilla
- E. is always accompanied by hypercementosis of teeth

1092. Fibrous dysplasia of the jaw
- A. is a very rapid growing lesion
- B. shows enlargement of maxilla primarily
- C. shows hypercementosis of teeth
- D. has a multicystic radiographic appearance
- E. contains granulation tissue

1093. Granulomas form at the apex of teeth
- A. with vital pulps
- B. with hyperemic pulps
- C. due to tuberculosis
- D. with chronic infection of the pulp
- E. due to histoplasmosis

1094. Mottled enamel is
- A. a defect in enamel matrix formation
- B. blue tooth covered by no enamel
- C. hypocalcification due to fluorosis
- D. an enameloma
- E. a hereditary defect

1095. Pulpitis may terminate readily in
- A. hyalinization
- B. calcification
- C. cyst formation
- D. granulomatous change in pulp
- E. pulp necrosis

1096. The most common tumor of salivary glands is
- A. adenocytic carcinoma
- B. adenoma
- C. Warthin's tumor
- D. pleomorphic adenoma
- E. onkocytoma

1097. Mucoceles
- A. are due to embryonic defects in excretory ducts
- B. are primarily lined by squamous epithelium
- C. arise from severance of duct
- D. are ranulas
- E. are none of the above

1098. Ranulas
- A. are retention cysts of the lips
- B. are due to severance of an excretory duct
- C. occur insidiously in the floor of the mouth
- D. occur at the exit of the parotid duct into the oral cavity
- E. do none of the above

1099. Paget's disease
- A. cannot take place in the jaw since these bones are unique
- B. shows an increased serum alkaline phosphatase
- C. shows slow rebuilding of resorbed bone tissue
- D. occurs under 35 years of age
- E. does none of the above

1100. Which of the following is NOT a form of lichen planus?
- A. Hypertrophy
- B. Filigree
- C. Pustular
- D. Linear
- E. Annular

1101. Allergic stomatitis
A. shows a plate-like distribution of lymphocytes
B. shows a histiocytic response
C. shows edema and neutrophiles in the oral mucosa
D. shows edema and eosinophiles
E. does none of the above

1102. Which of the following is NOT consistent with the histopathology of the ameloblastoma?
A. Cystic degeneration in epithelial masses
B. Epithelium shows marked cohesiveness
C. Capsule has limiting potential
D. Secondary inflammation
E. Loosely arranged stellate cells and atypical columnar cells

1103. The most common skin malignancy in humans is
A. melanocarcinoma (melanoma)
B. sebaceous adenocarcinoma
C. squamous cell carcinoma
D. transitional cell carcinoma
E. reticulum cell sarcoma

1104. A tongue biopsy, followed by a general examination, leads to the diagnosis of primary amyloidosis of the tongue. This means that the patient has
A. tuberculosis
B. syphilis
C. no known underlying diseases
D. chronic osteomyelitis
E. leprosy

1105. Which of the following usually does NOT spread by metastases?
A. Rodent ulcer
B. Ameloblastoma
C. Paget's disease of bone
D. Basal cell carcinoma
E. All of the above

1106. The center of an oral lesion is occupied by a small nest or aggregate of plumb, rounded cells. The centrally located cells have undergone necrosis. At the margin of this cell cluster and sometimes in the center of the cluster are multinucleated giant cells with peripherally located nuclei, creating a ring or horseshoe distribution Surrounding this cluster is a peripheral zone or lymphocytes and fibroblasts. The oral disease process is
A. gonorrhea
B. actinomycosis
C. lupus erythematosus
D. tuberculosis
E. lobar pneumonia

1107. If a sinus tract in the cheek extrudes yellow granules, this is suggestive of
A. cancer
B. yaws
C. furunculosis
D. actinomycosis
E. syphilis

1108. Oral foci of infection are of greatest clinical significance in
A. rheumatoid arthritis
B. subacute bacterial endocarditis
C. iritis
D. eczema
E. polycythemia vera

1109. Which of the following lesions cannot be classified as an odontogenic tumor?
A. Simple ameloblastoma
B. Myxoma
C. Acanthomatous ameloblastoma
D. Complex composite odontoma
E. Branchial cleft cyst

1110. Which of the following is NOT a classification of gingival hyperplasia?
A. Inflammatory gingival enlargements
B. noninflammatory fibrous enlargements
C. Gingivosis
D. A combination of inflammatory and fibrous enlargements
E. None of the above

22. ORAL ROENTGENOLOGY

DIRECTIONS: Each of the questions or incomplete statements below is followed by five suggested answers or completions. Select the ONE that is best in each case.

1111. Roentgenologic findings in the region of the mandibular symphysis represent
   A. an alveolus
   B. lingual cortical bone
   A. a radio-opaque circular area with a central dark spot in the midline
   D. spongy bone
   E. none of the above

1112. The lamina dura is
   A. a thin radiolucent line around roots
   B. a thin radiopaque line normally found in radiograph around roots
   C. a solid layer of bone forming the inner surface of socket
   D. a thick layer of solid cortical bone
   E. none of the above

1113. The lamina dura is actually
   A. cortical bone
   B. spongy bone
   C. immature bone
   D. a cribiform plate perforated by nutrient channels
   E. none of the above

1114. The roentgenogram is useful in periodontal disease to
A. locate calculus
B. determine amount of bone loss
C. determine type of infectious agent
D. measure the length of the root
E. do none of the above

1115. To locate the bottom of the pocket radiographically,
A. intraoral radiographic examination is sufficient
B. gutta percha point, periodontal probe or Hirschfeld point is useful
C. extraoral radiographic examination is sufficient
D. occlusal radiographic examination is sufficient
E. none of the above is done

1116. In modern dentistry the X-ray has become
A. infallible
B. a foremost aid in diagnosis
C. outlawed due to excessive radiation
D. unnecessary
E. none of the above

1117. The medullary bone underlying the lamina dura is distinguished because it is
A. radiopaque
B. radiolucent
C. radiolucent and radiopaque
D. cortical bone
E. none of the above

1118. In some individuals an anterior maxillary X-ray reveals a nasal fossa which
A. is very large
B. may closely approximate apices of central incisors
C. is very small
D. never approximates apices of central incisors
E. does none of the above

1119. The radiographic image of the incisive foramen is present
A. between the roots of upper incisors above their apices
B. between central and lateral roots below apices
C. between roots of upper centrals below their apices
D. between central and lateral roots above apices
E. in none of the above

1120. It is possible for inexperienced students to diagnose a wide and very radiolucent area in the midline suture for a
A. fracture
B. palatal cyst
C. granuloma
D. abscess
E. cementoma

1121. The maxillary antrum appears as
A. a radiolucent area extending into the alveolar process
B. a radiolucent and radiopaque area extending into the zygomatic process
C. a radiopaque area extending into the malar bone
D. a radiolucent area extending into the sphenoid bone
E. none of the above

1122. An important anomaly of the maxillary antrum is
A. bony partition of antrum
B. antral cysts
C. carcinoma of antrum
D. sinusitis
E. none of the above

1123. Nutrient canals are usually observed in the radiograph where
A. the sinus walls and alveolar bone are thin
B. the walls of the sinus are thick
C. the tuberosity is thick
D. the alveolar process is absent
E. none of the above is true

1124. If one cannot determine from a radiograph whether a radiolucency at the apex is osseous pathology or the mental foramen,
A. tracing the outline of the mandibular canal will help differentiate the two
B. biopsy the radiolucency immediately
C. do not repeat x-rays
D. leave it alone
E. do none of the above

1125. The occlusal radiography is the only type of x-ray examination that reveals
A. the mesial distal relationship of teeth
B. the buccolingual relationship between impacted tooth and other teeth
C. the anteroposterior relationship of teeth
D. the occlusal apical relationship of teeth
E. none of the above

1126. In the removal of anterior maxillary cysts
A. all the anterior teeth must be removed
B. only one incisor should be removed
C. the approach is via the palate
D. preoperative x-rays are valueless
E. none of the above is true

1127. When a dentist plans removal of an impacted tooth
A. a periapical film is all that is necessary
B. a bite wing examination is of little or no value
C. a lateral film is all that is necessary
D. an anteroposterior film is all that is necessary
E. none of the above is done

1128. Median anterior maxillary cysts occur
A. in the nasal bone
B. in the incisive canal and in the palatine process of the maxilla
C. in the zygomatic process of the maxilla
D. in hamular process
E. in none of the above

1129. Radiographically an important category of findings in the etiology of periodontal disease is
A. supernumerary cusps
B. incarcerated teeth
C. unerupted teeth
D. overhanging filling
E. none of the above

1130. When a radiograph reveals a radiolucent area at the apex of a root, the dentist should
A. diagnose it as cementoma
B. use the radiograph plus pulp vitality tester to establish diagnosis
C. diagnose it as a cyst
D. diagnose it as a granuloma
E. do none of the above

1131. In the maxilla it is possible for a rarefied area (granuloma) to be
A. always present in radiograph
B missing in radiograph
C. present at apex of vital tooth
D. due to increased exposure time
E. none of the above

1132. The nutrient canals in the jaws are visible radiographically because they
A. perforate the cortex
B. are radiolucent
C. are within cancellous bone
D. are radiopaque
E. are none of the above

1133. For proper localization of a foreign body in the jaws
A. a single radiograph is sufficient
B. the radiograph is of little value
C. multiple radiographs are necessary
D. multiple radiographs are not necessary
E. none of the above is done

1134. Oral manifestations of systemic disease produce jaw lesions which
A. never are visible radiographically
B. never cause pressure resorption from within
C. are visible if the kilovoltage is increased
D. erode the cortical-cancellous junction area and are visible as pseudocysts
E. do none of the above

1135. An acute alveolar abscess may be present clinically
A. always with a radiolucency in the radiograph
B. with an absence of pain
C. with no radiolucency in the radiograph
D. without any extrusion of affected tooth
E. none of the above

1136. In the early stages of multiple myeloma, radiographs of the jaws reveal
A. no bone alteration
B. punched out radiolucent lesions
C. punched out radiopaque lesions
D. a single punched out radiolucent lesion
E. none of the above

1137. In periodontal disease the infrabony pocket
- A. is always present in the radiograph
- B. may be absent in the radiograph
- C. is always absent in the radiograph
- D. is never diagnosed by means of the radiograph
- E. is none of the above

1138. In selecting x-ray equipment for the dental office, which of the following must be taken into consideration?
- A. The dentist can rarely afford the luxury of choosing individual pieces of equipment
- B. The entire system (radiation source, image receptor, devices used for processing the image, accessories or devices used for controlling or interconnecting the major components) should be considered as a unit
- C. The specific diagnostic needs of the practice should be identified
- D. There is a growing recognition that the risks associated with exposure to ionizing radiation may be significantly greater than have been estimated in the past
- E. All of the above

1139. The most common type of x-ray system used in modern-day dental practices employs
- A. a double-phase generator with self-rectified tube
- B. a single-phase generator using self-rectified tube and stationary anode
- C. a single-phase generator
- D. a self-rectified tube and double-phase generator
- E. none of the above

1140. Which of the following considerations should be involved in the dentist's choice of film for oral radiography?
- A. H and D curves should be available from the manufacturer
- B. H and D curves describe contrast
- C. H and D curves describe the relative sensitivity or speed of the film
- D. The latitude of the film can be determined by an examination of the range of exposures that yield an acceptable density
- E. All of the above

1141. Extraoral radiography involves which of the following considerations?
   A. This procedure is being performed in dental offices more frequently today
   B. Speed as well as contrast and resolution is a maıor factor
   C. In choosing a film-screen system, basic decisions are required concerning the type and amount of information necessary for the diagnostic task
   D. The common denominator in this procedure is the extraoral placement of the film or the image recorder; intensifying screens must be used and they are constructed of a semirigid base coated with a fluorescent material
   E. All of the above

1142. Filtration is another consideration in oral radiography since
   A. to obtain an energy spectrum that is both safe and compatible with the diagnostic task it is necessary to filter the beam
   B. the law requires a minimum amount of aluminum filtration in all x-ray machines to reduce patient exposure by eliminating unproductive low-energy x-ray photons
   C. some filters exclude high-energy photons that needlessly expose the patient and fail to contribute to the formation of an image
   D. the dentist can obtain photon energies more ideally suited for either soft tissue or hard tissue diagnosis and minimize exposure of the patient
   E. all of the above are true

1143. Extraoral collimators are
   A. fixed in panoramic x-ray machines as well as in most general purpose x-ray machines (by adjustable shutters made of lead or an absorber material)
   B. x-ray image receptors with postexposure processing
   C. semirigid bases coated with fluorescent material
   D. a new type of generator
   E. none of the above

1144. Image processing requires which of the following considerations?
A. All x-ray image receptors require postexposure processing
B. Each dentist has to determine whether to acquire a manual or machine processing system
C. Every film processing system has requirements related to time plus temperature
D. Overexposure and underprocessing yield a poor quality image
E. All of the above

1145. The quality of an image in oral radiography depends upon which of the following?
A. The size of the focal spot or target
B. There is a need to increase the target-to-object distance when using a long cone so that the relative distances between target, object, and film are more nearly in agreement with the principles of shadow casting
C. As the size of the focal spot and heat loading capacity are reduced, the quality of x-rays that can be generated per unit time is also reduced
D. The use of a small focal spot depends upon a reduction in the distance between the target and film and the use of faster recorder systems
E. All of the above

1146. The most common use of a contrast agent in dentistry
A. involves its incorporation into radiolucent filling materials
B. involves defining periodontal defects
C. involves its incorporation into otherwise radiolucent filling materials; defining periodontal defects with opaque materials; outlining pulpal morphology with iodinated material
D. involves outlining pulpal morphology with iodinated material
E. involves none of the above

1147. The process of xeroradiography involves which of the following?
A. Has features including pronounced edge enhancement, high contrast, a choice of positive and negative displays, good detail, and wide latitude
B. Does not require silver-halide containing films as required for intraoral and extraoral radiography
C. Is useful for studies that involve body parts with relatively low-subject contrast (as mammography)
D. Conventional x-ray sources are used in the production of xeroradiographs
E. All of the above

1148. Tomographic methods (body section radiography) in oral radiography involve which of the following factors?
A. It can be used to eliminate undesirable overlap (superimposition)
B. It produces an image of a layer within the body while whole images of structures above and below that layer are made invisible by blurring
C. Blurring or degradation of images of structures outside of the plane of interest is accomplished by simultaneous movement of the x-ray tube and the film during exposure
D. Overall sharpness depends upon the angle of movement and the distance of any point from the fulcrum
E. All of the above

1149. In nuclear medicine
A. dental, bone, and salivary gland scanning are useful in the detection and definition of diseases of the jaws and salivary glands
B. there are no limitations on the information obtained from bone and salivary gland scanning
C. the radiation burden to the patient is inconsequential
D. research has failed to produce a productive dental application of bone scanning using radiopharmaceuticals
E. none of the above are true

1150. Photographic coping procedures in oral radiograph
- A. provide projectable positive images (slides) for illustrating lectures
- B. provide negative intermediate images for production of paper prints to illustrate manuscripts
- C. provide same size (1 to 1) duplicates of original radiographs
- D. involve no substitute for a high quality original
- E. involve all of the above

1151. The interpretation of radiographic images must take which of the following factors into account?
- A. Anatomic variation within individuals and between individuals is rather large
- B. Calcified tissues (as teeth and bones) are dynamic structures capable of changing their size, shape, and density from time to time
- C. Three-dimensional biologic structures are reduced to two-dimensional images by radiography
- D. Radiography is not a precise science since its ability to demonstrate small alterations is very limited
- E. All of the above

23. PERIODONTICS

DIRECTIONS: Each of the questions or incomplete statements below is followed by five suggested answers or completions. Select the ONE that is best in each case.

1152. Diabetes mellitus
 A. does not affect the state of bone tissue
 B. does not cause periodontal disease per se
 C. does not affect the bone factor
 D. causes periodontal disease
 E. is none of the above

1153. The gingiva of a pregnant individual may
 A. undergo proliferation and enlargement
 B. undergo recession
 C. become ulcerated
 D. undergo hypertrophy
 E. do none of the above

1154. Gingivitis
 A. occurs after formation of calculus
 B. means interdental papilla are degenerated
 C. precedes calculus formation
 D. is due to trauma from occlusion
 E. is none of the above

1155. An infrabony pocket is
 A. an extra-alveolar pocket
 B. periodontal pocket
 C. a gingival pocket
 D. an intra-alveolar pocket
 E. none of the above

1156. Trauma from occlusion is a local factor in periodontal disease that causes
A. gingivitis
B. periodontal pockets
C. Vincent's infection
D. some changes in underlying tissues
E. none of the above

1157. Bacteria in relation to the etiology of periodontal disease are
A. primary factors
B. systemic factors
C. secondary factors
D. stress factors
E. none of the above

1158. Gingivectomy
A. is treating the disease
B. is symptomatic treatment of disease
C. does not influence the disease
D. is extending the disease
E. is none of the above

1159. Malocclusion
A. has no influence on periodontium
B. causes a distal drift
C. causes a lingual drift
D. adversely influences periodontium
E. is none of the above

1160. Calculus causes an altered
A. enamel
B. dentin
C. cementum
D. pulp
E. none of the above

1161. Curettage of the gingiva and periodontal pocket is
A. the removal of calculus
B. the removal of food debris
C. a debridement which converts the pocket into a shallow sulcus
D. the removal of cementum
E. none of the above

1162. Osteoplasty is shaping the
- A. cementum to desired contour
- B. alveolar bone to desired contour
- C. gingiva to desired contour
- D. periodontal ligament to desired contour
- E. none of the above

1163. Before therapy is undertaken in gingival hyperplasia, the dentist should
- A. surgically remove hyperplastic tissue
- B. apply phenol to hyperplastic gingiva
- C. find the etiology and remove same
- D. give intramuscular high doses of Vitamin C
- E. leave it alone and watch the lesion

1164. In the treatment of epilepsy, diphenylhydantoin sodium is very effective; however, it may produce gingival
- A. inflammation
- B. hyperplasia
- C. necrosis
- D. hypertrophy
- E. atrophy

1165. The periodontal tissues affected in vitamin C deficiency are
- A. bone marrow
- B. epithelial attachment
- C. nerves in ligament
- D. connective tissue
- E. musculature

1166. Migration of teeth is a symptom of
- A. gingivitis
- B. periodontosis
- C. gingivosis
- D. periodontitis
- E. none of the above

1167. Gingivectomy is a valuable method of
- A. curing dilantin hyperplasia
- B. obliterating pockets
- C. curing early periodontosis
- D. preventing recurrence of calculus
- E. doing none of the above

1168 Pregnancy gingivitis is due to
A. an alteration in the pH of the saliva
B. an exaggerated tendency of the gingiva to respond to local irritation
C. an excessive tissue response unrelated to local irritation
D. an increase in viscosity of the saliva
E. none of the above

1169. Gingivosis is classified as
A. hyperplastic pathologic process
B. atrophic pathologic process
C. degenerative pathologic process
D. hypertrophic process
E. inflammatory process

1170. Which of the following is NOT a type of pocket?
A. Periodontal pocket
B. Gingival pocket
C. Infrabony pocket
D. Cemental pocket
E. None of the above

1171. The etiology of periodontal disease includes which of the following intrinsic factors?
A. Blood impaction
B. Endocrinologic and nutritional influences
C. Trauma from occlusion
D. Calculus
E. Bacteria

1172. The most reliable guide for determining the presence of a pocket and measuring its depth is by
A. gross visual examination
B. radiographic examination
C. percussion
D. use of a probe, calibrated silver or gutta percha points
E. none of the above

1173. Periodontosis occurs more commonly in
A. young adult males
B. no age prediction
C. older individuals with long-standing chronic disease
D. young adult females when present at an early age
E. none of the above

1174. Uncomplicated chronic marginal gingivitis is due to
A. particles of calculus
B. oral physiotherapy
C. lack of food impactions
D. lack of materia alba
E. none of the above

1175. Mobility of normal teeth without any periodontal disease is related to
A. the primary cementum
B. the amount of alveolar bone
C. the physiologic state of the periodontal principal fibers
D. the amount of exposed crown
E. the cellular cementum

1176. A periodontal abscess originates in
A. a cyst of the gingiva
B. free gingiva
C. attached gingiva
D. a narrow deep end of a pocket cut off from the superficial part
E. alveolar mucosa

1177. A reliable sign indicative of traumatic occlusion is
A. periodontal pocket formation
B. gingivitis
C. increased tooth mobility
D. food impaction
E. calculus

1178. A 30-year-old white female, very nervous with a tendency to bruxism, developed a chronic suppurative periodontosis. The gingiva was pink and firm. The papillae were pointed and the attached gingiva stippled. There were deep pockets and a purulent exudate was present. Biopsy was taken of the area of the lingual upper right second molar. Histologically there was a localization of the inflammation to the free gingiva and along the pocket epithelium. Plasma cells, Russel-Fuchsin bodies, lymphocytes, and neutrophil leukocytes were present. The diagnosis is
A. acute gingivitis
B. gingivosis
C. chronic gingivitis
D. chronic desquamative gingivitis
E. dilantin hyperplasia

1179. A biopsy was taken from a hyperplastic gingiva of a 42-year-old male who showed signs of slight anemia and poor nutrition but without signs of definitive symptoms of deficiency. The marginal gingiva was swollen and irregular, the papillae blunted, both of turgid consistency with the presence of deep pockets and a purulent exudate. Histologically, there was lack of hornification, invasion of the epithelium by neutrophil leukocytes, acanthosis, the presence and distribution of neutrophil leukocytes, lymphocytes and plasma cells. The diagnosis is
A. hyperplastic gingivitis
B. atrophic gingivitis
C. pyogenic granuloma
D. eosinophilic granuloma
E. normal gingiva

1180. A 42-year-old south american, apparently in good health, never having been sick, noticed a change in his gingiva. The gingiva is red, swollen, the papillae are blunted, the surface is granular and the consistency of the gingiva is dense. There are deep pockets. A complete gingivectomy was performed. Histologically, extreme fibrosis was present in the reticular layer with a relatively low-grade inflammation. The diagnosis is
A. dilantin hyperplasia
B. fibrous hyperplasia of the gingiva
C. edema
D. pyogenic granuloma
E. acute necrotizing gingivitis

1181. In necrotizing ulcerative gingivitis the combustion products of tobacco
A. appear to be an irritating factor
B. are not an irritating factor
C. cause calculus formation
D. cause attrition
E. do none of the above

1182. After subgingival curettage
A. clinical recession never occurs
B. clinical recession may be expected
C. little recession always is the outcome
D. pronounced recession always is the outcome
E. none of the above is true

1183. Calculus
- A. never extends to bottom of the pocket
- B. always extends to bottom of the pocket
- C. extends half way to bottom of pocket
- D. extends to one-fourth of pocket depth
- E. does none of the above

1184. Infrabony pockets
- A. develop overnight
- B. develop in 2 weeks
- C. result from long-standing periodontitis with traumatic occlusion
- D. always progress rapidly
- E. do none of the above

1185. Splinting in periodontics
- A. is of no value
- B. is only useful in cases of periodontosis
- C. is useful if orthodontics is undertaken
- D. is useful during the healing period to stabilize teeth
- E. is none of the above

1186. After herpetic gingivostomatitis has become established, penicillin and aureomycin therapy are
- A. curative treatments
- B. palliative treatments to make the patient comfortable
- C. destructive to herpes simplex viruses
- D. useful if given with vitamin C
- E. none of the above

1187. One etiologic factor in periodontal disease that must be eliminated is
- A. contact between teeth
- B. correction of faulty contacts
- C. carbohydrates in diet
- D. vitamin C in diet
- E. none of the above

1188. Minor tooth movement in periodontics
- A. is impossible
- B. is useful in periodontosis
- C. makes periodontal therapy most lasting
- D. never maintains better gingival health
- E. is none of the above

24. ENDODONTICS

DIRECTIONS: Each of the questions or incomplete statements below is followed by five suggested answers or completions. Select the ONE that is best in each case.

1189. Diagnosis of an exposure in a tooth with vital pulp and an incompletely formed root is made by means of
   - A. roentgenographic evidence
   - B. clinical findings
   - C. clinical findings and roentgenographic evidence
   - D. subjective symptoms alone
   - E. none of the above

1190. Hyperemia may occur as a result of
   - A. hypersensitivity
   - B. fillings with proper bases
   - C. caries, deep fillings, trauma, fracture, abrasion, and erosion
   - D. cold but not heat
   - E. none of the above

1191. Acute pulpitis is caused by
   - A. fillings with proper bases
   - B. cold but not heat
   - C. deep fillings, carious lesions, trauma and fracture of crown
   - D. green stain on crown
   - E. none of the above

1192. The treatment for an acute apical abscess is
   A. pulp capping
   B. endodontic therapy or extraction
   C. sedative fillings
   D. incision and drainage alone
   E. none of the above

1193. The objective of pulp capping is to
   A. preserve vitality of the coronal pulp
   B. preserve the vitality of the entire pulp
   C. preserve the vitality of the radicular pulp
   D. regenerate a degenerated and necrotic pulp
   E. do none of the above

1194. The objective of pulpotomy is to
   A. preserve the vitality of the coronal pulp
   B. preserve the vitality of the radicular pulp
   C. preserve the vitality of the entire pulp
   D. regenerate a necrotic pulp
   E. none of the above

1195. Contraindications for pulp capping and pulpotomy consist of teeth
   A. with accidental exposures in vital young molars
   B. where inflammation of the radicular pulp is already present
   C. with greatly curved and tortuous roots
   D. with vital immature anterior teeth with wide open apices
   E. with none of the above

1196. Two successive negative cultures are
   A. absolutely necessary for successful endodontic treatment
   B. not always necessary for successful endodontic treatment
   C. not questioned today as a dogmatic rule in endodontics
   D. unquestioningly adhered to for successful endodontic treatment
   E. none of the above

1197. Indications for periapical surgery include
A. where endodontics is performed through existing restorations which may lead to fracture
B. when the endodontics is faulty
C. when there is danger of involving other structures
D. when the bony defect is so extensive that the edges of the incision will collapse
E. none of the above

1198. The root canal should be flooded with an antiseptic
A. in the absence of instrumentation
B. to prevent removal of shavings from root canal
C. to prevent removal of microorganisms
D. solution during instrumentation
E. in none of the above

1199. The main cause of endodontic failures is
A. broken instrument
B. canal overfilled
C. root perforation
D. incomplete obliteration
E. none of the above

1200. External resorption
A. continues after successful endodontic therapy
B. stops in most cases following successful endodontic therapy
C. continues only in mandibular incisors after successful endodontic therapy
D. stops in maxillary lateral incisors after successful endodontic therapy
E. does none of the above

1201. The concomitant periodontal-periapical lesion as the cause of endodontic failure
A. cannot be discovered prior to endodontic treatment
B. may be discovered prior to endodontic treatment
C. is most commonly found in the molar teeth
D. is most commonly found in the mandibular teeth
E. is none of the above

1202. Roentgenography is used in endodontics to
- A. aid in the diagnosis of periapical hard tissue lesions
- B. determine the number, location, shape, size and direction of roots and root canals
- C. confirm the length of the root canals
- D. evaluate the adequacy of the completed root canal filling
- E. do all of the above

1203. The purpose of the rubber dam in modern endodontics is to
- A. provide a dry, clean, and sterilizable field
- B. protect the patient from possible aspiration or swallowing of debris, bacteria, materials or instruments
- C. protect the patient from rotary and hand instruments, drugs and trauma
- D. eliminate the interference produced by lips, tongue and cheeks
- E. do all of the above

1204. To achieve optimum cavity preparation which of the following factors of internal anatomy must be considered?
- A. Outline form
- B. The size and shape of the pulp chamber and direction of individual root canals
- C. Internal-external relationship
- D. Intracoronal preparation
- E. None of the above

1205. The basic action of files or reamers is to
- A. Perforate root
- B. Ream out or drill the round, tapered apical cavity
- C. Remove cotton in the root canal
- D. Place medicaments in the root canal
- E. Do none of the above

1206. Irrigation should be undertaken prior to and at frequent intervals during instrumentation
- A. to remove cementum filling from the canals
- B. since noxious material may be forced through the apical foramen resulting in periapical infection
- C. to destroy all microorganism in the canals
- D. to stop the instruments from going through the apical foramen
- E. to do none of the above

1207. Total debridement of the pulp chamber and canals is
- A. not an important aspect of endodontic therapy
- B. a most important aspect of endodontic therapy
- C. accomplished by forcing air into the canal
- D. accomplished by forcing gas into the canal
- E. none of the above

1208. The length of a tooth is established by
- A. good, undistorted, preoperative roentgenogram
- B. adequate coronal access to all canals
- C. adjustable endodontic millimeter ruler
- D. definite repeatable plane of reference to anatomical landmark on tooth
- E. all of the above

1209. Pulpectomy is
- A. Always a total surgical removal of a vital pulp
- B. The surgical removal of a vital pulp from a tooth
- C. Never a partial surgical removal of a vital pulp
- D. Pulp cavity debridement
- E. None of the above

1210. Ideal root canal filling material requirements are that it should
- A. be easily introduced into root canal
- B. be preferably semisolid upon insertion and become solid afterwards
- C. fill the canal laterally and apically
- D. not shrink after insertion
- E. do all of the above

1211. Requirements of good root canal cements are that
- A. it should consist of fine particles of powder to mix readily with liquid
- B. it should not stain tooth structure
- C. it should not shrink
- D. set cement should be soluble in a common solvent
- E. all of the above are required

1212. Electric pulp testing
   A. cannot be accomplished when a tooth is fully covered by gold
   B. is not necessary when a tooth is fully covered by gold
   C. is absolutely essential for a tooth which is fully covered by gold or porcelain
   D. is not necessary when a tooth is fully covered by porcelain
   E. is none of the above

1213. Symptoms of chronic pulpalgia include
   A. mild discomfort
   B. pain which is a short, sharp shock
   C. excruciating pain
   D. a grumble or mild pain
   E. none of the above

25. DENTAL MATERIALS

DIRECTIONS: Each of the questions or incomplete statements below is followed by five suggested answers or completions. Select the ONE that is best in each case.

1214. Dental materials are generally solids. A true solid is characterized by
   A. its flow
   B. elasticity
   C. rigidity
   D. resilience
   E. none of the above

1215. The physical property measured in terms of the deformation of the structure per unit dimension is
   A. stress
   B. strain
   C. space lattice
   D. amorphous solid
   E. none of the above

1216. The principal constituent of dental plaster is
   A. beta-hemihydrate
   B. calcium sulfate hemihydrate
   C. alpha-hemihydrate
   D. soluble anhydrate
   E. none of the above

1217. Compared to dental plasters all dental stones
A. require less gauging water
B. require more gauging water
C. require the same quantity of gauging water
D. are beta-hemihydrate
E. do none of the above

1218. Impression plasters sometimes contain potato starch to
A. increase setting time
B. render them "soluble"
C. increase setting expansion
D. increase hardness
E. do none of the above

1219. The most effective manner for producing a hard surface on a cast is to
A. employ as much water as possible in mixing the stone
B. add 2% solution of borax to the mix of stone
C. add calcium tetraborate to the mix of stone
D. employ as little water as possible in mixing the stone
E. do none of the above

1220. When a dry cast is immersed in water saturated with calcium sulfate
A. there is contraction
B. there is negligible expansion
C. there is definite expansion
D. there is no change
E. none of the above happens

1221. Reversible hydrocolloid materials
A. are not strictly thermoplastic substances
B. harden by heat
C. harden by cold
D. are strictly thermoplastic substances
E. are none of the above

1222. A requisite of an impression compound is
A. it should be free of poisonous or irritating ingredients
B. it should harden completely at mouth temperatures
C. it should harden uniformly when cooled
D. it should be plastic at a temperature which will not cause discomfort to the patient
E. it should do none of the above

1223. Fusion temperature of impression compound should occur
A. before mouth temperature
B. at skin temperature
C. above mouth temperature
D. at room temperature
E. at none of the above

1224. An impression compound
A. should have a consistency suitable for use in the oral cavity at 37°C
B. should not be deformed or fractured when the impression is withdrawn from the mouth
C. surface should exhibit a smooth, glossy appearance after it has been flamed
D. when solidified should withstand trimming
E. should do all of the above

1225. A flow of the following percent is allowable for impression compound (type 1) at mouth temperature (37°C)
A. 6%
B. 10%
C. 2%
D. 20%
E. none of the above

1226. Disadvantages of heating compound in a water bath are
A. it may become brittle
B. lower molecular weight constituents are leached out by the water
C. the plasticity of the compound may be altered
D. it may become grainy
E. all of the above

1227. The zinc oxide-eugenol impression pastes harden
A. by heat
B. by cold
C. by pressure
D. by chemical reaction
E. by none of the above

1228. The mechanism of the reaction between zinc oxide and eugenol
A. is completely defined
B. is not complex
C. appears to be a chelation process
D. is that water is not essential to the reaction
E. is none of the above

1229. The composition of a zinc oxide-eugenol impression paste includes
A. zinc oxide, rosin, and magnesium chloride
B. oil of cloves or eugenol
C. gum rosin
D. olive oil, linseed oil, and light mineral oil
E. all of the above

1230. Prolonged setting of zinc oxide-eugenol impression paste
A. may result in inaccuracy due to movement
B. does not result in inaccuracy
C. is a desirable feature
D. results in an excellent impression
E. does none of the above

1231. A commonly used accelerator in zinc oxide and eugenol impression pastes is
A. zinc acetate
B. primary alcohols
C. glacial acetic acid
D. magnesium chloride
E. all of the above

1232. Generally there is a correlation in zinc oxide-eugenol impression pastes between flow and
A. working time
B. accelerator
C. setting time
D. composition
E. none of the above

1233. Two hours after mixing, the compressive strength of hardened zinc oxide-eugenol impression pastes is a maximum of
- A. 20 kg/sq cm
- B. 50 kg/sq cm
- C. 70 kg/sq cm
- D. 100 kg/sq cm
- E. none of the above

1234. Dental impression materials are hydrocolloids of
- A. the emulsoid type
- B. the suspension type
- C. the sol type
- D. the jel type
- E. none of the above

1235. The reversible hydrocolloid impression materials are manipulated by changing
- A. the gel to a sol with heat
- B. the fillers
- C. the modifiers
- D. the micelle network
- E. none of the above

1236. The basic constituent of the reversible hydrocolloid impression materials is
- A. magnesium chloride
- B. rosin
- C. agar-agar
- D. linseed oil
- E. none of the above

1237. Storage of the hydrocolloid impression to best preserve the impression should be in
- A. water
- B. a relative humidity of 80%
- C. a relative humidity of 100%
- D. dry air
- E. none of the above

1238. When all factors are taken into consideration, it is evident that there is
A. a satisfactory method for storage of a hydrocolloid impression
B. permanent dimensional stability of a hydrocolloid impression
C. a storage period of one year for hydrocolloid impressions
D. no satisfactory method for storage of a hydrocolloi impression
E. none of the above

1239. The chief ingredient of the irreversible hydrocolloid impression materials is
A. Agar-agar
B. borax
C. a soluble alginate
D. potassium sulfate
E. none of the above

1240. The irreversible alginate type of hydrocolloid impression material is
A. not used as much as the reversible type
B. used to the same degree as the reversible type
C. used far in excess of the reversible type
D. not used since agar-agar became available from Japan
E. none of the above

1241. An alginate is
A. a salt of alginic acid extracted from marine kelp
B. an impression material free of calcium sulfate
C. free of trisodium phosphate
D. free of diatomaceous earth
E. none of the above

1242. The possible composition of an alginate impression material includes
A. potassium alginate (12%)
B. diatomaceous earth (70%)
C. calcium sulfate-dehydrate (12%)
D. trisodium phosphate (2%)
E. all of the above

1243. The accuracy of the surface reproduction is dependent upon
A. the surface condition of impression only
B the dimensional behavior of material and surface condition of impression and mold
C. the surface condition of model only
D. the dimensional behavior of material
E. none of the above

1244. With irreversible hydrocolloid impression materials
A. an impression may be stored in a humidor
B. the cast should be poured immediately after impression is obtained
C. an impression may be stored in an atmosphere of 50% humidity
D. the cast may be poured at any time
E. none of the above is true

1245. In the reversible hydrocolloid impression materials, the gelation
A. begins adjacent to mouth tissues
B. starts in the middle of the impression material
C. begins adjacent to the cool tray
D. occurs simultaneously adjacent to the tray and mouth tissues
E. does none of the above

1246. Surface imperfections on stone casts may be minimized by
A. immersion of impression in water
B. immersion of impression in mouthwash
C. use of a mechanical vibrator when pouring in stone
D. an immerse-filled impression in water while the stone sets
E. none of the above

1247. Elastomers are
A. hydrophilic
B. hydrophobic
C. water-loving impression materials
D. potassium alginates
E. none of the above

1248. The polysulfide rubber impression materials are
A. not sensitive to temperature during curing
B. less sensitive to temperature than silicone rubber materials
C. of the same sensitivity to temperature as silicone rubber materials
D. quite sensitive to temperature during curing
E. none of the above

1249. The elastic properties of the rubber impression materials
A. improve with time
B. decrease with time
C. improve with temperature
D. decrease with temperature
E. do none of the above

1250. Which of the following are ideal requisites for a dental resin?
A. The material should exhibit a translucency or transparency
B. There should be no change in color
C. It should neither expand, contract, or warp during processing or use
D. It should possess adequate strength, resilience and abrasion resistance
E. All of the above

1251. The requirements of a dental resin include which of the following?
A. It should be impermeable to mouth fluids
B. Food should not cling to the resin
C. The resin should be tasteless, odorless, non-toxic and non-irritating
D. It should have a low specific gravity and a relatively high thermal conductivity
E. All of the above

1252. The types of resins of interest to dentistry are
A. vinyl resin only
B. polystyrene only
C. vinyl, polystyrene, and acrylic resins
D. acrylic resin only
E. none of the above

1253. The effect of the temperature rise above 100°C for a heat-curing denture base acrylic resins is
A. to produce porosity in the external portion of the resin
B. to produce porosity in the interior of the resin
C. to produce porosity in the surface of the resin
D. to prevent porosity in the interior of the resin
E. to do none of the above

1254. The principal cause of failure of amalgam restorations is
A. improperly prepared amalgam
B. improper cavity preparation
C. periodontal involvement
D. particles of the amalgam
E. none of the above

1255. Reduced occlusal area means
A. more fracture potential for amalgam
B. less fracture potential for amalgam
C. pulpal involvement
D. periodontal involvement
E. none of the above

1256. Amalgam is less prone to corrosion
A. if 25-27% is composed of tin
B. if 4-6% is composed of copper
C. if devoid of the detrimental gamma-2 phase, it contains tin in the form of copper-tin (Cu_6Sn_5)
D. when not weakened by zinc
E. for none of the above reasons

1257. Important physical properties of amalgam are
A. flow and creep
B dimensional change, strength, flow and creep, and corrosion
C. strength
D. dimensional change
E. none of the above

1258. The less mercury remaining in the condensed amalgam,
A. the stronger the restoration which contains fewer matrix alloys and fewer voids
B. the weaker the restoration
C. the more matrix alloys
D. the more voids
E. none of the above

1259. High-copper amalgams are superior
A. if the copper is available for a secondary reaction
B. if the copper is not available for a secondary reaction
C. if the copper is burnished
D. if the copper is fractured
E. for none of the above reasons

1260. Gold foil is produced in
A. gold foil (pellets, ropes, cylinders)
B. corrugated foil
C. platinum foil
D. laminated foil
E. all of the above

1261. Concerning condensation of restorative golds,
A. it may vary widely and has no influence on the final restoration
B. the degassing procedure is not important
C. it is the Achilles' heel of the direct gold restoration
D. clinical techniques are more important than the physical properties of restorative golds
E. all of the above are true

1262. Bonding
A. implies a force by which two substances are held in close contact with each other
B. implies physical bonds
C. implies chemical bonds
D. implies mechanical bonds
E. does none of the above

1263. The enamel surface
A. is a perfect substrate for bonding
B. does not conform to the bonding requirements; therefore, it must be modified if bonding is to take place
C. is for the most part inorganic, contaminated, and rough
D. is free from contamination and roughness
E. is none of the above

1264. Which of the following factors affect the establishment of adequate bonds in the clinical setting?
   A. The need for a dental prophylaxis prior to acid conditioning
   B. A dry field is extremely important to bonding
   C. The penetration of resin into enamel is affected by the type of enamel present
   D. It is not known whether prismless enamel bonds differently in vivo
   E. All of the above

1265. Acid conditioning of enamel and eroded dentin
   A. provides an atraumatic, conservative clinical approach to the bonding of restorative materials
   B. is a traumatic approach to bonding
   C. is not a safe and simple method of bonding
   D. bonding fails to produce a highly significant retention, good marginal integrity, and clinical durability
   E. does none of the above

1266. The effectiveness of the acid etch technique is dependent on which of the following factors?
   A. Materials must be used to clean the surface of the tooth prior to etching
   B. The effectiveness of the etchant
   C. The chemical and physical nature of the dental enamel
   D. The area and surface of the enamel to be etched; the properties of the resin materials used to seal and bond the restorative material to the tooth
   E. All of the above

1267. The pinledge retainers are indicated
   A. when the abutments are not in normal alignment
   B. where the abutment teeth are vital and free of restorations or carious lesions on facial, incisal, and proximal surfaces
   C. when the endentulous space is over four or five units wide
   D. when abutment teeth are nonvital
   E. in none of the above cases

ANSWERS AND COMMENTS

The author has made every effort to thoroughly verify the answers to the questions which appear on the preceding pages. However, in any text some inaccuracies and ambiguities may occur. Therefore, if in doubt, please consult your references.

The Publisher

PART I

BASIC DENTAL SCIENCES

Chapter 1 Anatomy

1. E. The cranium (skull) of vertebrates is adapted to support and contain the brain and special senses. The size of the human brain is related to the cerebral function of the skull. The skull without the mandible constitutes the cranium. The upper portion is termed the calvaria, and the remainder of the skull is the facial skeleton. The base of the skull (calva is removed) consists of the anterior, middle, and posterior cranial fossae. (REF. 1-p. 6)

2. E. The growth of the face occupies a long period compared with that of the calvaria. The ethmoid bone, orbital cavities, and upper part of the nasal cavities have practically completed their growth by the seventh year. Growth of the orbits and upper nasal region is achieved by sutural growth in their walls with deposition of bone on the facial aspects of the orbital margins. The maxilla is carried downward and forward by the expansion of the orbits, growth of the nasal septum, and sutural growth, especially at the fontanelles and at the zygomaticomaxillary and pterygomaxillary sutures. (REF. 1-p. 6)

3. E. The thorax (chest) is an osseocartilaginous framework encompassing the principal organs of respiration and circulation. Posteriorly the thorax includes 12 thoracic vertebrae and the posterior parts of the ribs. Anteriorly are the sternum, the anterior ends of the ribs, and the costal cartilages. Laterally the thorax is convex and is enclosed by the ribs. The inlet of the thorax is uniform in shape. The outlet is bounded by the twelfth thoracic vertebra behind, by the twelfth and eleventh ribs at the sides, and in front by the cartilages of the tenth, ninth, eighth, and seventh ribs. (REF. 1-p. 11)

4. E. The abdomen is the region of the trunk below the diaphragm. It consists of an upper part, the abdomen proper, and a lower part, the lesser pelvis. The abdomen is principally bounded by muscles. Thus its size and shape may vary greatly under different conditions. The tone of the latter muscles is an important factor in maintaining the abdominal and pelvic viscera in a normal position. The organs located in the abdominal and pelvic cavities are generally covered with a serous membrane, i.e., the peritoneum. (REF. 1-p. 11)

5. E. The skeleton of the upper limb consists of the scapula, a large, flattened, triangular bone on the posterolateral aspect of the thorax. The scapula has a costal surface, lateral border, inferior angle, spine, acromion, and coracoid process. The humerus is the longest and largest bone of the upper limb. The humerus has expanded upper and lower extremities and a shaft. (REF. 1-p. 12)

6. E. In the lower extremities the two axes are nearly parallel. The femoral head and the long axis of its neck are anteverted about 16° relative to the transcondylar axis of the lower end of the femur. (REF. 1-p. 12)

7. B. Fascia is a collection of connective tissue seen by the naked eye. Fascia develops as condensations on the surfaces of muscles, i.e., investing fascia. Deep fascia consists of collagen fibers indistinguishable from aponeurotic tissues. The deep fascia is well developed in the limbs. (REF. 1-p. 13)

8. B. The glabella may show the remains of the frontal suture, which in about 9% of skulls extends upward to the coronal suture. It indicates that the adult frontal bone is formed by the fusion of the right and left halves, which ossify independently of each other. (REF. 1-p. 15)

9. C. The bregma is the point of meeting of the sagittal and coronal sutures. (REF. 1-p. 15)

10. E. The fontanelles of the skull at birth are six in number; two, the anterior and posterior, are in the median plane; and two pairs, the sphenoidal and mastoid, appear on each side. The anterior fontanelle is the largest of the six and is located at the junction of the sagittal, coronal, and frontal sutures. (REF. 1-p. 15)

11. A. The external ear consists of the auricle or pinna and the external acoustic meatus. The auricle projects from the side of the head and collects the air vibrations which comprise the sound waves. The meatus leads inward from the bottom of the auricle, conducting the vibrations which are thereby transmitted to the tympanic membrane. (REF. 1-p. 16)

12. C. The conjunctiva is the transparent mucous membrane which passes over the inner surfaces of the eyelids and is reflected over the front part of the sclera and cornea. (REF. 1-p. 17)

13. B. The paranasal sinuses are the frontal, ethmoidal, sphenoidal, and maxillary sinuses. These sinuses vary in size and shape in different individuals and are lined with mucous membrane continuous with that of the nasal cavity. Nasal infections therefore may spread to the paranasal sinuses. (REF. 1-p. 17)

14. C. The parotid gland is the largest salivary gland and has an average weight of 25 g. It lies below the external acoustic meatus, between the mandible and the sterocleidomastoid. The parotid is enclosed within a capsule derived from the deep cervical fascia. (REF. 1-p. 18)

15. B. The mental nerve emerges at the mental foramen and divides beneath the depressor anguli oris into three branches. One branch descends to the skin of the chin, and two branches ascend to the skin and mucous membrane of the lower lip. The latter branches communicate freely with the mandibular branch of the facial nerve. (REF. 1-p. 19)

16. E. The anterior triangle of the neck is the area in front of the sternocleidomastoid muscle. The posterior triangle is the area behind the sternocleidomastoid. The carotid triangle of the neck is limited (behind) by the sternocleidomastoid muscle and (in front and below) by the superior belly of the omohyoid and (above) by the stylohyoid muscle. The muscular triangle (in front) is bounded, by the median line of the neck from the hyoid bone to the sternum and (behind and below) by the anterior margin of the sternocleidomastoid and (behind and above) by the superior belly of the omohyoid. (REF. 1-p. 22)

17. C. It should be noted that the neck contains many important structures, such as the internal jugular vein and the vagus nerve which both lie entirely subjacent to the sternocleidomastoid muscle and therefore are excluded from the carotid triangle. (REF. 1-p. 22)

18. E. The typical vertebrae consists of an anterior (ventral) part, the body, and a posterior (dorsal) vertebral arch which is extended by lever-like processes and encloses a vertebral foramen occupied in the living individual by the spinal cord, the meninges, and associated vessels. The opposed surfaces of adjacent vertebral bodies are strongly bound to each other by intervertebral discs of fibrocartilage (REF. 1-p. 147)

19. C. The outline of the skull varies greatly. It may be oval or more nearly circular, but its greatest width is usually nearer to the occipital than to the frontal region. This aspect of the skull is traversed by three sutures: the coronal, the sagittal, and the lambdoid. (REF. 1-p. 161)

20. D. The internal surface of the base of the skull shows a natural division into anterior, middle, and posterior cranial fossae. It is very irregular, partly due to the impressions for the cerebral gyri (conspicuous in the anterior and middle fossae). The dura mater is firmly adherent to the whole area, and through the numerous foramina and fissures its outer layer, the endocranium, is continuous with the periosteum on the exterior of the skull. (REF. 1-p. 169)

21. E. The occipital bone forms much of the back and base of the cranium and is trapezoid in shape and internally concave. It encloses basally a large oval opening, the foramen magnum, through which the cranial cavity communicates with the vertebral canal. (REF. 1-p. 183)

22. E. The hyoid bone is U-shaped and suspended from the tips of the styloid processes of the temporal bones by the stylohoid ligaments. It consists of a body and two greater and two lesser cornua. (REF. 1-p. 319)

23. D. Syndesmoses are slight movable joints such as the one between the inferior ends of the tibia and the fibula. In this form of articulation, closely apposed bony surfaces

are bound together by an interosseous ligament, affording a small degree of movement between adjoining bones (as the inferior tibiofibular joint). (REF. 1-p. 319)

24. C. A gomphosis, or peg-and-socket joint, is the specialized type of fibrous articulation restricted to the fixation of teeth in the mandible and maxilla. (REF. 1-p. 319)

25. C. The temporomandibular joint is a condylar joint and involves the articular tubercle and the anterior portion of the mandibular fossa of the temporal bone above and the condyle of the mandible below. The articular surfaces are covered with a variety of white fibrocartilage in which collagen fibers predominate and there are few cartilage cells. An articular disc divides the joint into upper and lower parts.. (REF. 1-p. 326)

26. C. The articular disc is a roughly oval plate which consists of fibrous tissue and completely divides the joint. Its upper surface is saddle-shaped or concavoconvex from before backward, accommodated to the form of the articular fossa and articular tubercle. Its inferior surface, in contact with the head of the mandible, is concave. (REF. 1-p. 327)

27. E. The muscles of mastication (and speech as well) include the masseter, temporalis, and pterygoid muscles. A strong layer of fascia (parotid fascia) covers the masseter and is firmly connected with it. The masseter elevates the mandible to occlude the teeth during mastication. The temporalis elevates the mandible, closes the mouth, and approximates the teeth. The lateral pterygoid assists in opening the mouth by pulling forward the condylar process of the mandible and the articular disc, while the head of the mandible rotates on the articular disc. The medial pterygoids assist in elevating the mandible. (REF. 1-p. 446)

28. E. The arteries supplying the heart are the right and left coronary branches of the aorta. Most of the veins of the heart are drained by the coronary sinus into the right atrium. The lymph vessels consist of the subendocardial, myocardial, and the subepicardial plexuses. The nerves of the heart are derived from the cardiac plexus. (REF. 1-p. 650)

29. D. The aorta is the major trunk of the system of blood vessels which carry oxygenated blood to tissues throughout the body. It begins at the upper part of the left ventricle and, after passing upward and to the right, arches backward and to the left, over the root of the left lung. Then it descends within the thorax on the left side of the vertebral column and enters the abdominal cavity through the aortic hiatus in the diaphragm. (REF. 1-p. 669)

30. E. The common carotid arteries differ in length and in mode of origin. The right artery begins at the bifurcation of the brachiocephalic trunk behind the right sternoclavicular joint and is confined to the neck. The left artery springs from the highest part of the arch of the aorta immediately behind and to the left of the brachiocephalic trunk and consists of a thoracic and a cervical portion. (REF. 1-p. 670)

31. E. The external carotid artery begins opposite the upper border of the thyroid cartilage, at the level of the disc between the third and fourth cervical vertebrae and, taking a slightly curved course, passes upward and forward and then inclines backward to a point behind the neck of the mandible. There it divides, in the parotid gland, into the superficial temporal and maxillary arteries. The branches of the external carotid artery are the superior thyroid, ascending pharyngeal, lingual, facial, occipital, posterior auricular, superficial temporal, and maxillary. (REF. 1-p. 672)

32. E. The maxillary (internal maxillary) artery is the larger terminal branch of the external carotid. It arises behind the neck of the mandible and at first is embedded in the parotid gland. It passes forward medial to the neck of the mandible and runs either superficial or deep to the lower head of the lateral pterygoid to enter the pterygopalatine fossa between the two heads of that muscle. The maxillary artery divides into the following: the first or mandibular portion, the second or pterygoid portion, and the third or pterygopalatine portion. The maxillary artery is distributed to the upper and lower jaws, teeth, muscles of mastication, palate, nose, and cranial dura mater. (REF. 1-p. 683)

33. E. The internal carotid artery supplies the greater portion of the cerebral hemisphere and the eye and its accessory organs and sends branches to the forehead and nose. It begins at the bifurcation of the common artery, where it

usually presents a localized dilatation, termed the carotid sinus. It ascends to the base of the skull and enters the cranial cavity through the carotid canal of the temporal bone. It then runs forward through the cavernous sinus, lying in the carotid groove on the side of the body of the sphenoid bone, and ends below the anterior perforated substance of the brain by dividing into anterior and middle cerebral arteries. (REF. 1-p. 687)

34. C. The pulmonary trunk conveys deoxygenated blood from the right ventricle of the heart to the lungs. It arises from the base of the right ventricle above and to the left of the supraventricular crest. It runs upward and backward in front of the ascending aorta. In the concavity of the aortic arch it divides, at the level of the fifth thoracic vertebrae, into right and left pulmonary arteries. All of the pulmonary trunk is contained within the pericardium. (REF. 1-p. 789)

35. D. The blood vessels supplying the liver are the portal vein, the hepatic artery proper, and the hepatic veins. The hepatic artery and branches follow a variable course in the porta hepatis. Hepatic veins carry blood from the liver to the inferior vena cava. Lymph vessels of the liver carry a very rich protein lymph fluid, and an obstruction of the venous drainage of the liver results in an increase of lymph in the thoracic duct. (REF. 1-p. 789)

36. A. The external jugular vein receives blood from the scalp and face, including its deeper parts. It begins level with the mandibular angle just below, or in the parotid gland, and runs down the neck from the angle toward the middle of the clavicle. It crosses sternocleidomastoid obliquely, and in the subclavian triangle perforates the deep fascia to end in the subclavian vein. (REF. 1-p. 795)

37. E. The internal jugular vein collects blood from the brain, superficial parts of the face, and neck. It begins at the base of the skull in the posterior compartment of the jugular foramen, as a direct continuation of the sigmoid sinus. At its origin is a dilatation, the superior bulb, below the posterior part of the floor of the tympanic cavity. The vein runs downward through the neck within the carotid sheath and, behind the sternal end of the clavicle, it unites with the subclavian to form the brachiocephalic vein. (REF. 1-p. 808)

38. E. The two maxillary sinuses are the largest accessory air sinuses of the nose and are pyramidal-shaped cavities within the bodies of the maxillae. The base is formed by the lateral wall of the nasal cavity; the apex extends into the zygomatic process of the maxilla. The roof is the orbital floor which is frequently ridged by the infraorbital canal. The floor is formed by the alveolar process. (REF. 18 - p. 200)

39. D. Ligaments are highly fibrous tissues formed into thick bundles. The direction of the connective tissue fibers in the thick bundles of ligaments is related to the stresses they experience. However, there is considerable interweaving of fibrous bundles within tendons or ligaments, which increases their structural stability. (REF. 18-p. 284)

40. B. The facial nerve possesses a motor and a sensory root; the latter is termed nervus intermedius. The motor root supplies the muscles of the face, scalp, auricle, buccinator muscle, platysma, stapedius, stylohyoid, and posterior belly of the digastric. The sensory root conveys from the chorda tympani nerve the fibers of taste for the presulcal area of the tongue and, from the palatine and greater petrosal nerves, the fibers of taste from the soft palate. (REF. 18-p. 937)

41. E. The pituitary gland (hypophysis cerebri) is continuous with the apex of the infundibulum, a hollow conical projection from the inferior aspect of the tuber cinereum. The pituitary lies in the hypophyseal fossa of the sphenoid bone, where it is overlapped by a circular fold of dura mater, the diaphragma sellae. The latter fold separates the anterior part of the superior surface of the hypohysis from the optic chiasma. On each side the hypophysis is related to the cavernous sinus and the structures it contains. The meninges blend with the capsule of the hypophysis and cannot be identified as separate layers in the fossa. (REF. 18-p. 1348)

Chapter 2 Microbiology

42. E. Microbiologists have long considered the possibility that a virus might be an inanimate poison capable of stimulating susceptible cells to replicate the virus. Viruses are

obligate intracellular parasites capable of infecting hosts in animals, plants, or insects. The structure of the virus particle (termed virion) ranges from simple through varying degrees of complexity to a quite elaborate structure (as in the smallpox virus). The simple virus is composed of an outer protein shell (the capsid) and an inner core of either DNA or RNA. (REF. 22-p. 649)

43. D. The blue-green algae are placed in the kingdom Procaryotae. The latter cells are characterized by having no nuclear membrane, mitotic apparatus, mitochrondria, or visible endoplasmic reticulum. Viruses, which are not cells, do not belong to the kingdom Procaryotae. (REF. 22-pp. 1, 27)

44. E. Bacterial taxonomy requires for classification the determination of as many characteristics as possible of the microorganism. Important characteristics include the following: size, shape, arrangement of aggregates, sporulation, capsules, flagella (cellular morphology), elevation, structure, color, transparency, topography, marginal characteristics, consistency, and changes induced in media (colonial appearance). (REF. 22-pp. 27-37)

45. E. Spirochetes which are parasitic and pathogenic for man are divided into three genera: Borrelia, Treponema, and Leptospira. They have either coarse or slender spirals, refractive indexes similar to those of bacteria, flexible or rigid cells, structureless protoplasm, and parasitic habitats in vertebrates. The diseases caused by the treponemata are yaws, syphilis, and pinta. Yaws is caused by T. pertenue, syphilis is caused by T. pallidum, and pinta is caused by T. carateum. (REF. 22-p. 544)

46. A. Sterilization means either to make incapable of reproduction or to destroy or remove all forms of life with reference to microorganisms. Germicide means to kill germs. Antiseptic means against putrefaction and is reserved for agents applied to the body. Disinfectant means free from infection and refers only to inhibition or destruction of pathogens. Asepsis means the avoidance of pathogenic microorganisms. (REF. 22-p. 89)

47. C. The operating room of a hospital is made aseptic in the use of sterile instruments, sutures, and dressings, and the wearing of sterile masks, caps, gowns, and rubber gloves by the operator. (REF. 22-p. 85)

48. C. Detailed physical methods of sterilization include moist heat, dry heat, radiant energy, ultrasonic vibration, filtration, osmosis, freezing, and drying. (REF. 22-p. 94)

49. C. The mode of action of useful chemotherapeutic agents include the following: inhibitors of cell wall formation, inhibitors of protein synthesis (at levels of transcription or translation), inhibitors of nucleic acid function, inhibitors causing cytoplasmic membrane damage, and metabolite antagonists. (REF. 2-p. 88)

50. E. In contrast to higher organisms, where the integument is capable of retaining water, the metabolism of bacteria is dependent on ambient water. (REF. 2-p. 62)

51. B. The most common cause of food poisoning is staphylococci. If broad spectrum antibiotics are used to treat human infections, they often upset the normal balance of the intestinal microbiota sufficiently for staphylococci to become the predominant intestinal bacteria. Individuals so treated often develop a pseudomembranous ulcerative enteritis related to the number of staphylococci present and to the action of the enterotoxin and staphylolysin. (REF. 22-p. 411)

52. E. The susceptibility of bacterial cells to disinfectants or to heat varies with their physiologic state. The cells in a young culture are generally more susceptible than those in a stationary phase culture, in which significant changes in the cell wall and membrane have been observed. (REF 2-p. 264)

53. E. Gastroenteritis, a disease confined to the gastrointestinal tract, is the most common kind of Salmonella infection. The most frequent cause in the United States is S. typhimurium. Symptoms begin 8 to 48 hours after consumption of contaminated food, with diarrhea ranging from mild to a fulminant form with sudden and violent onset of food poisoning. Headache, chills, and abdominal pain are followed by nausea, vomiting, and diarrhea, accompanied by fever lasting from 1 to 4 days. Blood cultures are rarely positive, but the organisms can usually be cultured from the feces. (REF. 2-p. 662)

54. D. The mechanism of action of most antibiotics as chemotherapeutic agents was a mystery until macromolecule synthesis became accessible to analysis. It is now possible to classify almost all these agents in terms of mechanism, origin, structure, or antimicrobial spectrum. (REF. 2-p. 116)

55. A. To stain the tubercle bacillus, in smears of tissues, methods must be used that promote penetration of the dye into the acid-fast bacteria. The Ziehl-Neelsen method is utilized to stain the acid-fast organism. Unlike most other pathogenic bacteria, the tubercle bacillus is an obligate aerobe. The bacillus can grow in simple synthetic media. Growth of tubercle bacilli in culture media is slow; the shortest doubling time observed, in rich media, is about 12 hours. (REF. 2-p. 724)

56. E. The nature of the penicillin produced can be influenced by the media: benzylpenicillin (penicillin G), the most satisfactory of the original penicillins, can be obtained in pure yield by providing an excess of the corresponding acyl donor (phenylacetic acid). It is still the most potent and inexpensive penicillin. (REF. 2-p. 116)

57. B. Drug resistance refers not to the natural resistance of a species but to acquired genotypic changes, which persist during cultivation in the absence of the drug. The change may be brought about either by mutation, which alters a cell constituent, or by infection by a plasmid, which brings together genes for new enzymes. The drug plays only a selective and not a directive role. (REF. 2-p. 123)

58. E. Tetracycline and chloramphenicol have an essentially identical antimicrobial spectrum: they were the first broad-spectrum antibiotics, effective against many gram-negative as well as gram-positive organisms. Both drugs reversibly block the ribosome and hence are bateriostatic. (REF. 2-p. 120)

59. D. Facultative organisms (many yeast and enterobacteria) can grow without air but shift in its presence to a respiratory metabolism. (REF. 2-p. 38)

60. B. Obligate anaerobes (such as clostridia or propionibacter) can grow only in the absence of oxygen. A subgroup, called microaerophilic, can tolerate, or even prefer, oxygen at low tension but not that of air. (REF. 2-p. 38)

61. C. Virulence (i. e., the degree of pathogenicity) is used to indicate two features of a pathogenic organism: its infectivity (ability to colonize a host) and the severity of the disease produced. Virulence varies not only among bacterial species but also among strains. (REF. 2-p. 552)

62. B. Gram-positive bacteria excrete a number of exoenzymes into the medium. Most of these enzymes convert impermeable substances into permeable foodstuffs; others destroy harmful substances (penicillinase) or serve as exotoxins (virulence factors) of pathogens. (REF. 2-p. 90)

63. C. The definitive diagnosis of diphtheria ordinarily can be made only by isolating toxigenic diphtheria bacilli from the primary lesion. Exudate from the lesion, taken from the membrane, should be immediately transferred to a Loeffler slant, a blood agar plate, and tellurite agar. After 24 hours incubation each culture should be carefully examined, and smears should be made from each type of colony that has grown out on any one of the media. (REF. 2-p. 591)

64. B. Delayed hypersensitivity may develop during the course of bacterial disease. The resulting accelerated and intensified tissue response to the infecting organism was first demonstrated in Koch's classic observations on the response to two successive injections of tubercle bacilli. (REF. 2-p. 567)

65. C. Lymphatic tissues are bombarded with antibodies from invasive or indigenous organisms and by those that enter the body of inhalation (e. g., pollens) and by ingestion (e. g., foods or drugs) and by penetration of the skin (e. g., poison ivy). Natural immunization results from the latter stimulation of the lymph nodes and spleen. Deliberate immunization is produced by immunogens being injected into skin or muscle, and the antibodies become distributed widely throughout the body via lymphatic and vascular channels. (REF. 2-p. 436)

66. E. Staphylococci appear in clusters similar to a bunch of grapes. Staphylococci have the following characteristics: spherical, gram-positive, irregular clusters, anaerobic growth, cell wall teichoic acid; pentaglycine cross-bridge in peptidoglycan, sensitivity to lysostaphin, and 30-40% DNA base composition. Staphylococci are among the hardiest of all nonspore-forming bacteria. They remain alive for months on the surface of agar plates stored at $4^{o}C$ and

may be cultured from samples of dried pus many weeks old. Some strains are relatively heat-resistant, withstanding temperatures as high as 60°C for 30 minutes. (REF. 2-p. 498)

67. E. Streptococci appear in chains or twisted patterns. Streptococci are gram-positive and characteristically grow in chains. The length of the chains tend to be inversely related to the adequacy of the culture media. All streptococci are lactic acid bacteria, which derive their energy primarily from the fermentation of sugars, regardless of whether they are growing aerobically or anaerobically. (REF. 2-p. 292)

68. D. Beta-hemolytic streptococci commonly occur as diplococci, in vivo. Streptococci chains are difficult to disrupt without killing the organisms. Hemolytic streptococci are grown in beef infusion media containing blood or serum. One potential surface antigen of group A hemolytic streptococcal cells, the hyaluronate of the capsule, is not immunogenic. The hyaluronate capsule is retained only by actively growing streptococci. (REF. 2-p. 291)

69. E. Neisseria species are essentially aerobic but will multiply under microaerophilic conditions. Neisseria genus includes two gram-negative cocci which grow in pairs or tetrads or clusters. (REF. 2-p. 338)

70. E. Clostridium tetani is a strict anaerobe without a capsule but with spherical terminal spores that give a characteristically "drumstick" appearance. It is present in the soil and in feces of various animals. In humans fecal carrier rates are extremely variable, suggesting that the organism is transient and dependent upon its ingestion. (REF. 2-p. 557)

71. E. The corynebacteria are gram-positive, rodlike organisms, which are arranged in palisades, possess club-shaped swellings at their poles, and stain irregularly. They are related to the mycobacteria and nocardiae. C. diphtheriae cause diphtheria and are lysogenized by a bacteriophage which causes synthesis of a potent, heat-labile protein toxin. (REF. 2-p. 559)

72. E. Mycobacteria are nonmotile rods that are defined by their distinctive staining property. They are relatively impermeable to various basic dyes, but once stained they retain dyes with great tenacity. They resist discoloriza-

tion with acidified organic solvents and therefore are termed acid-fast. Mycobacteria are found in soil and water and are responsible for tuberculosis and leprosy. Tubercle bacilli are typically slightly bent or curved slender rods, of uniform width but more often appear beaded with irregularly spaced, unstained vacuoles or heavily stained knobs. (REF. 2-p. 468)

73. D. The yeast Candida albicans is a frequent minor inhabitant of the oral cavity. It may grow out and cause lesions when the indigenous bacterial flora (such as S. salivarius, S. mutans, Bacteroides melaninogenicus, S. sanguis, or S. mitior) is suppressed by antibiotic therapy. (REF. 2-p. 468)

74. E. Spirochetes are motile, unicellular, spiral-shaped organisms, morphologically quite different from other bacteria. Physiologically the spirochetes range from obligate anaerobes to aerobes and from free-living forms to obligate parasites. Many are not yet cultivable. The genus Treponema causes syphilis, yaws, and pinta. (REF. 2-p. 485)

75. B. An antigen has two properties: immunogenicity and the ability to react specifically with the antibodies. Immunogenicity is the capacity to stimulate the formation of the corresponding antibodies. The term immunogen is generally used to indicate the substance that stimulates the formation of the corresponding antibodies. Substances termed haptens are not immunogenic but do react specifically with the appropriate antibodies. (REF. 2-pp. 18, 625)

76. C. Haptens react selectively with appropriate antibodies, but they are not immunogenic. Hapten may be a small molecule; however, some macromolecules also can function as haptens. (REF. 2-pp. 18, 610)

77. B. Antibody refers to the proteins that are formed in response to an antigen and react specifically with that antigen. All antigens belong to a special group of serum proteins, the immunoglobulins. (REF. 2-p. 610)

78. B. All proteins that function as antibodies or that have antigenic determinants in common with antibodies are called immunoglobulins. All immunoglobulins have a similar structural organization, but they are an immensely diversified family that can be arranged into groups and

subgroups on the basis of variations in antigenic properties and amino acid sequences. (REF. 2-p. 636)

79. E. Exotoxins of Corynebacterium diphtheriae, Clostridium tetani, Clostridium botulinum, and S. dysenteriae (Shiga's bacillus) are the most powerful poisons known. The pharmacologic actions of the known bacterial exotoxins are slow, some requiring several days. Most exotoxins are inactivated by heat, acid, or proteolytic enzymes (in GI tract). (REF. 2-p. 716)

80. E. Unlike the heat-labile protein exotoxins, endotoxins are heat-stable lipopolysaccharides, associated with the outer membranes of gram-negative bacteria. Their toxicity resides in the lipid portion of the molecule (lipid A). They are less potent and less specific than most exotoxins in their cytotoxic activities, and they do not produce toxoids. (REF. 2-p. 586)

81. E. Allergy and hypersensitivity should be considered synonymous. Both refer to the altered state, induced by an antigen, in which pathologic reactions can be subsequently elicited by the antigen or by a structurally similar substance. Allergy means altered action. (REF. 19-p. 961)

82. E. Anaphylactic reactions are due to special antibodies that bind with exceptionally high affinity to receptors on tissue mass cells and blood basophils. Ingestion of an antigen into a hypersensitive individual can cause an explosive response within 3 to 4 minutes. If the antigen is injected intravenously, the response (called systemic or generalized anaphylaxis) can lead to shock, vascular engorgement, and asphyxia due to bronchial and laryngeal constriction. If death does not follow promptly, recovery is complete within about one hour. (REF. 2-p. 811)

83. C. Arthus reactions occur in man and are not limited to the skin. These reactions can take place when antigens are injected almost anywhere (as the pericardial sac or synovial joint spaces). The principal requirement is the formation in tissues of immune aggregates that fix C. The resulting C fragments attract polymorphonuclear leukocytes. Their released lysosomal enzymes cause tissue damage, characteristically with destructive inflammation of the small blood vessels (vasculitis). (REF. 2-p. 752)

84. B. The dream of hybridization due to genetic engineering is approaching fruition. One application of genetic engi-

neering in dentistry is the prevention of viral hepatitis. (REF. 90-p. 30)

85. E. Microbiologists currently are evaluating the role of oral microorganisms, i. e., their components and products in activating host response systems leading to pathology. In evaluating a specific oral microorganism with regard to the biological correlation to disease it is necessary to utilize a crude, cell-free fraction prior to application of any purification procedures. (REF. 90, p. 47)

86. E. All five of these herpes viruses can become latent after a primary infection and are capable of being reactivated. The primary infection may be subclinical, but the clinical lesions appear in different ways. Investigation is currently ongoing with a chemotherapeutic agent (nucleosides) which shows some promise in the clinical management of herpetic disease, including herpes labialis. However, there is no drug in the United States with known efficacy against herpes labialis. (REF. 90-p. 95)

87. A. There is a great variation in the concentration of microorganisms in the oral cavity. The oral microbial flora is predominantly anaerobic in spite of the fact that the mouth is open to the air. However, the facial infections are commonly caused by aerobic microorganisms. (REF. 90-p. 111)

88. E. Most of the anaerobic microorganisms commonly associated with oral infection are highly sensitive to penicillin G. The exception to the latter is B. fragilis which, however, is sensitive to clindamycin. The treatment of facial infections involves the following: incising and draining the proper space and avoiding blood vessels and nerves, using antibiotics, and utilizing culture and sensitivity testing. Indiscriminant use of antibiotics has caused an increasing number of allergic patients and resistant microorganisms. (REF. 90-p. 53)

89. E. Some of the oral diseases produced are insidious. The microorganisms involved also may be infectious for the dental practitioner and dental office personnel. Spread of the infectious material can occur during the initial examination of the dental patient or during the performance of surgery and exodontia, operative dentistry, and oral hygiene procedures. Seventy-three diseases or oral manifestations of systemic diseases bear some direct or remote relationship to the oral cavity and to dental practice. (REF. 90-p. 78)

90. E. In general the oral tissues show excellent resistance to infection. The latter is due to the following protective mechanisms: irrigation of the oral cavity by saliva containing immunoglobulins, especially secretory IgA and lysozyme, and the crevicular fluid present in the periodontal diseases. Patients with diabetes, with poor nutrition, malignant lymphoma, with primary or secondary immuno-deficiency, or on cytotoxic drugs may develop oral infections that are very difficult to resolve. (REF. 90-p. 128)

91. E. Two species of lactobacilli are also cariogenic, i. e., L. acidophilus and L. casei. Two species of actinomycetes are cariogenic, Actinomyces viscous, and A. naeslundii. The lactobacilli and streptococci are homofermentative because they produce lactic acid during glucose metabolism. Dental caries are convergent biological phenomena. (REF. 90-p. 147).

92. E. By taking advantage of sucrose in the diet S. mutans becomes the dominant bacterium on certain locations on the tooth surface. It is the localized microcolonies of S. mutans that utilize the monosaccharides and disaccharides available in the diet to undergo proliferation and production of acid to attack the enamel surface. (REF. 90-p. 161)

93. B. Direct access occurs via pulp exposure and open dentinal tubules. Pulpo-periodontal pathways occur via lateral canals and the apical foramina. Bacteria gain access to the pulp via the bloodstream during transient bacteremias. Retrogenic pulp infection (apical invasion of bacteria from an adjacent infected tooth) is rarely observed. (REF. 90-p. 171)

94. E. The most frequently isolated organisms are streptococci (viridans). Staphylococci (epidermis) are the second most frequently isolated organisms from root canal cultures. The latter is a nonpathogenic species and thus is a contaminant. The remaining organisms listed under A, B, C, and D are the indigenous microbial flora of the oral cavity (REF. 90-p. 174)

95. C. Only approximately 7. 3% of dental practitioners culture the root canals routinely during endodontic therapy. Another 15. 3% culture root canals sometime when performing endodontic therapy. The significance of culturing root

canals remains an issue of controversy at the present time in spite of the fact that dental schools in the United States teach students that root canal cultures are important and worthwhile. (REF. 90-p. 175)

96. E. The advantages of culturing root canals include the following: the incidence of success is increased by 10%, a negative culture is the most reliable index of root canal sterility available to dentists, root canal cultures are a source of valuable information for the dentist, cultures make it possible to identify the antibiotic sensitivity of root canal organisms early in the course of therapy, and cultures are an important criteria used to determine when the canals are ready for filling. (REF. 90-p. 176)

97. E. Bacteria are held together in the plaque by an adhesive interbacterial matrix. Plaque may be measured in less than 1 hour after the teeth are thoroughly cleaned. Maximum accumulation occurs in one month. Small amounts of plaque are not clinically visible unless stained by pigments in the oral cavity or by disclosing solutions or wafers. (REF. 90-p. 198)

98. D. The following measures are available to control oral diseases: fluoride therapy, tooth extraction, breaking approximal contact points, banning sugar, and using antibiotics or chemical or natural biological properties to deny plaque adherence on the surface of teeth. In order to secure a fluoride effect on microbes in dental plaque, the frequency of application must be increased beyond 6 months. (REF. 90-p. 218)

99. C. It is not economically possible to routinely screen all dental patients or personnel to determine their carrier status. The best precaution is to assume that all blood and saliva are potentially infectious. In one study 12% of dental patients were found to be carriers of type B hepatitis. (REF. 90-p. 253)

100. D. The latter three procedures all remove, destroy, and prevent subsequent reentry of microorganisms into the root canal system. Microorganisms and their toxic products as well as pulp degradation products gain access to the apical periodontium by way of the apical foramina and thereby initiate periapical disease. (REF. 90-p. 169)

101. Practical methods of sterilization for endodontic instruments and materials include the following: the dry heat oven 160-170°C, the autoclave 121-123°C, or the hot salt sterilizer 220-240°C. The dry heat oven does not cause rust or corrosion. The autoclave has a short sterilizing time. The hot salt sterilizer is a fast chairside sterilization of one or only a few instruments. (REF. 90-p. 181)

Chapter 3 Physiology

102. E. The group of organelles bounded by a limiting membrane are the nucleus, endoplasmic reticulum, Golgi apparatus, lysosome, and mitochondrion. The group of organelles not bounded by a membrane include the chromosomes, nucleoli, microtubules, microfilaments, and centrioles. (REF. 3-p. 1)

103. E. Since particles do cross the cell membrane, one should seek an explanation for their transport in terms of special mechanisms of action as opposed to simple diffusion. (REF. 3-p. 19)

104. B. Pinocytosis is not simply the entrapment of extracellular fluids plus the uptake of solutes from the fluid. (REF. 3-p. 26)

105. E. The EPSP is monophasic and nonpropagating; it represents a hypopolarization localized to the soma of the motoneuron. (REF. 3-p. 52)

106. E. Acetylcholine has been shown to be a transmitter in autonomic ganglia, postganglionic parasympathetic terminals (sweat glands and vasodilator fibers), and motoneuron collateral-Renshaw cell synapses in the spinal cord. (REF. 3-p. 57)

107. D. The structural basis of electromyography is the motor unit. (REF. 3-p. 105)

108. E. All constituents of cells (except DNA in nondividing cells) are in a steady-state turnover but at different rates. (REF. 3, Ch. 4-p. 3)

109. E. The NPN of blood represents a balance between nitrogenous materials from the metabolism of ingested and tissue protein and the excretion of these products in the urine. (REF. 3-p. 348)

110. A. There is no direct method for measuring the volume or size of the intracellular fluid. Thus it is estimated as the difference between the total body water and the volume of extracellular fluid. (REF. 3, Ch. 5-p. 6)

111. E. Certain chemicals (such as arsenic or salts of heavy metals) and toxins of infectious diseases (such as diptheria or acute nephritis) act as capillary poisons, producing edema. (REF. 3, Ch. 4-p. 93)

112. B. The classification of the blood groups is based on the antigenic nature of red blood cell membranes. (REF. 3, Ch. 4-p. 50)

113. B. The long-lived lymphocytes are produced at a rate proportional to the growth of the body and are recirculated from blood to lymph. (REF. 3, Ch. 4-p. 98)

114. C. The law of Laplace applies to any membrane capable of distension into a spherical or cylindrical shape. (REF. 3, Ch. 3-p. 94)

115. D. The heart rate is temporarily increased in muscular exercise, emotional excitement, and high environment temperature and somewhat during digestion. (REF. 3-p. 144)

116. C. The control of coronary arterial resistance is exerted by intrinsic factors (local chemical milieu and mechanical compression secondary to myocardial contraction). (REF. 3-p. 134)

117. C. In addition to vasomotor control by way of nerves ending in, on, or in the region of blood vessels there is neurohumoral control that is autonomic in nature but acts upon vascular smooth muscle through catecholamines that circulate in the blood. (REF. 3-p. 169)

118. D. The splanchnic circulation plays an important role in the response of the organism to a reduction of circulating blood volume (an example is during hemorrhage). (REF. 3-p. 222)

119. D. Renal circulation is related to renal function. Renal blood flow in man is measured by the clearance technique. However, in certain renal diseases, when no urine is produced, renal blood flow cannot be evaluated by the clearance technique. (REF. 3-p. 223)

120. C. Poiseuille's equation applies to liquid flow when (1) the fluid is homogenous and its viscosity is the same at all rates of laminar flow, (2) the liquid does not slip at the wall, (3) the flow is laminar (liquid at all points moves parallel to the vessel wall), (4) the rate of flow is steady and not subject to cyclical acceleration or deceleration, (5) the tube is long compared to the section in which flow is studied, and (6) the tube is rigid. (REF. 3-p. 14)

121. E. At the region of transition between the AVN and bundle of His, the cells gather into fascicles and assume the characteristics of the typical Purkinje fibers. Together these Purkinje fibers are known as the bundle of His. (REF 3-p. 49)

122. B. The most important measurement in the circulation is the volume flow of blood, through the aorta or through any tissue or organ or region of the body. (REF. 3-p. 158)

123. A. Circulation time is the shortest time a particle of blood takes to go from any given point in the circulation through vessels of the systemic and pulmonary circulations and back to the point of origin. (REF. 3-p. 158)

124. D. Intravascular techniques for the measurement of blood pressure are useful in clinical dentistry only for experimental purposes, for diagnostic tests in cardiopulmonary laboratories, or during surgery. The palpatory, oscillatory, or auscultory methods may be employed to determine when the blood first escapes beneath the cuff. The first uses palpation of the radial pulse, the second the presence of oscillations in the manometer, and the third a sequence of sounds heard with a stethoscope over the peripheral part of the artery adjacent to the cuff. In all three procedures the value for the lateral pressure in the bronchial artery is obtained, whereas direct measures determine the end pressure. (REF. 3-p. 145)

125. E. Phases of the cardiac cycle are identified as (1) isovolumetric contraction (close of atrioventricular valves, rapid rise of intraventricular pressure), (2) maximum ejection (rapid outflow of blood from ventricles), (3) reduced ejection (declining flow of blood from ventricles), (4) protodiastole (rapid drop in intraventricular pressure, (5) isovolumetric relaxation (continued ventricular relaxation with no volume change), (6) rapid flow (rapid flow

of blood from the atria to the ventricles), (7) diastasis (continued slower flow from the atria to the ventricles), (8) atrial systole (increased flow from the atria to the ventricles). (REF. 3-p. 103)

126. E. Heart sounds or vibrations arising in the heart and great vessels are fundamentally the result of sudden displacement of blood (accleration) or abrupt stoppage of blood (deceleration) and turbulence. The first sound is of relatively long duration, soft in quality, and low in pitch. The first sound is heard most clearly and at maximum intensity over the fifth left intercostal space (an area centered over the apex beat). (REF. 3-p. 109)

127. A. Under the stimulus of gradual coronary occlusion, the coronary collateral vessels can expand their initial diameter tenfold, and collateral flow can increase from 0 to 200 m/min/100 g myocardium. The coronary arteries were regarded in the past as end arteries. However, they do have collateral channels that can enlarge in response to ischemia. (REF. 3-p. 143)

128. E. Cerebral blood flow is determined by two opposing sets of forces: the effective perfusion pressure and cerebral vascular resistance. The principal control of cerebral blood flow appears to be mechanisms of autoregulation mediated mainly by local pH changes. (REF. 3-p. 209)

129 C. The response of blood pressure to exercise depends upon physical conditioning, the mass of muscle involved, and the type of muscular work performed. At the transition from rest to heavy work, the pulse frequently rises very rapidly, reaching levels of 160-180/minute. During short bouts of near maximal exercise, heart rates as high as 240-270/minute have been recorded in normal young persons (perhaps due to an increase in pressure in the great veins and atria, causing acceleration of the heart). (REF. 3-pp. 121, 189)

130. E. The causes of chronic congestive heart failure are diseases of the myocardium, abnormalities that increase the work of one or both ventricles, conditions that cause a sustained increase in the output of one or both ventricles and conditions that interfere with cardiac filling. Failure develops gradually, and in the early stages only cardiac responses to excess demands, such as strenuous exercise, are compromised. (REF. 3-p. 242)

131. E. Ventilation is the process of getting gas to and from the alveoli of the lung. With each inspiration, 500 ml air enter the lung (the tidal volume of air). A very small volume of capillary blood is involved compared with alveolar gas. The anatomic dead space represents a small proportion of the total lung volume. (REF. 3, ch. 6-p. 7)

132. E. The molecules of a gas are in continuous motion and are only deflected from their course by collision with other molecules or with the walls of a container. When the molecules strike the walls and rebound, the resulting bombardment results in a pressure. The magnitude of the pressure depends on the number of molecules present plus their speed. (REF. 3, ch. 6-p. 5)

133. C. This is one of the most beneficial physiological responses to exposure to a low oxygen partial pressure. The cause of hyperventilation is hypoxic stimulation of the peripheral chemoreceptors. (REF. 3, ch. 6-p. 75)

134. B. Oxygen forms an easily reversible continuation with hemoglobin to form oxyhemoglobin. The maximum amount of oxygen that can be combined with hemoglobin is termed the oxygen capacity. It can be measured by exposing the blood to a very high Po_2 (600 mg mercury) and subtracting the dissolved oxygen. One gram of pure hemoglobin can combine with 1. 39 ml oxygen and, since normal blood has about 15 g hemoglobin/100 ml, the oxygen capacity is about 20. 8 ml oxygen/100 ml blood. (REF. 3, ch. 6-p. 14)

135. B. Oxygenated hemoglobin is bright red, but reduced hemoglobin is purple. Thus a low arterial oxygen saturation causes cyanosis. Several factors may shift the position of the oxygen dissociation curve, including changes in pH, PCo_2, temperature of the blood, and the concentration of organic phosphates within the red blood cells. (REF. 3, Ch. 6-p. 14)

136. D. Pulmonary ventilation in a normal subject at rest is relatively constant at a given level in response to the carbon dioxide tension, hydrogen ion concentration, and oxygen tension in specific sites. (REF. 3, Ch. 6-p. 63)

137. A. The anatomic dead space is the volume of the conducting airways. The normal value is in the region of 150 ml, and it increases with large inspirations because of the traction exerted on the bronchi by the surrounding lung parenchyma. (REF. 3, Ch. 6-p. 11)

138. B. Hypoventilation is a cause of hypoxemia. There is little variation in the level of oxygen uptake at rest. If for any reason the level of alveolar ventilation falls, so falls the Po_2 in the alveolar gas and therefore also in the alveolar blood. By the time that air has reached the alveolar gas, it has already lost one-third of the available oxygen pressure. (REF. 3, Ch. 6-p. 22)

139. E. The most important muscle of inspiration is the diaphragm. The latter is a thin sheet of muscle in the shape of a dome which is attached to the lower ribs, sternum, and vertebral column. During contraction of the diaphragm the abdominal contents are forced downward, thus enlarging the vertical dimension of the chest, and the rib margins are moved upward and outward. (REF. 3, Ch. 6-p. 36)

140. E. In respiratory muscles it appears that the role of the muscle spindles and the fusimotor innervation may be to adjust the strength of the contraction to achieve a given tidal volume on demand, despite the degree of resistance to movement of air. (REF. 3, Ch. 6-p. 36)

141. C. The immediate causes of dyspnea are (1) stimulation of the respiratory center reflexly from peripheral chemoreceptors, centrally by carbon dioxide excess, by impulses from cerebral centers, or by afferent impulses and (2) hypersensitivity of the Hering-Breuer reflex which brings about an earlier inhibition of the inspiratory phase and causes, as a consequence, a more rapid, shallow type of breathing. (REF. 3, Ch. 6-p. 71)

142. A. Hypoxia is known to be the most potent physiological coronary vasodilator; however, its mode of action is still obscure. Low partial pressure relaxes coronary arterial smooth muscle in vitro; in vivo this might account for the consistency of partial pressure in coronary sinus blood as a direct control of coronary arterial tone by arterial partial pressure (Po_2). Hypoxia is associated with high altitude where a remarkable degree of acclimatization occur. (REF. 3, Ch. 3-p. 3; Ch. 6-p. 20)

143. D. The body contains only small reserves of oxygen which can be called upon during complete asphyxia or anoxia. The total store of oxygen is only about 1500 ml, i. e., enough to maintain life for only 6 minutes provided it is properly distributed. Tissues vary greatly in their ability to withstand oxygen deprivation, depending on how easily they can utilize anaerobic glycolysis. (REF. 3, Ch. 6-p. 21)

Chapter 4 Pathology

144. D. Redness results from vascular dilatation and congestion. Swelling is due to edema and congestion in the area. Heat occurs because the dilated vessels bring a large quantity of warm blood to the area. Pain is due to swelling and tension caused by the exudate. The cells and tissues involved by inflammation have their normal function disturbed. (REF. 16-p. 63)

145. C. Suppurative (purulent) inflammations are those characterized by the development of pus (i. e., a creamy, semifluid, opaque substance containg mainly liquified necrotic material and numerous neutrophilic leukocytes or pus cells, both vital and necrotic). The abscess is an example of suppurative inflammation. (REF. 21-pp. 65, 66)

146. A. Active hyperemia is the result of increased arterial blood to a part. It is acute and characterized by dilatation of arterioles and capillaries. It develops during functional activity of a tissue, as a result of emotion or heat (flushing of the skin), and in the early stages of the inflammatory process. (REF. 21 -pp. 101, 102)

147. A. Red blood cells appear in the inflammatory exudate after their passage through permeable vessel walls in the area of inflammation by diapedesis. Small hemorrhages also result from ruptured blood vessels (as in anthrax) where an exudate of hemorrhage develops. (REF. 16-p. 60)

148. E. An acute inflammation may subside or proceed to subacute or chronic phases. Serous inflammation contains serous exudates. Catarrhal inflammation is a mild upper respiratory tract inflammation. Cellulitis is characterized by a diffuse spreading inflammation involving the tissue spaces and tissue planes and is frequently of a suppurative nature. (REF. 4-p. 64)

149. A. Resolution is the restoration of the inflammed part to a physiologic state. After recovery of the degenerated cells, the area is returned to normal. (REF. 16-p. 82)

150. B. Acute inflammation is a local reactive change in tissues following injury or irritation. The agents of injury may be microbial, immunological, physical, chemical, or traumatic in nature. It is the most common and fundamental pathologic process and, in general, it is a protective response on the part of the body, tending to localize or dispose of the injurious agent. (REF. 16-p. 62)

151. E. The causative organism of primary tuberculosis is Mycobacterium tuberculosis. The organism produces a specific granulomatous tissue reaction characterized by caseous necrosis, pale mononuclear "epithelioid" cells, and giant cells with multiple peripheral nuclei. The lung is the organ most frequently involved. Spread in the body occurs by direct extension, the lymphatics, the blood stream, and natural passages such as bronchi. (REF. 16-pp. 96, 97)

152. A. Acute miliary tuberculosis is the result of widespread dissemination of large numbers of tubercle bacilli by the blood stream. When the dissemination is massive, myriads of tiny miliary tubercles develop in the lungs, spleen, liver, kidneys, meninges, and other organs. The tubercles appear as grayish nodules, less than 2 mm in diameter, uniform in size, and studding the outer and cut surfaces of the affected organs. (REF. 16-p. 99)

153. D. Neoplasia (tumor) is an abnormal mass of tissue, the growth of which exceeds and is uncoordinated with that of the normal tissues and which persists in the same excessive manner after cessation of the stimuli which evoked the change. Tumors are composed of cells and intercellular substances such as may be found in embryonic or mature tissues. Growth of cells predominates over function, although the functional activity may be present. (REF. 16-p. 161)

154. D. Cancer ranks second among the causes of death in the United States (heart disease is first). Cancer deaths in males are due to cancers arising in (1) the lung, (2) the colon and rectum, and (3) the prostate. Cancer deaths in females are due to cancers arising in (1) the breast,

(2) the colon and rectum, (3) the lung, and (4) the uterus. Incidence of cancer of the lung in females is correlated with the increase in the number of women smokers. (REF. 5-p. 312)

155. E. Malignant tumors (cancer) generally are more rapidly growing than benign tumors, tend to infiltrate and extend into normal structures and, unless successfully treated, interfere with health and eventually cause death. They are composed of cells less differentiated than normal ones. (REF. 5-p. 325)

156. C. Malignant tumors show pleomorphism. The latter undifferentiated carcinomas show a variation in the size and shape of nuclei and mitotic figures, including abnormal tripolar mitoses, hyperchromatism of nuclei, enlargement of nuclei with increased nucleocytoplasmic ratio, clumping of chromatin, and prominent nucleoli. (REF. 16 -p. 164)

157. E. Hyperplasia is an increase in the number of the constituent cells. It occurs in tissues whose cells are capable of mitotic division. Hyperplasia is influenced by increased functional demand and endocrine stimulation. Hormones from the pituitary gland and gonads induce hyperplasia. Hyperplasia is a nonneoplastic process; however, it may also be the site of development of a neoplasm, particularly when the hyperplasia is abnormal or atypical in nature (as in areas of dysplasia). (REF. 16, pp. 150, 152)

158. C. The chancre (primary syphilitic lesion) appears at the point of inoculation of spirochetes following an incubation period of 1 to 6 weeks. The chancre develops on the genitalia in over 90% of infected patients; the second most common location is in the lips or in the oral cavity. In 20% of infected patients, no primary lesion develops or they are hidden and undetected. (REF. 16-p. 108)

159. C. A latent period of a few months to 5 to 20 years may occur from the secondary to the tertiary stage and lesions of syphilis. The gumma is the less common tertiary lesion and is characterized by great destruction of tissue while very few spirochetes are present. The gumma may develop in any organ or tissue in the body, and it consists of a solitary nodule of necrotic tissue. This

opaque necrotic material has an elastic or "gummy" consistency. The gumma is composed of coagulation and caseation necrosis, surrounded by lymphocytes, plasma cells, macrophages, and multinucleated giant cells which occur less in frequency than during tuberculosis. (REF. 16-p. 109)

160. E. Actinomycosis is a chronic suppurative infection produced by Actinomyces israeli in man. In cattle the mycotic infection is caused by Actinomyces bovis and is termed "lumpy jaw." Actinomyces organisms grow in the oral cavity, and the ray fungus (radiating projections or clubs) is present only in the tissues and not in cultures. The ray fungus (clubs) are considered to be a reaction of the organism to the surrounding tissues. When pus from a lesion is placed on a slide the actinomycotic colonies become grossly visible as "yellow sulfur granules." (REF. 16-p. 139)

161. B. The etiology of sarcoidosis is obscure. The clinical features depend upon the organs involved. The frequency of this disease appears to be greater in the southeastern area than in other parts of the United States. The incidence is also higher in black than in white patients and greater in women than in men. (REF. 16-p. 114)

162. A. Healing of injured tissue may occur by one or more processes: resolution or restoration of the part to normal, healing by granulation tissue or scar formation, or replacing of destroyed or lost cells by regeneration of cells of a similar type. Healing and repair are synonymous. When tissues without the ability to regenerate are destroyed, repair takes place by connective tissue or, in the central nervous system, by neuroglial cells. (REF. 16-p. 85)

163. D. Metaplasia is a change from one type of cell to another. It results from chronic inflammation or irritation, impairment of nutrition and function, or demand for altered function. Metaplasia is common in cells of connective tissue, with formation of cartilage or bone in scars, arteriosclerotic blood vessels, injured or sightless eyes, or degenerated areas of a goiter. (REF. 16-pp. 156, 158)

164. A. Chronic passive congestion of the liver leads to the "nutmeg" liver. Grossly, the liver shows a contrasted pattern of red areas (blood filled vessels) and yellowish brown areas (fatty change in liver cells) which are responsible for the nutmeg appearance. The liver is highly susceptible to circulatory alterations. (REF. 4-p. 59)

165. E. Primary carcinoma of the lung is mainly bronchogenic in origin. It ranks as the leading cause of death from cancer in males. It is more common in men than women; however, the incidence in women has been constantly increasing. A mass of statistical evidence indicates that cigarette smoking is the cause of lung carcinoma. Other carcinogenic agents include atmospheric pollution in cities or tarring of roads and the late effects of pneumonitis of viral origin. (REF. 17-pp. 22, 23)

166. B. The breast is the most common site of carcinoma in women, but it is a rare site in males. Carcinoma of the female breast may occur at any adult age but commonly develops between 40 and 60 years of age. The etiology of the tumor is unknown. The following factors may play a role in the development of breast carcinoma: hereditary predisposition, hormonal influence, oncogenic viruses, and irradiation. It has been stated that the urinary estrogen profile in women is the determinant of their breast cancer risk. (REF. 5-p. 362)

167. E. Carcinoma of the prostate gland is the third most frequent cause of cancer deaths among United States males. Lung cancer is the most frequent, and cancer of the colon and rectum combined is the second most frequent cause of cancer deaths in males. Carcinoma of the prostate gland occurs after 50 years of age. About 14 to 46% of males over 50 years of age have prostatic carcinoma. (REF. 17-p. 263)

168. A. Leukemia is the overgrowth of white blood cells proceeding to eventual death, although therapy may favorably affect the clinical course in some patients. The cause of leukemia is obscure in humans. The leukemias are classified according to the type of white blood cell involved, i.e., myelocytic (granulocytic), lymphocytic, and monocytic. All three forms have acute or chronic clinical pat-

terns. The acute types are difficult to distinguish from each other. The occurrence of leukemia in persons over 50 years of age is increasing. (REF. 16-p. 53, 194)

169. A. Fungi are cellular filamentous plants belonging to a division called Thallophyta. Fungi may be saprophytic or parasitic. Superficial involvement of the skin or mucous membrane is a common type of fungal infection (as is athlete's foot or thrush). (REF. 16-p. 139)

170. E. Malaria is an infection with a protozoan parasite that has an asexual cycle in man and a sexual cycle in the *Anopheles* mosquito. Three species infect man, i. e., *Plasmodium vivax* (causes tertian or vivax malaria), *Plasmodium malariae* (causes quartan malaria, and *Plasmodium falciparum* (causes falciparum, estivoautumnal, or malignant tertian malaria). (REF. 5-p. 280)

171 D. Penumoconiosis is the pulmonary alteration that takes place as the result of inhalation of dust. The alterations depend on the type and amount of dust inhaled, the size of the dust particles, the length of time of exposure, and the failure of eliminative mechanisms of the lung. The most important types are nonoccupational anthracosis, silicosis, coal workers' pneumoconiosis, asbestosis, silicosiderosis, pneumoconiosis from graphite dust, and berylliosis caused by beryllium dust. (REF. 16-p. 34)

172. B. Granulomatous lesions or granulomas may occur as a result of microorganisms and are known as infectious granulomas. The lesions of tuberculosis, the tubercle, is characteristic of the granulomas, being composed of epithelioid cells, lymphocytes, and Langerhans' giant cells. Syphilis, leprosy, and certain fungal infections, produce similar lesions (tuberculoid granulomas). (REF. 16-pp. 106, 108)

173. D. Viruses and rickettsiae grow only within cells, often within certain types of cells and in certain species of animals, i. e., they show host and cell specificity. There may be a formation of inclusion bodies. Many viruses lie dormant in tissues for long periods of time, producing neither symptoms nor lesions. Viruses are sensitive to environmental conditions. Viral and rickettsial infections tend to pave the way for bacterial infections. (REF. 16-pp. 131, 138)

174. D. Infectious hepatitis (hepatitis A) is seen in children and young adults and is generally transmitted orally but may be acquired by the parenteral route following inoculations. Early in the disease no clinical manifestations are present, and a biopsy of the liver discloses only minor cell necrosis, enlargement and increase in the number of Kupffer cells, and an increased number of lymphocytes in the sinusoids. Symptoms are present at the height of the disease accompanied by a generalized parenchymal liver damage. (REF. 5-p. 292)

175. B. Pyemia refers to that type of septicemia in which pyogenic organisms spread by way of the blood stream and result in multiple abscesses in distant sites. Pathologic changes associated with septicemia include the following: degenerative changes in parenchymal organs, foci of necrosis and reticuloendothelial hyperplasia in lymph nodes, acute splenitis, congestion and hemorrhage, thrombi in small vessels, hemolysis of erythrocytes, and acute inflammation in various organs. (REF. 5-p. 224)

176. E. Various systemic diseases are characterized as primary disturbances of connective tissues of the body. The latter possess certain clinical and morphologic similarities. Thus they have been grouped together as diffuse collagen diseases. The collagen diseases are not necessarily related to the same cause. Lesions of the blood vessels accompany the changes in connective tissue. Hypersensitivity or autoimmunity plays an important role in the pathogenesis of these diseases. (REF. 16-p. 274)

177. C. Bronchiectasis is a dilatation of the bronchi (local or generalized). The dilatation may be cylindrical, fusiform, or saccular if localized to one area. The lower lobes are more commonly involved than the upper lobe, and the left lower lobe is involved more frequently than the right. This disease is associated with chronic bronchitis or with multiple abscess formation resulting from the invasion of pyogenic and fusospirochetal organisms. (REF. [illegible]-p. 263)

178. A. Emphysema is the most common chronic [illegible]se of the lungs and a major cause of pulmonary disturbance. It is a nonspecific, chronic, obstructive pulmonary disease. Emphysema is frequently associated with chronic bronchitis, and this relationship is referred to as the em-

physema-bronchitis complex. However, chronic bronchitis may occur without the latter pulmonary complications. Emphysema is inflation of the lung. (REF. 4-p. 269)

179. C. In anemia there is a quantitative deficiency of hemoglobin, generally accompanied by a corresponding decrease in the number of red blood cells. The different types of anemia show varying degrees of dissociation between the reduction of hemoglobin and of red blood cells. Characteristic findings of anemia include pallor of the skin, mucous membranes, fat, and muscle and fatty change in the heart and liver. In severe anemias, fatty degeneration of the myocardium is often of extreme degree and is especially prominent on the endocardial surface (thrush-breast markings). (REF. 17-p. 75)

180. E. Subacute glomerulonephritis is a rapidly progressive diffuse glomerular disease. The glomeruli may be injured by physical agents such as ionizing radiation, chemical agents, anoxia, and bacterial toxins. A major cause of inflammatory disease of the glomeruli is immunologic in character, i. e., antiglomerular basement membrane disease, immune complex disease, and alternative complement pathway disease. (REF. 17-pp. 25, 27)

181. E. Microorganisms may reach bone tissue through a wound, may spread to bone from adjacent tissues, or may be transported to bone tissue by way of the blood stream, producing osteomyelitis. Both bone and marrow tissue and periosteum are infected during osteomyelitis. Osteomyelitis is caused by bacteria and only occasionally by fungi and nonbacterial organisms. Staphylococci is the most common organism to produce osteomyelitis. However, streptococci (in infants) and gram-negative bacilli may be causative organisms. Salmonella spreads by way of the blood stream to cause osteomyelitis in patients with sickle cell anemia. (REF. 17-pp. 122, 123)

182. C. Ulcerative colitis or proctocolitis is of controversial etiology. The etiology postulated includes infection, immunologic derangement, lack of protective enzymes in the bowel wall, neurogenic and psychogenic disturbances, mucolytic and proteolytic enzymes acting on the mucosa, and alterations in the ground substance of the connective tissue. Many patients reveal a family history of ulcerative colitis. Immunologic factors, sensitivity to foods,

and autoimmunity have been postulated in the pathogenesis of colitis. Ulcerative colitis is a mucosal disease which involves the submucosa but not the muscularis or serosa. (REF. 17-p. 72)

183. C. Acute gastritis may result from various irritant foods, alcoholic beverages, aspirin and other drugs, and poisons. Various ingested corrosives are capable of provoking a severe inflammatory reaction in the stomach. (REF. 17-p. 61)

184. E. Chronic peptic ulcers is of obscure etiology. The action of acid-pepsin gastric content is one known factor in the etiology of the peptic ulcer. The chronic peptic ulcer develops only in areas exposed to acid-pepsin secretion such as the duodenum, the stomach, the lower part of the esophagus, the jejunum at the site of a gastrojejunostomy, and Meckel's diverticulum containing gastric mucosa. Duodenal ulcers are much more common than gastric ulcers. Patients with duodenal ulcers secrete a greater than normal amount of gastric acid and have a greater than normal number of acid-secreting parietal cells in the stomach. (REF. 17-p. 62)

185. E. Diverticulitis is inflammation of a true diverticulum (as congenital Meckel's diverticulum). The inflammation is promoted by the lodging of fecal matter in the sacs which contain all layers of the bowel in its wall. The inflammatory reaction may spread to the surrounding tissue, resulting in peridiverticulitis. The gross appearance of diverticulitis may simulate that of a carcinoma of the colon. (REF. 17-p. 56)

Chapter 5 Oral Histology and Embryology

186. D. There are three distinct population of embryonic cells that arise largely through division and migrations. Migrations create new associations between cells which allow unique possibilities for subsequent development through interactions between the cell populations. (REF. 6-p. 1)

187. A. The union of the ectoderm and endodermal layers produces the buccopharyngeal membrane. At approximately 27 days this membrane ruptures and the stomodeum establishes a connection with the foregut. (REF. 8-p. 24)

188. D. There are six bronchial (visceral) arches, of which the fifth is rudimentary. The proximal portion of the first arch (mandibular) becomes the maxillary process. As the heart recedes caudally, the mandibular and hyoid arches develop at their distal surfaces to consolidate in the ventral midline. (REF. 6-p. 15)

189. E. Upon completion of the crest cell migration and vascularization of the derived mesenchyme, a series of outgrowths or swellings called facial processes initiates the next stages of facial development. The growth and fusion of the upper facial processes produce the primary and secondary palates. (REF. 8-p. 8)

190. D. New growths from the medial edges of the maxillary processes form the shelves of the secondary palate. The palatal shelves grow downward beside the tongue, with the tongue partially filling the nasal cavity. At the eighth gestational week, the shelves elevate, make contact, and fuse with each other above the tongue. (REF. 6-p. 13)

191. D. The tongue forms in the ventral floor of the pharynx after arrival of the hypoglossal muscle cells. The anterior two-thirds of the tongue is covered by ectoderm, whereas endoderm covers the posterior one-third. (REF. 8 - p. 18)

192. C. The salivary gland is formed through the growth of a bud of oral epithelium into the underlying mesenchyme. The primordia of the parotid and submandibular glands of humans appear during the sixth week, and the primordium of the submandibular glands (human) appear after 7 to 8 weeks of fetal life. (REF. 8-p. 361)

193. D. The crest mesenchymal cells of the visceral arches give rise to skeletal components such as the temporary visceral arch cartilages (Meckel's cartilage), middle ear cartilages, and mandibular bones. (REF. 6-p. 18)

194. D. The mandible appears as a bilateral structure in the sixth week of fetal life as a thin plate of bone lateral to, and at some distance from, Meckel's cartilage. The greater part of Meckel's cartilage subsequently disappears without contributing to the formation of the bone of the mandible. A small portion of the cartilage, at a distance from the midline, is the site of endochondral ossification. (REF. 8-p. 243)

195. A. The formation of a band of epithelium that runs along the outline of the future dental arches is called the dental lamina. At the sixth week of embryonic life the oral epithelium consists of a basal cell layer of high cells and a surface layer of flattened cells. It is the primordium of the ectodermal portion of the teeth that is called the dental lamina. (REF. 8-p. 25)

196. D. The bell stage consists of an invagination of the epithelium, which deepens, and the margins continue to grow. The enamel organ thus forms a bell shape. The bell stage consists of the following structures: inner enamel epithelium, stratum intermedium, stellate reticulum, outer enamel epithelium, dental lamina, dental papilla, and dental sac. (REF. 8-p. 33)

197. A. As the tooth bud proliferates, it undergoes unequal growth in the different parts of the bud, leading to the formation of the cap stage. The cap stage consists of a shallow invagination on the deep surface of the tooth bud. The cap stage contains the following structures: outer and inner enamel epithelium, stellate reticulum (enamel pulp), dental papilla, and dental sac. (REF. 8-p. 27)

198. B. Odontoblasts are integral parts of mature dentin and represent highly specialized connective tissue cells that differentiate from the peripheral cellular layer of the dental papilla. The beginning of differentiation of odontoblasts takes place only in the presence of the inner enamel epithelium. (REF. 8-p. 136)

199. C. Before the ameloblasts are fully differentiated and produce enamel, they interact with adjacent mesenchymal cells. The ameloblasts enter their formative stage after the first layer of dentin has been produced. The presence of dentin appears to be necessary for the beginning of enamel matrix formation. (REF. 8-p. 80)

200. A. Two processes are involved in amelogenesis: organic matrix formation and mineralization. The beginning of the mineralization of enamel does not await the completion of the matrix of the enamel. The ameloblasts begin their secretory activity when a small amount of dentin has been laid down. (REF. 8-p. 85)

201. B. The first mineralization of the enamel matrix occurs in the form of crystalline apatite. Chemical analysis reveals that the initial mineralization amounts of 25-30% of the eventual total mineral content. However, the second stage (maturation) is characterized by gradual completion of the mineralization. (REF. 8-p. 46)

202. A. The first sign of predentin development is the appearance of bundles of fibrils between the differentiating odontoblasts. Korff's fibers are a major constituent of the first-formed matrix of the predentin. Korff's fibers occur in a fanlike arrangement and are composed of collagen. (REF. 8-p. 133)

203. B. The cervical loop is located at the border of the wide basal opening of the enamel organ, where the inner enamel epithelium reflects onto the outer enamel epithelium. When the crown of the tooth has been formed, the cells of the cervical loop give rise to Hertwig's epithelial root sheath. (REF. 8-p. 80)

204. B. The enamel organ plays an important role in root development by forming Hertwig's epithelial root sheath, which is responsible for molding the shape of the roots and initiates dentin formation. Hertwig's root sheath consists of the outer and inner enamel epithelia, without a stratum intermedium and stellate reticulum. (REF. 8-p. 37)

205. A. Enamel of deciduous teeth develops partly before and partly after birth. The line or ring between the two portions of enamel in deciduous teeth consists of an incremental line of Retzius or the neonatal line or ring. In the first permanent molars the dentin is formed partly before and partly after birth. The line separating the prenatal from postnatal dentin is an accentuated contour line or neonatal line in dentin. (REF. 8-p. 82, 115)

206. D. Enamel is composed of enamel rod (prisms), rod sheaths, and a cementing interprismatic substance. About 5-12 million enamel rods are present in the lower lateral incisors to the upper first molar respectively. Enamel rods have a clear crystalline appearance so light may pass through the rods. The enamel rods in the cusps are longer than those located at the cervical areas of the teeth. (REF. 8-pp. 48, 56)

207. D. Mineralization of enamel matrix occurs in two stages. With age, the total amount of organic matrix is either believed to increase, to remain unchanged, or to decrease. Localized increases of nitrogen and fluorine have been found in the superficial enamel layers of older teeth, suggesting a continuous uptake from the oral environment during aging. There is evidence demonstrating that enamel becomes harder with age. (REF. 8-pp. 46, 48)

208. C. The dental follicle is reserved for the thin layer of cells that is continuous with the cells of the dental papilla and lies adjacent to the dental organ. The cells of the dental follicle give origin to the fibroblasts of the developing periodontal ligament. Formation of the periodontal ligament occurs after the cells of Hertwig's epthelial root sheath have separated, forming the strands of cells termed the epithelial rests of Malassez. (REF. 8-p. 206)

209. B. Connective tissue fibers present in the periodontal ligament pass between the cementoblasts into the cementum. Their embedded portions are called Sharpey's fibers. Each Sharpey fiber consists of numerous collagen fibrils passing well into the cementum. (REF. 8-pp. 188, 221)

210. B. There are two kinds of cementum: acellular and cel lular. Some layers of cementum do not incorporate cells (cementocytes), whereas other layers contain cementocytes in lacunae. However, cementum as a unit is composed of cementoblasts, cementoid, and fully mineralized cementum. (REF. 8-p. 182)

211. C. The surface of the dentin at the dentinoenamel junction is pitted. Rounded projections of the enamel fit into the depressions, assuring a firm hold of the enamel on the dentin. The dentinoenamel junction is a scalloped line, not a straight one. A hypermineralized zone about 30 micromicrons thick is present at the dentinoenamel junction and is most prominent before mineralization is complete. (REF. 8-p. 18)

212. A. A delicate membrane called Nasmyth's membrane (primary enamel cuticle) covers the entire crown of the newly erupted tooth. The membrane is soon removed by mastication. The latter membrane is a typical basal lamina present in most epithelia. The erupted enamel is

normally covered by a pellicle, formed by precipitation of salivary proteins. The pellicle becomes colonized by microorganisms in a day or two to form the bacterial plaque. (REF. 8-pp. 63, 303)

213. B. Enamel lamellae are thin, leaflike structures that extend from the enamel surface toward the dentinoenamel junction. They may penetrate the dentin. They are composed of organic matter and little mineral content. The enamel lamellae may be predisposing locations for caries, because they contain a high content of organic matter (REF 8-pp. 59, 67)

214. A. The surface of enamel consists of a structureless layer of enamel in 70% of permanent teeth and in all deciduous teeth. The structureless enamel is most often present over the cusp tips and most commonly toward the cervical areas of the enamel surface. No prism outlines are visible in this surface layer, and all apatite crystals are parallel to one another. (REF. 7-p. 118)

215. A. The most effective means for mass control of dental caries to date has been adjusting the fluoride level in communal water supplies to 1 part/million. The mechanism of action of fluoride involves changes in enamel resistance, brought about by incorporation of fluoride during calcification, and alterations in the environment of the teeth, particularly with respect to the oral bacterial flora. (REF. 7-p. 124)

216. D. As dentin calcifies the hydroxyapatite crystals mask the collagen fibers so that they are no longer visible. The odontoblasts are arranged in a layer on the pulpal surface of the dentin, and only their cytoplasmic processes are embedded in the mineralized matrix. (REF. 8-pp. 105, 140)

217. D. The projections of the ameloblasts into the enamel matrix are called Tomes' processes (fibers). The surfaces of the ameloblasts facing the developing enamel therefore are not smooth. There is an interdigitation of the cells and the enamel rods that they produce. Ameloblasts cover maturing enamel. These cells are shorter than the ameloblasts over incompletely formed enamel. (REF. 8-p. 120)

218. B. Dentinal tubules of primary and secondary dentin contain dental lymph (tissue fluid) surrounding the processes of the odontoblasts. (REF. 8-p. 107)

219. H. The imbrication or incremental lines of von Ebner appear as fine lines, which in cross sections run at right angles to the dentinal tubules. These lines correspond to the incremental lines in the enamel and reflect variations in the structure and mineralization that takes place during formation of dentin. (REF. 8-p. 130)

220. F. Neonatal lines in dentin represent a contour line where dentin is partly formed before and partly after birth. This line separates the prenatal from the postnatal dentin. The neonatal line is due to incomplete calcification and abrupt changes in the environment and nutrition that occurs at birth. (REF. 6-p. 123)

221. A. Mineralization of the dentin begins in small globular areas that normally fuse to a uniform calcified layer of dentin. If fusion fails to occur, interglobular dentin results due to unmineralized or hypomineralized regions between the globules. (REF. 8-p. 115)

222. C. The interface between the peritubular and the intertubular dentin stands out very clearly, and this boundary is due to the presence of the sheath of Neumann. (REF. 8-p. 106)

223. D. Acellular cementum occurs in some layers of cementum that do not incorporate cells (spiderlike cementocytes) in lacunae. However, it is better to consider cementum as a living tissue comprised of cells (cementoblasts), cementoid, and mineralized tissue. Acellular cementum covers the root dentin from the cementoenamel junction to the apex. However, it is often missing on the apical one-third of the root. (REF. 8-p. 185)

224. G. Secondary cementum is cellular cementum consisting of collagen fibrils which make up the bulk of the organic portion of this tissue. Cementocytes are incorporated into cellular cementum and are similar to osteocytes. Cellular cementum is more frequently located on the apical half of the root. Cellular cementum is frequently formed on the surface of acellular cementum, but it may comprise the entire thickness of the apical cementum. (REF. 8-p. 196)

225. A. Sharpey's fibers are connective tissue fibers which are embedded in the cementum and serve to attach the tooth to the surrounding bone. They are composed of numerous collagen fibrils that pass well into the cementum. (REF. 2-p. 206)

226. E. Canaliculi are fine extensions or canals that extend from the lacunae of cementum which house the cementocytes. The cytoplasmic processes of the typical cementocyte are present in fine canals (canaliculi) radiating from the cell body. These processes may branch and anastomose with processes of adjacent cells. (REF. 8-p. 208)

227. B. Cementoid tissue can be observed on the surface of cementum lined by cementoblasts. Cementoid is the uncalcified matrix of cementum. As a new layer of cementoid is formed, the old layer calcifies. (REF. 8-p. 202)

Chapter 6 Biochemistry

228. E. Biochemistry is not an isolated biological science. It has become the very language of biology, basic to an understanding of phenomena in the medical sciences. The correlation of biological function and molecular structure is the basis of biochemistry. (REF. 9-p. 1)

229. B. In chemical equilibria, the phenomenon of diffusion demonstrates that the free energy of a solute in solution increases with its concentration. Solutes in a concentrated solution placed in contact with a dilute solution diffuse into the latter until a uniform concentration is achieved. The free-energy change for the dilation by such diffusion must be negative. (REF. 9-p. 13)

230. D. K is the ionization or dissociation constant of the acid. The equation indicates that K is a measure of the strength of the acid. The higher the value of K, the greater is the number of hydrogen ions liberated per mole of acid in solution and, hence, the stronger is the acid. Different acids therefore may be compared in terms of their K values. This equation applies only to activity values. (REF. 9-p. 18)

231. C. According to the Bronsted definition, an acid is a substance, charged or uncharged, that liberates hydrogen ions (H^+) or protons in solution. A base is a substance that can bind protons and remove them from a solution. For example, ammonia, acetate ions, and sulfate ions are bases, whereas ammonium ion, acetic acid, and bisulfate ion are acids. (REF. 9-p. 21)

232. C. Many substances that are weak electrolytes exist in characteristically colored or colorless forms in different pH regions. These are useful as indicators of the pH of a solution. The indicator is a weak electrolyte and may be written as the acid HIn, which can exist in two chromogenic forms (color A and color B). At any pH, In^-/HIn will give color B/color A. The mixture of color A and color B permits a visual comparison with color standards and, hence, a rapid determination of pH. (REF. 9-p. 40)

233. A. Buffered solutions resist the changes in hydrogen ions that otherwise would result from the addition of an acid or base. Buffer action is exhibited by ions of weak acids or bases. Strong acids and bases are almost completely dissociated in water and have no reservoir of undissociated acid or base. (REF. 9-p. 35)

234. B. The best buffer action is exhibited by a mixture of a weak acid and its salt. Salts are completely dissociated. Weak acids and bases exert their buffer action from pH 2 to pH 12, and this buffering capacity represents an important means of maintaining constant pH. (REF. 9-p. 44)

235. C. L are protein molecules which do not pass through semipermeable membranes. However, water and low molecular weight solutes readily pass through. Most biological membranes are impermeable to proteins but allow small molecules and water to pass through freely. Osmotic pressure is the force required to oppose the osmotic flow (which occurs when a semipermeable membrane separates a protein solution from pure water). Water flows until its concentration on both sides of the membrane is equal. (REF. 9-p. 71)

236. C. The effect of temperature on an equilibrium constant for a chemical reaction is given by the van't Hoff equation. This equation describes the data for ordinary chemical

reactions in a satisfactory manner. Increased temperatures favor the formation of active molecules (those with sufficient energy of activation to react). (REF. 9-p. 73)

237. D. The viscosity of a solution depends on the molecular weight and shape of the solute molecules at a given solute concentration. Highly asymmetrical molecules show a high intrinsic viscosity as compared with spherical molecules of the same molecular weight. (REF. 9-p. 108)

238. E. Numerous factors regulate the rates of fatty acid synthesis, the conversion of excess carbohydrate to fatty acids, and the storage of lipid. The initial entry of glucose (dietary carbohydrate) into the cells is dependent upon the action of insulin which controls the availability of excess carbohydrate for glycogen synthesis. A key enzyme for regulating the rates of fatty acid degradation and synthesis is isocitrate dehydrogenase of the citric acid cycle. (REF. 9-p. 123)

239. E. Fatty acids are abundant in either ester or amide linkage in several classes of compounds (lipids containing glycerol, lipids not containing glycerol, lipids combined with other classes of compounds, and fatty acids). Saturated fatty acids occur naturally. The fatty acids dissociate in aqueous solution. The mixture of fatty acids obtained by hydrolysis of lipids derived generally contains both saturated and unsaturated fatty acids. The most abundant saturated fatty acid is palmitic, with stearic second in amount. (REF. 9-p. 126)

240. E. Oleic acid is the most widely distributed and most abundant fatty acid in nature. Fatty acids containing more than one double bond also are commonly found and are said to be in conjugation. The fatty acids most frequently found in mammalian biochemistry showing multiple unsaturation are linoleic acid (containing two double bonds) and linolenic acid (containing three double bonds). (REF. 9-p. 134)

241. E. Fats are insoluble in water but soluble in nonpolar solvents. Saturation plus increasing chain length tends to result in elevation of the melting point. Vegetable fats or oils exhibit diversity in their fatty acid composition and in regard to both chain length and degree of unsatura-

tion of the constitutent fatty acids. Many are liquids at room temperature. Hydrolysis of neutral fats yields three molecules of fatty acid and one of glycerol. (REF. 9-p. 138)

242. A. The name "wax" is given to a naturally occurring fatty acid ester of any alcohol other than glycerol. The principal lipid of many marine plankton organisms, one of the food sources of the ocean, is classified as a wax. (REF. 9-p. 137)

243. E. Glycerol ether derivates of lecithin (phosphatidylcholine) are widely distributed in animal tissues. The glycerol ether derivatives occur in erythrocytes and bone marrow. (Ref. 9-p. 148)

244. A. Sphingomyelins are found primarily in nervous tissue but are also present as lipids of the blood. Brain sphingomyelin contains polyunsaturated sphingosines (dehydrosphingosines). (REF. 9-p. 152)

245. D. Glycosphingolipids (gangliosides) are found in nerve and certain selected tissues, such as the spleen. Their structure is related to that of cerebrosides since gangliosides contain a ceramide linked to carbohydrate (containing several additional moles of carbohydrates). (REF. 9-p. 158)

246. E. Cholesterol occurs in all samples of animal lipid, blood, and bile. In the blood two-thirds of the cholesterol is esterified, chiefly to unsaturated fatty acids. The remainder occurs as free alcohol. (REF. 9-p. 161)

247. E. Alterations in the level of blood cholesterol have been noted in response to changes in the degree of saturation of dietary fatty acids. The more saturated the fatty acids of the diet, the higher the serum cholesterol concentration. The reason for the latter is obscure. Cholesterol synthesis and degradation are influenced by a number of hormones. The formation of cholesterol calculi occurs in the biliary tract. The pathological deposition of cholesterol-containing plaques in the intima of the aorta is the characteristic lesion of atheromatosis present during arteriosclerosis. (REF. 9-p. 162)

248. E. Dietary carbohydrate provides the raw material for synthesis of a great variety of organic compounds in mammalians: steroids, amino acids, purines, pyrimidines, complex lipids, and polysaccharides. Glucose has one principal fate: phosphorylation to glucose-6-phosphate. The consecutive reactions are a pathway, e. g., glucose-6-phosphate via pathways 8, 9, 10, 12, 13, and 14 to lactate. All pathways proceed with a loss of free energy. The major form of utilizable energy in all cells is ATP. Cells generally cannot store either glucose or glucose-6-phosphate. The major storage form of energy is in the fatty acids of neutral triacylglycerols. (REF. 9-p. 173)

249. E. All cells that can metabolize glucose contain some form of a hexokinase (MW/52, 000) constructed of two nonidentical polypeptide chains. D-glucose exists in more than one modification resulting from the specific rotation of a freshly prepared glucose solution that changed under observation in the polarimeter. (REF. 9-p. 174)

250. C. Monosaccharides containing four carbon atoms are termed tetroses, five carbon atoms are pentoses, six carbon atoms are hexoses, and seven carbon atoms are heptoses. Derived monosaccharides include compounds structurally very similar to monosaccharides but deviating from the aldoses and ketoses. (REF. 9-p. 175)

251. C. Oligosaccharides yield, on hydrolysis, per molecule, 2-10 monosaccharide residues. Most naturally occuring oligosaccharides occur in plant (as opposed to animal) sources. (REF. 9-p. 227)

252. D. Sucrose is the common sugar of the home and restaurant. Maltose is the most common sugar that on hydrolysis yields two identical fragments. Maltose is the major product of the enzymic hydrolysis of starch. Lactose of mammalian origin is found in milk in about a 5% concentration. Upon hydrolysis lactose yields an equimolar mixture of galactose and glucose. Lactose is a reducing sugar and reacts with carbonyl reagents. (REF. 9-p. 227)

253. E. Polysaccharides are carbohydrates that exist in nature in the form of molecules of high molecular weight, which on hydrolysis yield chiefly monosaccharides or products related to monosaccharides (D-glucose). Various poly-

saccharides differ from one another not only in constituent monosaccharide composition but also in molecular weight and other structural features. Some polysaccharides are linear polymers, while others are highly branched. (REF. 9-p. 235)

254. C. Dextrin is a polysaccharide fragment that remains after incomplete hydrolysis of amylopectin. Dextrin is the limit of attack of alpha, 1, 4-glucan maltohydrolase upon amylopectin, and thus is termed a limit dextrin. (REF. 9-p. 241)

255. E. Cellulose is the most abundant organic compound in the world, constituting 50% or more of all the carbon in vegetation. It is predominantly a plant polysaccharide but is present in certain tunicates. The purest source is cotton, which contains at least 90% cellulose. On complete hydrolysis cellulose yields the disaccharide cellobiose. (REF. 9-p. 245)

256. E. Heparin is a saccharide containing glycosyl bonds present in the blood in metachromatic granules of mast cells of the tissues. Heparin prevents the coagulation of blood plasma. Heparin has a molecular weight of 17,000 and has been isolated from lung and liver as the crystalline barium salt. The repeated sulfate polymer structure of heparin is apparently responsible for its biological activity. Heparin acts in vivo as well as in vitro to prolong the clotting time of blood by interfering with the conversion of prothrombin to thrombin. Heparin does not act alone since it has no influence on purified prothrombin. Therefore, a serum protein cofactor is necessary for heparin action. Heparin inhibits activation of the Christmas factor by activated Factor XI. Heparin also inhibits the activation effect of antihemophilic factor with the activated Christmas factor. (REF. 9-p. 251)

257. E. Proteins have molecular weights ranging from 5000 to millions. Each protein is a macromolecule with repeating units consisting of amino acids. Twenty of the amino acids are commonly present in proteins and are linked together by peptide bonds. A protein molecule consists of one or more polypeptide chains. Each chain is composed of approximately 20 to several hundred amino acid residues. (REF. 9-p. 262)

258. E. The same 20 amino acids have been found in the proteins of all species of microorganisms, plants, and animals. Amino acids that have been isolated from protein hydrolysates are generally primary alpha amino acids, i.e., the carboxyl and amino groups are attached to the same carbon atom. (REF. 9-p. 270)

259. B. Albumins are readily soluble in water and coagulable by heat. The albumins represent a large group, of which egg albumin and serum albumin are examples. (REF. 9-p. 298)

260. A. Globulins are insoluble or sparingly soluble in water However, their solubility is increased by adding neutral salts such as sodium chloride. Globulins are coagulable by heat. Many globulins are prepared from animal or plant tissues, being readily extracted by salt solutions (as 5-10% sodium chloride) and are precipitated from the salt solution by dilution with water. Examples are serum globulins, globulins of muscle and other tissues, and globulins of plant seeds. (REF. 9-p. 298)

261. E. Myoglobin is a respiratory pigment present intracellularly in mammalian muscle. It has a molecular weight of 17,000, has one atom of iron per molecule of myoglobin, has an hyperbolic dissociation curve, and lacks the Bohr effect. (REF. 9-p. 317)

262. E. Hemoglobins (mammalian) have a molecular weight of approximately 65,000 and are tetramers of four peptide chains, to each of which is bound a heme. Hemoglobin molecules are constructed by combining two alpha chains with two beta, gamma, or delta chains. Normal adult hemoglobin, Hb/A, contains two alpha and two beta chains. (REF. 9-p. 317)

263. E. Collagen is the major protein of connective tissue. Collagens are insoluble in water and resistant to animal digestive enzymes. However, they are altered to easily digestible, soluble gelatins by boiling in water, dilute acids, or alkalies. Approximately 30% of the total protein in the mammalian body is collagen. Collagens contain a high content of hydroxyprolines. They also contain hydroxylysine. (REF. 9-p. 321)

264. E. Nucleic acids are linear polymeric molecules that are the hereditary determinants of living organisms. Nucleic acids also are naturally occurring, associated with proteins (as nucleoproteins). Nucleic acids contain approximately 15-16% nitrogen and 9-10% phosphorus. Complete hydrolysis of a nucleic acid yields a mixture of substances called purines and pyrimidines, ribose or deoxyribose sugars, and phosphoric acid. (REF. 9-p. 356)

265. B. Enzymes are natural catalysts. They are responsible for the great rapidity of biochemical reactions. Enzymes are universally present in living organisms. All physiological functions (i. e., muscular contraction, nerve conduction, excretion by the kidney, as well as life itself) are all linked to the activity of enzymes. Muscular contraction is complex and involves a series of enzyme-catalyzed reactions associated with energy. (REF. 9-p. 419)

266. B. Saliva is primarily secreted by three pairs of salivary glands. The parotid gland (all serous type cells) and the submaxillary and sublingual glands (mixed type cells) produce the saliva. Parotid saliva is nonviscous in nature, whereas sublingual and submaxillary saliva are viscous due to their mucoprotein content. At low rates of secretion, saliva is markedly hypotonic, whereas at maximum secretory rates the saliva is almost isotonic. (REF. 9-p. 494)

267. E. Secretions enter the stomach from ducts of 10-30 million gastric glands. These glands are composed of chief cells and parietal cells. The parietal cells are not present in the glands of the pyloric or cardiac portions of the stomach or in the lumen of the gland. Chief cells secrete pepsinogen. The parietal cells secrete a solution of 0. 16 M HCl and 0. 007 M KCl, with traces of other electrolytes and little or no organic material. (REF. 9-p. 497)

268. E. The hydrogen ion concentration of gastric juice is 10^6 times greater than that of plasma. Secretion of 1 liter of gastric juice requires the expenditure of at least 1500 calories if the process were 100% efficient (assuming plasma to be the source of hydrogen ions, potassium ions, and chloride ions). (REF. 9-p. 499)

269. B. The daily volume of pancreatic secretion in human adults is 500-800 ml/day. Pancreatic secretion contains the following proteins of importance to the digestive process: trypsinogen, chymotrypsinogen, proelastase, and procarboxypeptidases. Secretion of pancreatic juice is under both neural and hormonal control. (REF. 9-p. 505)

270. E. Bile is elaborated by polygonal cells of the liver passing through bile canaliculi and hepatic and cystic ducts to reach the gall bladder. Bile is stored in the gall bladder and concentrated there, entering the intestines through the common bile duct. Cholecystokinin is released into the circulation by the duodenum and is responsible for stimulating contraction of the gall bladder, with release of its contents into the duodenum. (REF. 9-p. 509)

271. D. Porphyrin contains four pyrrole-like rings linked by four CH groups or bridges in an alternating double-bond, resonating ring system. The porphyrins are all weak bases because of the tertiary nitrogens in the two pyrrolene nuclei in each porphyrin. The most striking physical property of the porphyrins is their color. Solutions of porphyrins in organic solvents exhibit a strong red fluorescence when illuminated with ultraviolet light. (REF. 9-p. 518)

272. E. The blood volume in the vascular system is approximately 8% of the body weight. The solutes of the blood plasma consist of approximately 10% of the volume; proteins, 7%; inorganic salts, 0. 9%; plus organic compounds other than protein. The quantity of any particular blood component is the result of the rate of addition of the component to the blood and the rate of utilization or removal of the substance from the blood by various tissues. The total protein content of the plasma is 5. 7-8. 0 g/100 ml. (REF. 9-p. 554)

Chapter 7 Nutrition

273. B. Dietary counseling should be considered in terms of who, what, when, how, and why. Dietary counseling is an integral part of preventive and therapeutic dentistry. Nutrition interviews are concerned with the patient's present food intake and food habits. (REF. 10-p. 9)

274. E. The caloric requirement consists of the following factors: amount of energy required to maintain the organism in its minimal state; amount of energy required for the specific dynamic action of foods; and energy required for growth, repair, and physical activity. (REF. 10-p. 22)

275. E. Carbohydrates may be classified in terms of the number of saccharide units of which it is composed: monosaccharide (cannot be broken down to simpler sugars by acid hydrolysis), disaccharides (formed by condensation of two monosaccharides), and polysaccharides (polymers of many monosaccharides). (REF. 10-p. 25)

276. B. Glucose is the only hexose known to exist in free form in the fasting human. Most glucose is present in a combined form and is found in nearly all foods. (REF. 10-p. 25)

277. C. Starch is the energy stored up in most plants and seeds. Upon digestion, starch is broken down to form maltose and glucose ultimately. Glycogen is the animal equivalent of starch. (REF. 10-p. 32)

278. D. W. D. Miller (1890) established that carbohydrate substrate was necessary for oral bacterial action and that anaerobic glycolysis by microorganisms provided the acids which decalcify the mineral portions of teeth. The only available substrates from which acids can be formed in the mouth are carbohydrates (sucrose and glucose). (REF. 10-p. 35)

279. E. Lipids constitute a heterogeneous group of compounds that have the following characteristics: are insoluble in water but soluble in organic solvents; contain or combined with one or more fatty acids; and include only compounds utilizable by or occurring in biological systems. (REF. 10-p. 39)

280. D. Proteins are large, complex, colloidal molecules formed from simple units (amino acids). Amino acids have an NH_2 group and a carboxyl group (COOH) attached to the same carbon atom. The rest of the molecule varies with the specific amino acid. Proteins contain nitrogen and various combinations of other elements (sulfur, phosphorus, iron, iodine, copper, manganese, and zinc) in addition to carbon, hydrogen, and oxygen. (REF. 10-p. 48)

281. B. Animals have limited powers of converting one amino acid into another; they must obtain some of the amino acids they require from the diet. These are called essential amino acids. A dietary supply of eight amino acids is essential to humans. They include lysin, tryptophan, phenylalanine, leucine, isoleucine, threonine, methionine, and valine. (REF. 10-p. 49)

282. E. About 99% of body calcium is present in bones and teeth and 1% in the soft tissues and body fluids. Readily mobilized calcium is present in bone trabeculae to be called upon in times of stress (as lactation). Little if any calcium is lost from molars when the diet is low in calcium. (REF. 10-p. 68)

283. C. Iron deficiency anemia is found in 12% of females and 5% of males over age 65. It can be prevented or corrected by the adequate intake of liver, red meats, and green vegetables (such as brussel sprouts, cabbage, peas, beans, and lentils). (REF. 10-p. 92)

284. C. An increase in recrystallization of apatite occurs in the presence of fluoride. As little as 0. 2 parts/million fluoride significantly increased the rate of precipitation of hydroxyapatite from supersaturated solutions of calcium and phosphate in the pH range of 6. 2 to 7. 4. (REF. 10-p. 114)

285. B. Fluorosis is seen only at fluoride concentrations exceeding 1. 5 parts/million. When the drinking water contains 1 part/million fluoride or less, the index of dental fluorosis is normal to questionable. Dental fluorosis develops pre-eruptively since the calcification of teeth is generally completed prior to tooth eruption. (REF. 10-p. 122)

286. D. An understanding of the metabolic functions of the fat-soluble vitamins (A, D, E, and K) is fragmentary. Natural and synthetic sources of all of the fat-soluble vitamins are universally available. (REF. 10-p. 125)

287. B. Vitamin A deficiency individuals are prone to infection. Vitamin A does not affect pathogens or the immune response. Vitamin A maintains the integrity of the mucous membranes; thus it can be considered to play a protective role against infection. (REF. 10-p. 128)

288. A. The pathology of vitamin D deficiency is related directly to its effect on bone formation. Vitamin D affects calcium absorption from the gastrointestinal tract and likewise on phosphorus absorption. (REF. 10-p. 136)

289. D. Vitamin K is found in green vegetables. Vitamin K deficiency causes a defect in blood coagulation. The plasma of vitamin-deficient animals shows a deficiency in the amount of prothrombin and several factors needed for its conversion to thrombin. (REF. 10-p. 141)

290. A. Ariboflavinosis also involves the eyes, skin, and tongue in addition to the lip lesions. Ocular alterations include conjunctivitis, blepharitis, photophobia, lacrimation, burning and itching of the eyes, changes in pigmentation of the iris, and visual disturbances. (REF. 10-p. 150)

291. B. Pernicious anemia is characterized by a slick, denuded tongue demonstrating striking atrophy of the lingual papillae and discoloration of the tongue. Vitamin B_{12} therapy produces regrowth of the lingual papillae and disappearance of the abnormal color of the tongue in 2 to 3 weeks. (REF. 10-p. 158)

292. E. Ascorbic acid (vitamin C) plays a direct role at the site of collagen synthesis rather then indirectly through some type of systemic effect. Scurvy arises as a result of continued deficiency in the diet of vitamin C (common in vegetable and citrus fruits). Humans are unable to synthesize L-ascorbic acid. An enlargement of the marginal gingiva, enveloping the crowns of the teeth, is an oral manifestation of scurvy. (REF. 10-p. 179)

293 E. About 15 mineral elements are required in the metabolism of the body. Calcium and iron are the two most important minerals from the latter group of mineral elements. Iron intake is important during the growth period of children and during the reproductive period of the adult female. Calcium utilization and body requirements are influenced by previous levels of calcium intake. (REF. 10-p. 192)

294. D. Older persons differ from the adult or young and middle-aged person in their caloric requirements, which are are 10-20% lower. The older person should reduce caloric

intake. Sweets and desserts very often furnish 20% of the day's calories. Some senior citizens fail to eat enough green and yellow vegetables and milk. (REF. 10-p. 205)

295. C. The caloric allowances for infants and children of both sexes should be provided to the individual child after observation of growth rate, appetite, and body build. The amount of calories for boys and girls differs after the age of 9. (REF. 10-p. 203)

296. D. Adolescents or teenagers have special psychological characteristics with regard to nutrition. The latter are at an age of self-concern and want one to be interested in them, not their problems. Adolescents are the great imitators who live for the moment and want quick results. (REF. 10-p. 203)

297. B. Fad diets are especially dangerous to young women since they improverish the reserve which is called upon during physical stress in the reproductive period. (REF. 10-p. 203)

298. D. During pregnancy the need for protein, minerals (calcium), and the vitamins is increased. Caloric requirements may be 10-20% greater than for the nonpregnant woman. Any basic increase in the need for calories is generally offset by a decrease in activity. A gain of 15-20 pounds is acceptable during pregnancy. (REF. 10-p. 204)

299. D. During the period of lactation, the amount of output of milk in a single month is greater than the increased mass of the whole 9 months of pregnancy. A mother who nurses and produces 850 cc milk a day requires 1000 additional calories in order to produce this milk. (REF. 10-p. 205)

300. E. Vitamin A, ascorbic acid, and folic acid are more sensitive than minerals, amino acids, and niacin with regard to their stability. Some nutrients are destroyed simply by processing because they are sensitive to acids or alkalies. Some nutrients are sensitive to oxygen and others to light. (REF. 10-p. 213)

301. E. Chronic vitamin A deficiency is associated with night blindness. The cells (cones and rods) of the retina contain several proteins conjugated with vitamin A aldehyde. Rhodopsin (visual purple) is found in the cones and is the main photosensitive material in the rods, being responsible for vision in dim light. (REF. 10-p. 243)

302. C. The most important nutrient to the surgical patient is protein. Protein supplies the amino acids required for the growth and repair of tissues, for the transport of lipids, and for the maintenance of blood volume, serum protein, and total circulating blood cell mass. (REF. 10-p. 243)

303. B. Decreased appetite and decreased tolerance for food are the consequences of infection. The ingestion of protein and other nutrients may be decreased at the moment when metabolic losses are increased. Changes in the diet to less solid and more liquid food are common therapeutic measures which depreciate the nutritional value of the diet during infection. (REF. 10-p. 249)

304. C. Obesity is a state of excessive fatness. The diagnosis of obesity may be easy or require body densitometry. Unless the causal factors which initated and maintain the obese state are identified and corrected or the faulty diet patterns of the individual are permanently corrected by appropriate dietary counseling, weight loss will be transient. (REF. 10-p. 253)

305. D. The dentist may aid in the initial diagnosis of Cushing's syndrome, hypothalamic brain tumor, and insulinoma by observing obesity and referring the patient to an internist. Obesity is generally not diagnostic by itself. However, it may be suggestive of possible Cushing's syndrome and others and be responsible for medical referrals. (REF. 10-p. 254)

306. C. Virtual elimination of galactose from the diet can be effectively accomplished by the use of milk substitutes and will prevent all of the sequelae of this severe condition. No special dietary need for galactose exists since ll of this hexose (galactose) necessary for galactolipid formation in the central nervous system can be synthesized from glucose. (REF. 10-p. 269)

307. B. Alveolar bone is altered by hydrocortisone administration, low protein diets, and other dietary regimens producing marked bone loss in the alveolar process of the jaws. Alveolar bone is richer in alkaline phosphatase activity than other bone tissue as well as in ability to incorporate various bone-seeking isotopes. (REF. 10-p. 283)

308. A. Dentin contains about 3.5% nitrogen; all of it is present in the collagen. About 18% of the dentin is collagen, assuming that 95% of the protein present is collagen. The collagen of dentin is similar to that of skin and bone in the proportion of amino acid present and also by the finding that on heating it liquifies to form gelatin. (REF. 10-p. 285)

309. A. The purpose of cementum is to furnish the attachment for fibers of the periodontal membrane. The pulpless tooth has a vital cementum for the attachment of periodontal fibers. (REF. 10-p. 285)

310. A. More fluoride concentrates in the ash of bone compared to the ash of enamel and dentin. Dentin contains higher concentrations of magnesium than bone and enamel. Carbonate content is highest in bone and lowest in enamel. (REF. 10-p. 286)

311. B. Calculus from salivary glands is made up of calcium and phosphorus in a weight ratio of 1.97. Because of the high ash and calcium concentration, the salivary calculi are expected to accumulate high quantities of fluoride. (REF. 10-p. 289)

312. E. Saliva contains bacteria and cellular debris from the oral mucosa and gingiva. Resting saliva is saliva obtained under minimal stimulation. Saliva is secreted at the rate of 1.0-1.5 liters/day. (REF. 10-p. 312)

313. B. Fluorides ingested at optimal levels are by far the most effective caries-inhibiting nutrient discovered for humans. Since fluoride deposition is dependent on the period of time that fluoridated water is consumed, the resistance to dental caries is based on lifelong continuous fluoride exposure, prenatal fluoride exposure, postnatal fluoride exposure, and posteruptive fluoride exposure.

About 1 part/million fluoride in the water supply represents the optimal level for caries inhibition. (REF. 10-p. 333)

314. C. Fluoride may be acquired by dissolution of calcium and phosphorus and reprecipitation with extraneous fluoride, or fluoride derived from dissolved material (fluorapatite). The latter process is vital during the incipient carious lesion. Complete saturation of enamel with fluoride does not take place in vivo. Fluoride is confined to the surface of the crystals and does not involve the body of the crystal. (REF. 10-p. 341)

Chapter 8 Dental Anatomy

315. B. The temporomandibular joint (TMJ) is the articulation of the condyloid process of the mandible and the interarticular disk with the mandibular fossa of the temporal bone. The TMJ has received more attention and study than any other joint in the human body. The pathology of the TMJ (i. e., functional disorders) has led to focusing attention on the extrinsic influences that are involved in these movements. (REF. 11-p. 147)

316. C. The glenoid fossa is located anteriorly and inferiorly to the auditory meatus. The bony roof of this glenoid fossa is thin, and this indicates that the surface is not an articulating one. (REF. 11-p. 23)

317. B. The articular disc is a flat, circular or approximately circular, dense, fibrous connective tissue plate. Islands of cartilage and fibrocartilage occur in the disc in the older age groups. The disc varies in thickness from its thickest posterior to thinnest center portion to thicker anterior portion. The superior surface of the disc is concave, and the inferior surface is concave (a biconcave structure). (REF. 11-p. 147)

318. B. The articular capsule is a loose, thin sack of fibrous connective tissue attached to the border of the articulating surface of the temporal bone and to the neck of the condylar process. It is attached to the skull as follows: to the posterior end of the zygomatic process, the anterior margin of the articular process, the medial edge of the mandibular fossa, and the posterior edge of the mandibular fossa anterior to the petrotympanic fissure. (REF. 11-p. 151)

319. D. The sphenomandibular ligament arises from the angular spine of the sphenoid bone and inserts into the mandibular ligament just superior to the mandibular foramen. The stylomandibular ligament extends from the styloid process and stylohyoid ligament to the region of the mandibular angle. (REF. 11-pp. 151, 152)

320. D. Mandibular movements differ in nature from the movements of any other joint in the skeleton. The presence of the articular disc allows two types of movement, diarthrodial (sliding) and ginglymus (hinge). Thus the TMJ is a diarthrodial ginglymus joint. (REF. 11-p. 159)

321. C. The term centric is an adjective, and it should be used in conjunction with nouns (e.g., centric position, centric jaw relation, or centric occlusion. (REF. 11-p. 164)

322. A. The muscles that are important in dentistry are skeletal muscles (from their site of origin or attachment), striated muscles (from their morphology), and voluntary muscles (controlled by the will). Skeletal muscles are controlled by the central nervous system and do not have automatic action. (REF. 11-p. 164)

323. E. The muscles of mastication generally have their origins and insertions in bone. One exception is the uppermost fibers of the upper head of the external pterygoid, which inserts into the mandibular articular capsule and indirectly into the anterior border of the articular disc. (REF. 11-pp. 120, 164)

324. D. An interesting phenomenon of muscles is their power to undergo contracture. When a muscle length becomes shortened, the fibers of the elevator muscles shorten and reestablish new muscle lengths approximately equal to the maximum length of the lever system itself. The latter reestablishes optimum force of contracture by the muscle. (REF. 11-p. 164)

325. D. The parotid duct empties through Stensen's duct with its orifice in the cheek. The parotid glands secrete only serous (thin and watery) secretion containing the enzyme ptyalin for the digestion of starch. However, saliva is primarily a lubricating and protective agent. (REF. 11-p. 192)

326. B. The oral mucosa is the soft tissue of the mouth supporting dentures in the edentulous patient. The oral mucosa in the edentulous individual does not have the same resiliency as the oral mucosa of individuals with a full dentition. An uneven displacement of the soft tissues takes place in the edentulous individual and must be taken into consideration in the construction of dentures. (REF. 11-pp. 179, 197)

327. A. The mucosa of the soft palate is a transitional tissue between the fixed and loosely attached tissues. Some soft palates provide a very desirable posterior palatal seal, whereas others do not. A cushion type of soft palate can be displaced rather easily. However, the soft palate will return to a normal position once the displacing forces are withdrawn. (REF. 11-p. 181)

328. E. The muscles of mastication are the masseter, temporalis, internal pterygoid, and external pterygoid, and all have their origins from the bones of the skull and are attached to the mandible. These muscles provide both masticatory movements of the mandible and nonmasticatory functions. The muscles of mastication are extremely powerful muscles. (REF. 12-p. 47)

329. B. The horizontal plates of the palatine bones articulate with the posterior rough border of the horizontal palatal processes of the maxillae. The posterior border of the horizontal plates of the palatine bones unite at the midline to form a sharp spine (posterior nasal spine). Processes of the maxillary bone arise as horizontal plates from the body of the maxilla. The two horizontal plates unite in the midline to form a suture, the midpalatal suture. The palatal torus (hyperplasia of bone) may be seen on the palatine processes as on exostosis. (REF. 12-p. 29)

330. A. The mental foramen occupies a more superior position if the loss of the residual ridge is extensive. The denture base must be relieved over the foramen since the force of the denture base may occlude some blood vessels and cause irritation to the mental nerve passing out of the foramen. (REF. 11-p. 47)

331. E. The mylohyoid line is an irregular, rough, bony crest extending from the third molar region to the lower border of the mandible in the region of the chin. (REF. 11-pp. 120, 164)

332. B. If a muscle contracts slowly or if rapid contraction occurs, the efficiency to accomplish work is decreased. Maximum efficiency is developed when the velocity of contraction is about 30% of maximum. The source of the energy for muscle contraction is adenosine triphosphate. (REF. 11-p. 130)

333. D. The incisive glands empty through individual ducts at their incisive location. The salivary glands are stimulated by the parasympathetic nervous system. (REF. 11-p. 191)

334. H. Labial salivary glands are small accessory glands siutated in the labial mucosa. (REF. 11-p. 196)

335. F. Submandibular glands are located in the submandibular fovea. (REF. 11-p. 196)

336. B. Buccal glands are small accessory glands located in the buccal mucosa. (REF. 11-p. 196)

337. A. The parotid gland is controlled principally by the inferior salivary nuclei, which sends impulses to the glands. (REF. 11-p. 192)

338. C. Sublingual glands empty along the sublingual fold in the floor of the mouth. (REF. 11-p. 196)

339. G. The infraorbital nerve block anesthesizes the following nerves: the infraorbital, anterior, and middle superior alveolar nerves and the inferior palpebral, lateral nasal, and superior labial nerves. (REF. 11-p. 354)

340. D. The maxillary nerve (sensory nerve) is the second division of the trigeminal nerve. It arises between the ophthalmic above and the mandibular nerve below. It begins at the middle of the semilunar ganglion as a flat band and passes forward, leaving the skull via the foramen rotundum. (REF. 11-p. 423)

341. H. The frontal nerve is the largest of the three branches of the ophthalmic division which arises from the semilunar ganglion. It enters the orbit via the superior orbital fissure and passes between the orbital periosteum and the levator palpebrae superioris muscle. (REF. 11-p. 351)

342. A. The trigeminal nerve has both sensory and motor fibers. Three large nerves arise from the semilunar ganglion, i. e., the ophthalmic nerve, the maxillary nerve, and the mandibular nerve. The motor root of the trigeminal nerve consists of fibers originating in the motor nucleus of the upper pons. (REF. 11-p. 359)

343. C. There are three branches of the semilunar ganglion. As the ophthalmic division passes forward from the cavernous sinus, it divides into the lacrimal, frontal, and nasociliary branches (nerves). (REF. 11-p. 359)

344. B. The lacrimal nerve is the smallest of the three branches of the ophthalmic division. It passes into the orbit at the lateral angle of the superior orbital fissure, below and lateral to the frontal nerve of the ophthalmic division. (REF. 11-p. 351)

345. B. The degree to which the lymphatic vessels provide nourishment and drainage of the lips, tongue, and soft and hard palates is not completely known. (REF. 11-p. 341)

346. D. The degree to which the lymph vessels contribute to draining the dental pulp is somewhat obscure. (REF. 11-p. 342)

347. B. The trigeminal nerve is the largest of the cranial nerves. It has both sensory and motor fibers and is involved in conveying afferent fibers from stretch receptors in the muscles of mastication. Visceral afferent fibers are present that innervate the muscles of mastication, the tensor tympani, and the tensor veli palatini muscles, eye muscles, and facial muscles. (REF. 11-p. 349)

348. B. The ophthalmic nerve is the first division of the trigeminal nerve. It is a sensory nerve and the smallest of the three divisions of the trigeminal nerve. The ophthalmic nerve originates from the semilunar ganglion, passes forward, and enters the orbit through the superior orbital fissure. (REF. 11-p. 351)

349. B. The mesencephalic nucleus of the trigeminal nerve is an encapsulated mass of gray matter which lies outside of the central nervous system. This nucleus serves the function of an afferent station that supports proprioceptive impulses from the temporomandibular joint. (REF. 11-p. 349)

350. B. The ophthalmic division of the trigeminal nerve passes forward from the cavernous sinus and divides into the following branches: lacrimal, frontal, and nasociliary nerves. The three branches of the ophthalmic division are located in the cranial cavity just before they enter the orbit through the superior orbital fissure. (REF. 11-p. 351)

351. C. The maxillary nerve is the second division of the trigeminal nerve. It is an entirely sensory nerve that arises between the ophthalmic nerve above and mandibular nerve below. It passes subdurally to the foramen rotundum of the great wing of the sphenoid bone. It traverses the pterygopalatine fossa, giving off branches to the sphenopalatine ganglion, the posterior alveolar nerve, and the zygomatic branches. It then enters the inferior orbital fissure to pass into the orbital cavity and through the infraorbital foramen, where it divides into its terminal branches. (REF. 11-p. 354)

352. D. The infraorbital nerve, a branch of the maxillary division of the trigeminal nerve, is located in the infraorbital groove and canal. From the infraorbital canal, several of the fibers separate from the infraorbital nerve and descend to form the middle superior alveolar nerve and the anterior superior alveolar nerve. The superior dental plexus is formed in the bony alveolar canals by the three superior alveolar nerves. (REF. 11-p. 357)

353. D. The mandibular division is the first division of the trigeminal nerve. It has both sensory and motor fibers. The motor division fails to arise from the Gasserian ganglion but joins the sensory branch after the latter leaves the Gasserian ganglion. The anterior division gives rise to the following branches: external pterygoid nerve (motor branch), masseter nerve (motor branch), temporalis muscle nerve (motor branch), and long buccal nerve (sensory branch). The posterior division gives rise to the auriculotemporal nerve and the lingual nerve. (REF. 11-p. 349)

354. D. The long buccal nerve is a sensory nerve that passes downward, anteriorly, and laterally between the heads of the external pterygoid muscle. It divides into terminal branches that supply the mucosa of the cheek, the skin of the cheek, the retromolar triangle region, the molar buccal gingiva, and the mucosa in the lower part of the buccal vestibule. (REF. 11-p. 362)

355. E. The inferior alveolar nerve is the largest branch of the posterior division of the mandibular branch of the trigeminal nerve. Within the mandible the inferior alveolar nerve descends in the alveolar canal and gives off branches throughout the body of the mandible. It gives off branches to the mandibular teeth in the form of apical fibers that enter the apical foramina of the mandibular teeth. (REF. 11-pp. 364, 365)

PART II

CLINICAL DENTAL SCIENCES

Chapter 9 Oral Diagnosis and Treatment Planning

356. C. Oral diagnosis is the ability of a dental clinician to detect or note the presence of an abnormality in the oral and maxillofacial regions plus the ability of the clinician to recognize or identify a specific oral abnormality and to know the nature of the pathologic process. (REF. 13 -p. 1)

357. D. To be successful in oral diagnosis, the dental clinician must not only be acquainted with the oral signs of a disease, but with related facets such as the causes, pathogenesis, roentgenologic, and histopathologic findings. The ultimate basis of an oral diagnosis is to suggest and provide an accurate basis for the plan of treatment. (REF. 13 - p. 1)

358. A. Laboratory tests are an adjunct to diagnosis. They are of value only when the dental clinician knows what test or tests to order and is able to interpret the results. (REF 13-p. 3)

359. D. Clinical features are enlarged maxilla (bilaterally in all directions), teeth lingually placed, bony elevations over the roots of anterior maxillary teeth, spacing, and movement of teeth. Radiographic features include the following: "cotton-ball" pattern (irregularly shaped radiolucent areas), linear trabecular striations, "ground-glass" or stippled pattern, and partially or totally absent lamina dura. Laboratory findings include elevated alkaline phosphatase and normal serum calcium and phosphorus concentrations. (REF. 13-p. 3)

360. D. Differential diagnosis implies the employment of extensive and all-inclusive diagnostic procedures. A thorough familiarity with the pathologic process as it affects the oral and maxillofacial tissues is necessary if a correct differential diagnosis is to be made. (REF. 13-p. 4)

361. B. Knowledge of the cause or causes of the disease process is essential. A knowledge of the cause of the oral disease is a prerequisite to successful treatment. (REF. 13-p. 5)

362. B. Pathogenesis is that body of knowledge concerning the entire oral disease process, i. e., how the disease begins, step-by-step progression, its variances, its behavior patterns, and its final outcome. (REF. 13-p. 5)

363. B. Medical history includes all significant facts about the disease process. The patient should be at ease during the taking of a medical history. (REF. 13-p. 7)

364. A. Enlargement of the thyroid gland may or may not be associated with overactivity of the thyroid gland. During hyperthyroidism there may be a bruit (sound) audible over the gland. (REF. 13-p. 13)

365. D. Angina pectoris is characterized by a steady pressing or constricting pain in the chest, often radiating to the neck, or left arm. The pain is brought on by exertion or emotion and relieved promptly by rest or nitroglycerin. (REF. 13-p. 13)

366. C. Exophthalmos or prominence of the eyes may occur alone or associated with other eye signs. Hyperthyroidism, exophthalmos, and thyroid enlargement are present in a syndrome termed toxic goiter (Graves' disease). (REF. 13-p. 17)

367. B. Bence-Jones protein is an abnormal, low molecular weight protein sometimes present in patients with multiple myeloma. A specific test is required for its detection. (REF. 13-p. 21)

368. D. Glucose (urine) occurs in diabetes mellitus and is rarely due to renal glycosuria. Salicylic acid produces a false position reaction for glucose in the urine. (REF. 13-p. 20)

369. E. The differential white blood cell count of the leukocytes identifies the various cell types. The values are expressed as percentages of the total number of leukocytes. (Normal: neutrophils, band-forms, 1-5%; neutrophils, segmented, 50-65%; eosinophils, 0-4%; basophils, 0-1%; lymphocytes, 25-40%; and monocytes 0-8%). (REF. 13-p. 21)

370. A. The Rh (Rhesus) factor is important because transfusion of Rh positive blood to a Rh negative person may induce antibody formation. In a pregnant female these antibodies can traverse the placenta and cause hemolysis in a Rh positive fetus. Erythroblastosis fetalis is commonly due to Rh incompatibility between the mother and the infant thus affected. (REF. 13-p. 23)

371. A. Dry socket (alveolar osteitis, septic alveolitis) is characterized by deep-seated, throbbing, radiating pain, beginning 48-hours following the extraction of a tooth and lasting 7-10 days. It is vital to distinguish the pain due to dry socket from that caused by a fracture or deformed bony plate. (REF. 13-p. 30)

372. A. This disease refers to osteomalacia, osteoporosis, and osteitis fibrosa generalisata (the bone disease of hyperparathyroidism). (REF. 13-p. 36)

373. C. Osteoporosis is the most common metabolic bone disease. The decreased density leads to weakness of the affected bone(s) and is due to an inadequate or depressed formation of matrix and a decreased rate of bone formation. The rate of bone resorption exceeds the rate of bone formation, leading to a decrease in bone density. Osteoporosis per se is not a definitive diagnosis. One must describe the bone disease as protein-deficiency osteoporosis and the like. (REF. 13-p. 39)

374. E. Long-standing hypoparathyroidism results in an abnormally dense maxilla and mandible in the presence of a low serum calcium level. The number of bone trabeculae are increased so that the jaws appear highly calcified. The developing roots of permanent teeth tend to be shorter than normal and the apices are blunted or flat. (REF. 13-p. 40)

375. E. Early findings in diabetes mellitus are dryness and burning of the tongue and gingival tenderness. Uncontrolled diabetics have gingival hypertrophy, plus periodontal manifestations that include gingival hemorrhages, pocket formation in children, and increased tooth mobility. Controlled diabetics have microangiopathy in the gingival and periodontal tissues. (REF. 13-p. 5)

376. B. Pregnancy gingivitis begins as a gingival change from the second month of gestation, reaching a maximum in the eighth month. A decrease in gingivitis is present during the last month of gestation. The gingivitis of pregnancy consists of a firey red color to the marginal gingiva and interdental papillae. The gingiva is enlarged mainly in the interdental papillae. There is pain and an increased tendency for bleeding. Good hygiene should be practiced to prevent the gingivitis. (REF. 13-p. 58)

377. B. Histiocytoses (reticuloses) are characterized by proliferation of reticulocytes or histiocytes of the reticuloendothelial system with cells accumulating in masses within one or more areas. Three varieties are distinguished under histiocytoses (acute or subacute, chronic disseminated, and localized). Histiocytosis-X is another term for the three varieties of histiocytoses. The clinical and radiographic findings for the three varieties of histiocytoses are frequently so similar that one may not be able to differentiate the varieties by clinical and radiographic means. (REF. 13-p. 65)

378. E. Letterer-Siwe disease is an acute, severe, widespread proliferation of reticuloendothelial cells forming granulomatous masses and infiltrating cells in a number of tissues and organs (liver, spleen, lymph nodes, lungs, bone marrow, and skin). This disease occurs in the first 2 years of life and is fatal in a short period of time. (REF. 13-p. 65)

379. E. Hand-Schuller-Christian disease is a chronic disseminated reticulosis with infiltration by reticuloendothelial cells in the first five years of life and, occasionally, later. Prognosis is good with fatalities occurring in 10-15% of patients. (REF. 13-p. 66)

380. E. Amelogenesis imperfecta is an heredity disorder transmitted as a non sex-linked, mendelian-dominant trait. It is characterized by agenesis or hypoplasia of

the enamel of the deciduous and permanent teeth. The hypoplastic enamel is very thin and discolored with various shades of brown. (REF. 13-p. 76)

381. E. Dentinogenesis imperfecta is a heredity induced tooth abnormality transmitted as a nonsex-linked, mendelian-dominant trait. The teeth are discolored due to the dentin alteration and range from gray to yellowish-brown. The teeth may contain "opalescent dentin," i.e., a translucent or opalescent hue to the teeth. (REF. 13-p. 80)

382. D. Periodontosis may be a distinct and specific disease of obscure etiology or merely an infrequent variation of the common periodontitis (a sequela to marginal gingivitis). The periodontal symptoms are more of a degenerative type than of an inflammatory alteration (migration and loosening of the teeth). (REF. 13-p. 93)

383. E. Osteomyelitis is an inflammation of both the bone tissue and bone marrow. Osteomyelitis is characterized by resorption, sequestration, and simultaneous repair of bone. All three of the latter alterations are visible radiographically. Separated dead bone (sequestrum) is produced by choking off the vascular channel of bone tissue. Long-standing osteomyelitis produces new reparative bone termed an involucrum. (REF. 13-p. 88)

384. E. The dental practitioner must rule out the possibility of focal infection, i.e., pathogenic organisms or toxins disseminating by way of the blood stream, lymphatics, nerves, or direct passage to the oral tissues. The dental foci include periodontal disease, pericoronal infection and third molar flaps, periapical infections, retained areas of infection, radicular cysts, and residual cysts and devitalized teeth. (REF. 13-p. 102)

385. E. The more common signs and symptoms of mandibular fracture are the U-shaped mandible with bilateral fractures which may result from a single blow; the amount of edema which depends on the force of impact and the degree of fragment displacement; the pain which is elicited by palpating over the fractured site and upon chewing; the masticatory force which is markedly reduced in cases of complete fracture; salivation and drooling which are increased, and possibly guarded speech. (REF. 13-p. 104)

386. E. Acute rheumatic fever is a late nonsuppurative complication of infections with group A streptococci (a hypersensitivity reaction appears to be the cause). Subacute bacterial endocarditis is a microbial infection affecting the heart valves. It is generally encountered in patients with congenital or acquired lesions of the heart valves. (REF. 14-p. 10)

387. E. The skin and mucous membranes may be altered by drugs or diagnostic agents. The skin is subject to allergic reactions (cross sensitization and contact dermatitis), photosensitivity reactions, fixed drug eruptions, and toxic reactions. Systemic manifestations also produce cutaneous reactions associated with blood dyscrasias such as leukopenia, hemolytic anemia, and thrombocytopenic purpura. (REF. 14-p. 25)

388. A. White lesions of the buccal mucosa are termed lichen planus, leukoplakia, or moniliasis (fungus). Whenever the oral lesion (white) feels indurated and becomes deeply fissured, the dentist should suspect squamous cell carcinoma. For instance, chronic, indurated, and fissured white lesions on the lateral margin of the tongue or in the floor of the mouth in the anterior segment on either side of the midline near the orifices of salivary glands are frequently squamous cell carcinomas. (REF. 14-p. 33)

389. E. Allergic reactions of the supporting tissues to denture base materials appear to occur fictionally. However, a patient and the dentist can develop a sensitivity to methyl methacrylate resin and other materials used in dentistry. (REF. 14-p. 40)

390. E. Two types of radiographs used for recording maxillomandibular relations include cephalometric profile and when the condyles are in the fossae. The inaccuracies of the technique or the method of comparing findings makes the methods somewhat unreliable. (REF. 14-p. 47)

391. E. Local factors may be evaluated by roentgenographic study combined with accurately articulated study casts and visual and digital examination. Diagnosis, radiology, and treatment planning are so closely related that they should be considered together. (REF. 14-p. 48)

392. E. Diagnosis of odontogenic lesions of the jaws is the determination of the nature, location, and the cause of the disease. It represents a complete investigation that should be conducted prior to formulating a treatment plan. Treatment planning is the consideration of all diagnostic findings that have a bearing on the preoperative treatment, maxillomandibular relation records, occlusion, surgical procedures, and the postinsertion treatment. (REF. 14-p. 65)

393. E. It is advisable to divide diagnosis of odontogenic lesions into two phases: the patient examination and consultation interview for existing systemic conditions appraised. In the diagnostic procedure it is often necessary to seek professional assistance from the medical diagnostician and pathologist (oral) before an oral treatment plan can be instituted. (REF. 14-p. 65)

394. D. Bruxism (grinding of teeth) and clenching (elevating and closing of teeth firmly) are acts caused by powerful masticatory muscles. The results of the latter actions are damaging to the teeth and denture-supporting structures and tissues. (REF. 14-p. 160)

395. C. There are many accepted intraoral methods for correcting occlusal disharmony. The intraoral methods are more accurate if the uneven contacting of the teeth has been corrected first. The intraoral methods include the following: articulating paper, central-bearing devices, occlusal wax, abrasive paste, patient remount, and selective grinding for dentures, and selective grinding procedures. (REF. 14-p. 163)

396. E. Bisected articulated plaster diagnostic casts demonstrate the desired cusps fossae relations of the posterior teeth in centric occlusion. (REF. 14-p. 168)

397. E. Treatment planning for patients with a full complement of teeth is the consideration of all of the diagnostic findings, systemic and local, which influence the surgical preparations of the mouth, maxillo-mandibular relation records, occlusion to be developed, and form and material in the teeth. (REF. 14-p. 171)

398. E. The factors in treatment planning are governed by the patient's mental attitude, past dental history, and local oral conditions. (REF. 14-p. 171)

399. B. Balanced occlusion means an occlusion of the teeth which presents a harmonious relation of the occluding surfaces in all centric and eccentric positions within the functional range of mastication and swallowing. It is the simultaneous contacting of the maxillary and mandibular teeth on the right and left and in the posterior and anterior occlusal areas in centric and eccentric positions, developed to lessen or limit a tipping or rotating of denture bases in relation to supporting tissues. (REF. 14-p. 176)

400. A. Vertical dimension (vertical opening) is the length of the face as determined by the amount of separation of the jaws. (REF. 14-p. 177)

401. E. An appreciation of the influences of local factors is based on the anatomy and physiology of the supporting tissues, the functions of the muscles of mandibular movements, and the temporomandibular joint. (REF. 14-p. 180)

402. A. Palpation is part of the act or process of deciding the nature of a diseased condition by oral examination. Palpation is frequently necessary to undertake a careful investigation of the facts to determine the nature of oral tissues or to determine the nature, location, and causes of oral diseases. (REF. 14-p. 193)

403. B. Percussion may aid in evaluating pathologic, nonpathologic, normal, and abnormal conditions. (REF. 14-p. 298)

404. E. Overlay denture, overdenture, telescoped denture, and biologic denture are the numerous terms applied to the tooth-supported complete denture. (REF. 14-p. 182)

405. A. The tooth-supported complete denture should be considered for patients who face the loss of the remaining natural adult dentition. The younger the patient, the greater the indication for the treatment, even though the prognosis for lengthy retention of the modified teeth may not be too favorable. It also should be considered when the complete denture will be opposed by retained mandibular anterior teeth. (REF. 14-p. 182)

406. E. Surgical and prosthodontic approaches to the management of patients who have extensive loss or an absence of the residual ridge or ridges include the following: cobalt chromium alloys, cobalt chromium buttons, attracting

magnets, opposing magnets, and in recent years there has been clinical research in augmentation to increase basal bone in a vertical and horizontal direction for denture base stability. Generally, autogenous bone has been preferred by most dentists. (REF. 14-p. 184)

407. E. Long-term studies with augmentation techniques of the mandible show a high percentage of vertical height loss of the graft material. There is clinical evidence of mass alterations, specifically in the buccal lingual dimension which allows an increase in basal support for the lower prosthesis. (REF. 14-p. 184)

408. E. Any effort in implant dentistry should be based on sound anatomic, physiologic, histologic, surgical, and prosthodontic procedures that will help the implant patient should be fostered. (REF. 14-p. 184)

409. C. Diagnostic procedures should be continuous with the past dental history furnishing valuable information as to the mental attitude of the patient toward dentistry. (REF. 14-p. 186)

410. E. During the consultation and history taking, the following important factors should be revealed: the patient's behavior pattern, personality, temperament, and ability to communicate (hearing is essential to communication), and the medications (if any) that he or she is taking including nonprescription drugs. (REF. 14-p. 186)

411. D. Surgical trauma occurs in the removal of the mandibular teeth for patients who are to undergo irradiation therapy for a malignant neoplasm. The teeth may have been quite serviceable. However, because of the periodontal situation or location adjacent to the site of irradiation, they must be condemned to extraction. (REF. 14-p. 199)

412. B. Saliva is a major factor in evaluating the physical influences that contribute to denture retention. The physical forces in which saliva are involved are adhesion, cohesion, capillarity, and atmospheric pressure. Thin, watery saliva of high surface tension affords enough retention that patients do not have a problem with denture retention if all other retentive factors are acceptable. Patients who have ropy saliva do have problems with denture retention as do those who have profuse watery saliva. (REF. 14-p. 209)

413. E. Alveolar residual ridge lost as a result of a pathologic condition, an accident, or surgical procedures does not undergo regenerative reconstruction. When the natural teeth are removed or lost, the tensile stimulation provided by the periodontal attachments is lost. Bone resorbs in response to pressure, and complete dentures are capable of producing pressure sufficient to interfere with the blood supply. (REF. 14-p. 210)

414. C. Systemic factors affect the oral tissues. Many systemic diseases have local manifestations with no apparent systemic symptoms, and others have both local and systemic reactions (debilitating diseases, diseases of the TMJ, cardiovascular diseases, diseases of the skin, neurologic disorders, and oral malignancies). (REF. 14-p. 211)

415. C. Case presentation should be conducted in a private room in pleasant surroundings, devoid of any equipment. Begin educating the patient in his or her responsibilities as early as possible. For the chronically ill patient treatment may be primarily palliative in nature. (REF. 14-p. 205)

416. A. Oral pain in the geriatric patient may be caused by the following: osteoporosis, bone sore mouth, diminished blood supply; metabolic (thiamine deficiency); or a lack of estrogen resulting in tissue tone loss (to be differentiated from psychogenic facial pain). (REF. 14-p. 125)

417. A. The psychologic problems influencing behavior can be divided into reactions to physiologic changes, reactions to social changes, changes in the environment, and changes in mental capacity. (REF. 14-p. 125)

418. C. Occlusal force is the product of muscular force applied on opposing teeth. (REF. 14-p. 125)

419. E. Errors in registering maxillomandibular relations may be the result of one or more of the following: record bases that do not fit accurately, shifting of the record bases over displaceable tissues, excessive pressure exerted by the patient during the registering of maxillomandibular relations, unequal distribution of stress during the registering of maxillomandibular relations, record bases placed on soft tissues that have been deformed by

ill-fitting dentures, patients not registering centric relation because of systemic factors (muscle spasm), abnormalities of the TMJ, and impairment of muscle tonus or failure of mental, aged, or senile patients to understand instructions. (REF. 14-p. 127)

420. A. Vertical opening (vertical dimension) is the length of the face as determined by the amount of separation of the jaws. (REF. 14-p. 132)

421. C. The freeway space (interocclusal clearance, interocclusal distance, interocclusal gap, and interocclusal rest space) is the distance between the occluding surfaces of the maxillary and mandibular teeth when the mandible is in its physiologic rest position. This may be determined by the difference between the rest vertical dimension and the occlusal vertical dimension. (REF. 14-p. 132)

422. B. The temporomandibular syndrome is composed of the various symptoms of discomfort, pain, or pathosis stated to be caused by loss of vertical dimension, lack of posterior occlusion (malocclusions), trismus, muscle tremor, arthritis, or direct trauma to the temporomandibular joint. (REF. 14-p. 133)

423. D. Balancing contacts take place between the maxillary and mandibular natural or artificial teeth at the side opposite to the working side. (REF. 14-p. 136)

424. C. The condylar hinge position is the position of the condyles of the mandible in the glenoid fossa at which hinge axis movement is possible. (REF. 14-p. 134)

425. A. The terminal hinge position is the position of the mandible in relation to the maxilla from which hinge axis movement can be accomplished. (REF. 14-p. 135)

426. B. Centric jaw relation is the jaw relation when the condyles are in the most posterior, unstrained position in the glenoid fossae at any given degree of jaw separation from which lateral movement can be made. It is the most posterior relation of the mandible to the maxillae at the established vertical dimension or the relation of the mandible to the maxillae when the condyles are in their most posterior position in the glenoid fossa from which unstrained lateral movements can be made at the occluding vertical dimension normal for the individual. (REF. 14-p. 135)

427. C. Centric occlusion is the centered contact position of the occlusal surfaces of the mandibular teeth against the occlusal surfaces of the maxillary teeth. Centric relation record is the registration of centric relation made at the established occlusal vertical dimension. (REF. 14-p. 135)

428. C. Centric relation is anteroposterior bone-to-bone relation of the maxillae and mandible. It is an unstrained position whereby the individual can assume the most posterior relation voluntarily and by reflex action without stretching the muscles to their utmost to reach the position. (REF. 14-p. 137)

429. A. Protrusive record is a registration of a forward position of the mandible with reference to the maxillae. A position of the mandible forward of or lateral to centric position. (REF. 14-p. 137)

430. D. Selective grinding has the following advantages: it reduces patient participation; it permits the dentist to see better what he is grinding; it provides a stable working foundation (bases are not shifting on resilient tissues); the absence of saliva makes possible more accurate markings with the articulating paper or tape; and corrections can be made away from the patient, thus preventing occasional objections when patients see their dentures being ground. (REF. 14-p. 138)

431. D. Prematurity is a condition of tooth contacts which diverts the mandible from a normal path of closure (REF 14-p. 150)

432. A. Premature contact is the initial contact of the teeth prior to closure of the mandible to the maxilla (as deflective occlusal contact). (REF. 14-p. 150)

433. C. Alveolectomy is the surgical removal of part of the alveolar process of the upper or lower jaw. An alveolectomy is necessary in the alveolar fracture and where uneven interseptal or interproximal spines exist. (REF. 14-p. 239)

434. D. Opposing undercuts present obstacles to the path of insertion and removal of the denture. These undercuts should be eliminated by surgical removal. Bilateral removal is not always necessary. (REF. 14-p. 239)

435. A. Denture hyperplasia is an abnormal multiplication or increase in the number of normal cells in normal arrangement in a tissue. It is caused by an ill-fitting denture. (REF. 14-p. 245)

436. C. One of the problems of aging is the failure of some of the bodily functions that do not maintain their efficiency. (REF. 14-p. 300)

437. E. The changes in the geriatric patient are classified as follows: physiologic, psychologic, and pathologic. Not all patients can be classed into these strict groupings. The dentist should analyze the aging process and describe the effects of the changes on the patient to understand this classification better. (REF. 14-p. 300)

438. C. The psychological problems influencing the behavior of the aging can be related to the reactions to physiologic changes and to social changes, changes in environment, and changes in mental capacity. (REF. 14-p. 300)

439. E. The changes influencing one's appearance seem to affect females more than males. Women complain more about the loss of hair and face height, wrinkling of the skin, changes in tooth appearance, and the loss of the natural teeth. (REF. 14-p. 301)

440. E. A dentist should know what behavior or personality changes occur with aging and recognize them during his clinical examination of the patient. The dentist should examine the geriatric patient for the following: pathologic changes, facial expression, complexion, posture and walking pattern, voice, breathing pattern, local factors, pain, and intraoral changes. (REF. 14-p. 302)

441. E. Intraoral aging changes include the following: marked resorption of the residual alveolar ridge; ill-fitting dentures with inflammatory hyperplasia; white lesions of the buccal mucosa; and painless, nonulcerated, poorly defined firm mass covered by pink mucosa (may be a fibrosarcoma). (REF. 14-p. 305)

442. C. Physiologic factors that alter salivary flow are agreeable taste stimuli resulting in profuse salivation; smooth object in the mouth results in increased salivation; during dehydration, salivation decreases, and with aging the saliva

becomes more ropy in consistency; emotions and other psychic effects excite the autonomic nervous system and in turn the organs are altered. (REF. 14-p. 307)

443. A. The dentist should question the patient with pain for the following: renal disease, gall bladder pain, bowel obstruction, chest pain, glossodynia, paroxysmal pain, pain of tic douloureux, pain over maxillary sinuses, and psychogenic facial pain. (REF. 15-p. 129)

444. E. The radiation therapist and the prosthodontist will have to determine how long a time should elapse after radiation therapy prior to subjecting the tissues to the stresses of a denture. The tumor prognosis, the amount of radiation, and the tone and appearance of the tissues govern the time factor. The radiation therapist should be consulted and no denture should be constructed unless approved by the therapist. (REF. 20-p. 8)

445. E. The temporomandibular joint syndrome is associated with bruxism and clenching or gnashing of the teeth, with secondary tension, spasm and pain in the muscles of mastication. (REF. 20-p. 242)

446. E. Glossopharyngeal neuralgia is a disorder producing paroxysms of severe pain in the tonsils, posterior pharynx, back of the tongue, and middle ear. Atypical facial neuralgia has the following forms: cluster headache, "lower-half" headache, and psychogenic facial pain. (REF. 20-p. 246)

447. E. There are likewise many keratotic diseases of the mouth. These include hyperkeratosis, leukoplakia, lichen planus, chronic discoid lupus erythematosus, psoriasis, and keratosis follicularis (Darier's disease). (REF. 20-p. 258)

448. E. Scleroderma (progressive systemic sclerosis) frequently involves the skin, gastrointestinal tract, lungs, and heart. Scleroderma is an overproliferation of fibrous connective tissue with inflammation of blood vessels and connective tissue. Induration and atrophy of the skin are prominent features. (REF. 20-p. 272)

449. E. In the parotid glands the most common malignant neoplasm is the mucoepidermoid carcinoma, followed by the malignant mixed tumor. The adenoid cystic carcinoma (cylindroma) is the most common submaxillary malignant tumor. Thought should be given to the possibility that a rapid rate of growth in a salivary gland neoplasm indicates that the mass is a malignant transformation of a benign tumor. (REF. 20-p. 289)

450. E. Xerostomia is the sequel to a decrease in salivary secretion, from both the major and minor salivary glands. The decrease in salivation leads to complaints of dryness and burning of the mouth. Ascending infections are facilitated and serve to further complicate the dry mouth. (REF 20-p. 296)

451. E. Macroglossia (enlarged tongue) occurs more frequently than aglossia or microglossia. Primary macroglossia results from an overdevelopment of the muscles of the tongue which may be related to a generalized muscular hypertrophy affecting the entire body. Secondary (acquired) macroglossia results from relaxation of the tongue musculature, regardless of its etiology. (REF. 20-p. 342)

452. E. Multiple myeloma (plasma-cell myeloma) is a malignant neoplasm which generally arises in multiple bone marrow sites of the skeleton. Its characteristic cells resemble plasma cells which are thought to originate from the reticuloendothelial cells of the marrow. This myeloma leads to radiolucencies in bone. (REF. 20-p. 356)

453. D. During respiratory emergencies (shallow or labored breathing) place the patient flat on his back. Make certain the airway is clear. Administer oxygen, being sure there is an exchange. Send for help. If the above does not restore adequate respiration, then breathe for the patient (oxygen, mouth to mouth, or mechanical resuscitation). Be sure the chest moves (check for pulse). If the airway is blocked, establish an emergency airway. (REF. 20-p. 423)

454. C. It is extremely important for the dentist to develop a treatment plan for each patient. The plan should include allocation of time for performance of individual procedures. The procedures should be sequenced according to user-defined criteria. The most important use of the

treatment plan is in the management of a dental practice, which along with sequence and allocation of time will improve patient care. (REF. 91-p. 8)

455. D. The three broad categories are not necessarily mutually exclusive or completely inclusive. Moral responsibility is the relationship of the dentist to others. It includes the sharing of knowledge and experience with family, community, and profession. (REF. 91-p. 21)

456. E. The practice of dentistry is extremely complicated, requiring in special circumstances the services of people who have special training. The dentist who practices comprehensive care must possess and exercise a wide range of managerial skills to select, employ, and utilize the services of a diverse group of individuals. (REF. 91-p. 28)

457. A. The most effective way to instill attitudes in dentists that are supportive of comprehensive care is probably by role models. The degradation of attitudes among dentists would appear to be related more to increased age and experience with the system than to any other identifiable variable. (REF. 91-p. 39)

458. A. One of the most difficult tasks of the dentist is to be able to subdue his feelings sufficiently and to make constant adjustments in his reactions to different personalities The dentist must be willing and able to deliver dental care and recognize the need and make appropriate referrals. (REF. 91-p. 54)

459. E. A group practice is generally a dental practice consisting of three or more dentists who share, on whatever basis they select, pooled income from the practice. We exclude those groups composed of individual general practices sharing some facilities. (REF. 9-p. 59)

460. E. Total patient care has been increasing because of the deficiencies of the point and block system in dental education and due to automatic data processing methods to assist in the management of such programs. (REF. 91-p. 67)

461. E. The most vital record keeping in a dental office is a rather significant expense. It has been estimated to be one-third of the total overhead expense. This is a realistic estimate. (REF. 91-p. 69)

462. E. The law requires that the records must be permanent, accurate, and complete. The records must clearly state income, justifications for deductions, explanations of credit, and information on employees. (REF. 9-p. 71)

463. E. It is unlikely to find a dental record today which contains all of these requirements in an optimal degree. (REF. 9-p. 79)

464. E. Improving dental records will be stimulated by the insurance industry and government requirements and probably not from within the profession. There is little pressure from dentists to improve record keeping. (REF 91-p. 81)

465. E. The average dental record in the United States fails to provide the answers to these four questions. We generally find some but not all of the data recorded. (REF. 91-p. 92)

466. E. The ideal dental record has never been developed in the United States. (REF. 91-p. 92)

467. E. The problem list is the most important part of a problem-oriented record. The dentist should construct a list so that each problem is numbered, titled, and dated. (REF. 91-p. 97)

468. E. The simple implementation of any system will not solve the basic organizational or clinical management problems. (REF. 61-p. 127)

Chapter 10 Operative Dentistry

469. C. Restorative dentistry requires the treatment of dental caries at the earliest time the lesions can be detected. The initial attack of dental caries is on enamel; therefore, early diagnosis of enamel caries is vital in determining the appropriate treatment. (REF. 28-p. 48)

470. B. Smooth surface enamel caries begins as a white spot of demineralization. The area may become stained and present some cavitation in the enamel. Enamel caries of the gingival third of a tooth is diagnosed by clinical examination. (REF. 28-p. 51)

471. E. Radiographs seldom show occlusal caries before the condition is clinically evident. Interproximal enamel caries is diagnosed by periapical and bite-wing radiographic examination. Some interproximal caries will appear confined to the enamel. (REF. 28-p. 53)

472. E. Enamel caries need not progress into the dentin. Fluorides applied topically to the tooth surface can inhibit enamel caries and arrest the progress of the incipient lesions. Fissure sealants can prevent the extension of enamel caries into the dentin. (REF. 28-p. 73)

473. D. The success of operative dentistry is preventive treatment of enamel caries and the response of the patient to preventive therapy. More and more carious enamel lesions remain confined to the enamel. (REF. 28-p. 75)

474. B. The preferred treatment for enamel caries is not operative dentistry. Treating enamel caries should involve the following: removing bacterial plaque from all enamel surfaces, impregnating the enamel with flourides, obturating pits and fissures with a fissure sealant, helping the patient to reduce the ingestion of cariogenic foods, teaching the patient a method of effective home care, and continuing the therapy through periodic recall. (REF. 28-p. 77)

475. B. Placing the margins of a restoration in relatively caries-immune areas is axiomatic for extension for prevention. It is a valid principle for all dentists to follow. (REF. 28-p. 77)

476. E. Inadequate extended occlusal fissures provide a common site for the attack of dental caries. (REF. 28-p. 77)

477. B. Recurrent caries is a major cause for the failure of restorations. Once dental caries has attacked the tooth at the margins of restorations, there is no good alternative to increasingly complex operative dentistry. (REF. 28-p. 81)

478. B. The dentist's role in preventing recurrent caries continues in the restorative phase of operative dentistry. Restorations must be placed that will not invite recurrent caries. Sound operative dentistry principles coupled with current primary preventive measures can virtually eliminate recurrent caries. Underextended proximal margins invite recurrent caries. (REF. 28-p. 89)

479. E. Pits and fissures are normally considered to be caries-prone. The margin of a restoration located in a fissure increases the hazard of recurrent caries. Therefore, a cavity preparation should be extended to include all fissures so that the margins of the preparations do not terminate in fissures. (REF. 28-p. 91)

480. A. Special attention should be paid to the enamel walls of the cavity preparation. Properly prepared enamel walls provide a firm foundation for the adaptation of the restorative material. Rough enamel margins present unsupported enamel rods that may subsequently break away. (REF. 28-p. 94)

481. D. Amalgam failures occur when the underextended buccal proximal margins of the premolars and molars have a marginal breakdown, displaced restoration, poor contour and contact, and poor finish of the restoration. (REF. 28-p. 95)

482. E. The enamel walls should first be smoothed in the direction of the enamel rods. The cavosurface angle should be beveled for those restorations that permit beveling. (REF. 28-p. 97)

483. E. The routine use of hand instruments in practice may initiate better preparation of the enamel walls. The findings that hand instruments are a mental hazard in our age of ultraspeed may be due to influence of dull instruments. (REF. 28-p. 98)

484. E. The protective effect of topical fluorides on enamel is well documented. Topical fluorides have been shown to have a similar protective effect on freshly cut dentin. In addition, 10% stannous fluoride remineralized carious dentin left in the depths of a cavity. (REF. 28-p. 100)

485. B. Hand instruments of value include the following: side-cutting hatches, Wedelstaedt chisels, and spoon excavators. (REF. 28-p. 109)

486. A. The dental assistant, using an electric instrument sharpener, should be taught to quickly provide hand instruments that are sharp, efficient, and pleasant to use during cavity preparation. (REF. 28-p. 117)

487. E. The exclusion of saliva is necessary for the proper placement of all restorative materials. An isolated operating field provides the optimum working environment for restorative procedures and therefore is basic to preventing the failure of restorations. (REF. 28-p. 197)

488. E. The dentist interested in improving dental practice should return to the use of the rubber dam. The rubber dam can be turned from a mental hazard into a most helpful tool in operative dentistry. (REF. 28-p. 201)

489. E. Disadvantages of any rubber dam can be eliminated by relearning to use the rubber dam; beginning with easy cases; isolating a minimum of teeth; not trying to be perfect; ligating only if absolutely necessary; using a simple rubber dam holder such as Young's rubber dam frame or Nuggaard-Ostby rubber dam holder; and not letting the psychic trauma of unassisted fumbling deprive you of the advantages of the rubber dam. (REF. 28-p. 201)

490. E. Amalgam is adapted directly to the cavity walls during the condensation procedure. Saliva or blood contamination adversely affects the physical properties of amalgam and all other filling materials. The condensing force for amalgam should be directed toward all walls and line angles of the cavity preparation. (REF. 28-p. 235)

491. E. Undercondensation is likely to occur at the walls and margins when the amalgam is simply plugged into the preparation. Spherical alloys require less condensing force than that required by conventional alloys. (REF. 28-p. 244)

492. D. Grossly carious teeth can now be saved for patients who cannot or will not accept cast gold restorations for economic reasons. There is little or no evidence to suggest that properly placed pin amalgams are any more a liability to the patient than large cast gold restorations. (REF. 28-p. 234)

493. E. Sufficient bulk of the restorative material is achieved at the margins of restorations by providing a cavosurface with no bevel or flare. Marginal fracture is prevented by removing the small spurs of the restorative material that may extend over the margin. (REF. 28-p. 261)

494. E. Cast gold restorations do not fracture. Therefore, resistance form for inlays is concerned with protecting weakened tooth structure. Cast gold inlays must be adapted to the walls of a cavity preparation by cement. The zinc phosphate cement used for inlays is soluble in mouth fluids. (REF. 28-p. 279)

495. E. Restorations fail when they initiate or contribute to periodontal disease. Gold inlay restorations can prevent this kind of failure by providing good margins, contour, and occlusion. The conservative extension of preparations helps to prevent gingival irritation. (REF. 28-p. 303)

496. C. The occlusion should be checked before operative dentistry is begun and also at the completion of the restorative therapy. Shiny wear facets can be detected on restorations in areas of premature occlusal contact. Prematurities should be relieved before they cause trouble. (REF. 28-p. 304)

497. A. The conservative extension should be followed with radical patient education and primary preventive measures. Conservatism is a cardinal principle of operative dentistry and of cavity preparation. (REF. 28-p. 316)

498. D. Endodontic therapy provides the means for saving teeth that were once destined for extraction. (REF. 28-p. 325)

499. D. Endodontic therapy is indicated only after vital pulp therapy has failed or when the patient presents an already nonvital pulp. When there is vital pulp tissue, there is hope of recovery. Therefore, the first attempt should be to maintain the vitality of the pulp. (REF. 28-p. 325)

500. D. Periodontal splinting, especially provisional splinting, may be accomplished by means of etched enamel retention. Tooth stabilization after various surgical procedures may be similarly accomplished. (REF. 28-p. 322)

501. E. Direct golds are adapted to the cavity walls by the condensing force. The force for cohesive gold should be directed toward the walls and line angles. Each increment must be completely condensed with overlapping steps of the condenser before the next increment is added. (REF. 28-p. 407)

502. E. Powdered golds may be adapted by hand condensation, as long as the rules of magnitude and direction of forces are observed. (REF. 28-p. 408)

503. C. Silicate cements and restorative resins are best adapted to cavity walls in relatively small increments. Poor adaptation may occur when large bulks of material are forced into the preparation by the matrix strip. (REF. 28-p. 438)

504. E. The adaptation of restorative resin materials to cavity walls may be enhanced by acid etching of the enamel margins of the preparation. The dye penetration is significantly reduced at the enamel-restoration interface of composite restorations by acid etching. (REF. 28-p. 439)

505. E. However, only the dentin wall should have a lining of cavity varnish for silicate cement restorations. The enamel walls should be in direct contact with the silicate cement. The fluoride flux in the silicate cement can then exert its anticariogenic effect on the enamel. (REF. 28-p. 443)

506. E. Because silicate cement is a friable filling material, the silicate cement preparations should not be beveled. A nonserrated fissure bur running at slow speed is effective for finishing the enamel walls. The bur should be held perpendicular to the enamel surface. (REF. 28-p. 443)

507. E. Etched surface enamel is particularly receptive to the retention of acrylic and composite resins. Methyl methacrylate restorative resins bond well to etched enamel. However, their low resistance to abrasion and tendency to discolor leave much to be desired. (REF. 28-p. 462)

508. B. Acid-etched enamel retention provides the means of conserving tooth structure in various restorative situations. Phosphoric acid (50%) has become the clinical choice for etching of enamels. After a 1-to-2-minute etch, the enamel provides a microscopically rough and retentive surface. (REF. 28-p. 463)

509. B. Smooth surface enamel caries begins as a white spot of demineralization. The area subsequently becomes stained and presents a cavitation in the enamel. (REF. 42-p. 1)

510. B. Detection of dental caries while the lesion is in enamel is advantageous. The treatment for the less extensive lesion is simpler and is associated with less morbidity. (REF. 42-p. 7)

511. D. Therefore, teaching the dental patient to exercise control over his oral environment is a major factor in prevention. Dentists must develop skills in teaching and motivating patients. (REF. 42-p. 11)

512. E. The treatment should therefore consist of topical fluoride therapy and a continued reduction of the cariogenic flora in the patient's mouth. (REF. 42-p. 12)

513. A. In the mouth, acid dissolution is influenced by saliva. Saliva is normally supersaturated with respect to fluorapatite and hydroxyapatite and the driving force is in favor of depositing rather than dissolving enamel mineral. As the pH is lowered by the addition of acid, saliva becomes undersaturated with hydroxyapatite at about pH 5. It remains supersaturated with fluorapatite until the pH falls below 4. (REF. 42-p. 12)

514. C. Dental plaque is mainly composed of living bacteria. Antimicrobial agents have been tested for their plaque-inhibiting capacity such as 1% vancomycin in an adhesive paste, a 0.25% tetracycline rinse, and a macrolide antibiotic (1232) all of which reduced plaque in humans. However, there is no doubt of the potential danger in the use of such drugs because of production of resistant strains, sensitization, and undesirable side effects of long-term administration. (REF. 42-p. 14)

515. E. Preventive dentistry consists of many interrelated procedures with microbial plaque control as the keystone in the prevention of caries and gingival diseases. Every patient who forms microbial plaque in every dental practice should be on a plaque control program. (REF. 42-p. 25)

516. C. Gold alloy castings require meticulous attention to the impression and preparation of the die (in the indirect technique) coupled with an understanding of the physical interactions between the pattern and the investment (as temperature rise and setting expansion forces) to result in a clinically acceptable casting. (REF. 39-pp. 527, 575)

517 D. Cast gold inlays by the direct method are fracture-free restorations. The resistance form for gold inlays is concerned with protecting weakened tooth structure. (REF. 39-p. 416)

518. A. Use the minimum number of pins that will provide adequate retention. Although the retention increases with the number of pins, each pin is potentially hazardous to the pulp. Pins should provide retention when retentive tooth structure is not present. (REF. 39-p. 91)

519. E. Wax is probably the most dimensionally unstable material used in clinical dentistry. There are two types of inlay wax: Type I wax for use in the direct technique and Type II wax for use in the indirect technique. (REF. 39-p. 577)

520. D. To minimize dimensional changes, wax should be softened with dry heat at a constant temperature and inserted into the prepared cavity at as high a temperature as possible and under pressure. (REF. 39-p. 573)

521. D. Impression compound, still used by dentists, does not reproduce surface detail with the same degree of accuracy as do some of the hydrocolloid and elastomeric impression materials. Alginate hydrocolloids and silicone rubbers also can be used as impression materials. (REF. 39-p. 545)

522. C. Amalgam restorations are retained by frictional resistance between the restorative material and the walls of the preparation. Therefore, both proper preparation of the cavity walls and good adaptation of the material to the walls are important factors in retention. (REF. 39-p. 279)

523. B. A box form of the preparation, finished cavity walls, undercuts, and grooves provide adequate retention for silver-amalgam restorations. (REF. 39-p. 295)

524. C. The fracture of most amalgam restorations can be prevented by sufficient bulk of the restorative material. The latter is achieved by the proper depth of cavity preparation. The optimal depth in sound tooth structure is 0.5-1.0 mm pulpal to the dentinoenamel junction. Preparations at this optimal depth need no intermediate base. (REF. 39-p. 296)

525. D. Moisture produces defective restorations. The magnitude of the problem of defective restorations is not known. More than one-third of the operative dentistry was consumed by replacing defective restorations. An isolated, dry operative field provides the optimum working environment for restorative procedures and therefore is basic to preventing the failure of amalgam restorations. (REF. 39-p. 268)

526. C. The goal in finishing a restoration is to provide smooth and polished surfaces and margins that may be kept clean with ease. Poorly finished surfaces and interproximal overhangs make flossing and cleaning difficult if not impossible. Unpolished occlusal margins trap debris. (REF. 39-p. 340)

527. E. Large cutting instruments invite the excessive removal of tooth structure. For conservative preparations, a number 34 inverted cone bur or a number 56 nonserrated bur is indicated for roughing out the cavity. Large burs produce large preparations. (REF. 31-p. 59)

528. C. Eccentric cutting instruments invite the excessive removal of tooth structure. The destructive action of eccentric instruments on tooth structure has been studied with high-speed photography to show tooth structure being blasted away by the action of the bur. Diamond instruments are more efficient than burs for the controlled removal of tooth structure. (REF. 31-p. 67)

529. A. The dentist should have a thorough knowledge of the directions of the enamel rods on various tooth surfaces so that he or she will finish all enamel walls so that all of the enamel rods forming the enamel wall have their

inner ends resting on sound dentin. Enamel rods that do not run uninterrupted from the cavity margin to dentin tend to split off resulting in a V-shaped defect along the margin of the restoration. (REF. 31-p. 182)

530. A. Resistance form refers to the form of a cavity preparation that enables the tooth and the restoration to resist the forces of mastication. Fracture of the restoration and/or tooth structure results when sufficient resistance form is not provided. (REF. 31-p. 188)

531. C. The occlusal divergence of the vertical walls in cavity preparations for gold inlays also should be considered as convenience form. (REF. 31-p. 191)

532. E. In pit and fissure cavities the rule is to extend the cavity margin until solid tooth structure is obtained and no unsupported enamel is left. The objectives of cavity preparation are to eliminate all decay and provide pulpal protection, to locate the margins of the restorations in relatively immune areas of the tooth to prevent recurrent caries, and to form the cavity so that the tooth or the restoration or both will not undergo fracture during mastication. (REF. 31-p. 171)

533. E. In gingival cavities, the outline form should extend gingivally beneath the free margin of the gingiva; mesially and distally to, or past, the respective line angles of the tooth; occlusally or incisally to the height of contour of the tooth surface; and be shaped so as to present an esthetically harmonious effect. (REF. 31-p. 173)

534. E. Diamond and carbide instruments perform best at the highest speeds available. The increased speeds produce more effective cutting. The speed at which an instrument is rotated is measured in revolutions per minute. Of equal importance in rotational speed is the diameter and width of the cutting instrument surface that contacts the tooth in a given time. (REF. 31-p. 256)

535. E. Matrix band should be easy to apply and remove: rigid to provide resistance against pressures during insertion of the filling; and capable of providing proper contour (REF. 31-p. 284)

536. E. Operative dentistry consists of those operations on natural teeth performed in order to repair damage inflicted by caries as well as for prevention of future caries. Some procedures (as restoration of eroded and abraded areas of teeth and treatment of fractured teeth) may go beyond caries treatment and prevention. However, operative dentistry is the restoration of lost tooth structure to near normal function and appearance. (REF. 31-p. 302)

537. E. Every tooth should be provided with some thermal insulating material between the pulp and metal restoration. In cavities of normal depth, cavity varnish should be applied to the dentin walls before the silver amalgam is placed. In deeper cavities, a thin layer of zinc oxide-eugenol cement should be flowed into place in order to insulate the pulp from rapid thermal changes plus act as an obtundent. (REF. 31-p. 308)

538. E. Gold foil is one of the most versatile restorative materials available. It is excellent for filling many incipient and moderately carious areas in both anterior and posterior teeth. Gold foil comes in the following forms: sheet foil in book form, gold foil ropes, gold foil pellets or cylinders, matt gold, and cohesive and noncohesive gold. (REF. 31-p. 357)

539. E. Cohesive gold is pure gold foil or crystal gold that will weld at room temperature under pressure. (REF. 81-p. 360)

540. C. Some patients will not be convinced that a small esthetic sacrifice is worth the reward of a lasting restoration. For patients who are unwilling to make this adjustment, an esthetic material will have to be used to restore the teeth. (REF. 81-p. 361)

541. E. Gold inlays are useful restorations for the following classes of cavity preparations: Class I cavities, Class II cavities, Class IV cavities, Class V cavities, and Class VI cavity preparations (pinledge restorations). (REF. 81-p. 364)

542. B. A one-surface wax pattern should receive an investment that expands more than the investment for the multiple-surface inlay wax pattern (facioocclusal). The one-surface casting will generally be too small or loose-fitting. (REF. 81-p. 418)

543. B. In the indirect technique (inlays) if the sprue is to be attached to the occlusal, the U-wire need not be of gold alloy, because it can be readily removed from the wax pattern before attaching the sprue and investing. (REF. 31-p. 433)

544. E. The technique for using reversible hydrocolloid impression materials is based upon the ability of the material to be liquefied and then cooled to temperatures compatible with the oral tissues while liquid, then readily chilled to a stiff gel with elasticity to permit removal of the impression without distortion. (REF. 31-p. 470)

545. A. The securing of an impression includes the following: liquefying, storing, lowering the temperature of the tray by tempering, injecting fluid hydrocolloid into the cavity preparation, placing the tray in the mouth, and changing the sol into a gel by circulation of tap water through the tray. (REF. 31-p. 472)

546. D. Retention for resin in Class IV cavities may be obtained by one or a combination of the following: undercuts, dovetail extension, and cementation of stainless steel threaded pins. (REF. 31-p. 485)

547. E. Porcelain inlays are the finest restorations for Class V cavity preparations when esthetics is of paramount importance. Porcelain inlays have a low thermal conductivity, a glazed surface, a coefficient of thermal expansion close to tooth structure, relative insolubility in oral fluids, and a hardness sufficient to resist abrasion. (REF. 31-p. 499)

548. B. Cemented, threaded, stainless steel pins (0.025 inches in diameter) judiciously placed to evade the pulp and its horns, offer excellent auxiliary retention. Preparation of the holes removes only a small quantity of tooth structure. (REF. 46-p. 7)

549. C. The pin amalgam is more retentive if the pinholes are not parallel. Low speed should be utilized when cutting pinholes to improve retention of the restoration. (REF. 46-p. 9)

550. E. The dangers of incorrect angulation of retention pins are pulp exposure and root perforation. Before cutting the pinholes, not only angle the drill correctly but also position it so that 0. 7 mm of tooth structure (equal to the diameter of the twist drill) will be between the hole and the parallel root surface. (REF. 46-p. 15)

551. C. The pins must be placed in positions that will allow adequate clearance for amalgam between them and any tooth structure or proposed base. The ends of the wire pins should be rounded to aid entry into the holes during the cementing procedure. (REF. 46-p. 31)

552. A. The pinledge restoration is a three-pin hood or a partial veneer casting for incisors and canines. The pinledge is highly retentive and does not depend upon the length of the tooth crown for retention compared to a three-quarter crown. (REF. 46-p. 51)

553. A. The pinledge is useful for treatment of a fractured anterior tooth and for arresting and correcting abnormal lingual surface erosion or additional wear. It is used as a unit in a splint and is useful as a retainer for an abutment tooth whose clinical crown is short. (REF. 46-p. 52)

554. B. The pinlay is useful when treating a fractured anterior tooth and for arresting and correcting abnormal lingual surface erosion or attritional wear. (REF. 46-p. 52)

555. B. The principle known as extension for prevention occurs in smooth surface caries. The restoration should be extended to areas that are normally self-cleansing in order to prevent a recurrence of the caries lesion. The principle is generally broadened to encompass the removal of enamel defects such as pits and fissures on occlusal surfaces of premolars and molars and on the occlusal two-thirds of the facial and lingual surfaces of molars. (REF. 46-p. 55)

556. D. Preparing a cervical cavity and restoration to stop abrasion in the gingival one-third of the crown is often indicated when the exposed dentin in the abraded region is

sensitive and this sensitivity fails to respond to sodium silico-fluoride or where the pulp is in jeopardy if additional dentin is lost due to tooth brushing. (REF. 46-p. 55)

557. D. The use of pinholes or slots in the dentin helps to provide the desired retention form for gold inlay preparations which must cap all of the cusps. Pinholes are cut by a 0.6 mm twist drill with the lip of each hole beveled by the No. 2 bur. (REF. 46-p. 69)

558. B. A 0.6 mm twist drill is used at ultra low speed (500-1000 rpm) for cutting the pinholes which should be cut to depth of 2 mm. The holes should be started with a No. 1/2 or No. 1/4 carbide bur. (REF. 46-p. 73)

559. F. Often it appears necessary for retention purposes to prepare a pinhole on the gingival floor in addition to the incisal pinhole. The gingival pinhole should be cut parallel to the incisal pinhole and have a depth of 1 mm. The gingival pinhole is cut in dentin and must never undermine the enamel on the gingival floor. The axial wall of the cavity preparation must be properly positioned and deep enough pulpally to allow the correct location of the pinhole. (REF. 46-pp. 77, 78)

560. B. The proper position and shallowness of the pinhole should eliminate any danger of perforating the pulp or root surface. (REF. 46-p. 81)

561. E. Moisten the teeth slightly with saliva, and fill the tray with alginate. Apply the alginate tray over the region. After the alginate is set, remove the impression in a quick pull in the direction of draw of the cavity preparation. Pour this impression with fast-setting plaster. (REF. 46-pp. 88, 92)

562. E. Operative dentistry relates to diagnosis, prognosis, and treatment of teeth with vital or nonvital pulps and to maintenance or restoration of the functional and physiologic integrity of the teeth including the adjacent hard and soft tissue structures of the oral cavity. (REF. 56-p. 114)

563. D. Teeth may not be recognized immediately as being fractured. However, they will present a history of discomfort brought on by mastication. Positive findings are

absent after repeated oral examinations. Pain may be mild to severe depending upon the degree of pulpal inflammation. The diagnosis of the fractured tooth is frequently made after all other conditions have been eliminated. (REF. 46-p. 138)

564. E. Pain upon release of a fractured tooth is a noteworthy symptom of a fracture. This test must be repeated several times and upon different areas of the occlusal surface of the tooth before pain is produced. (REF. 46-p. 139)

565. B. In the case of a severe tooth fracture, pain is elicited upon prying into the fracture line, and the one portion of the tooth will move away from the other. In some cases, it is necessary to employ a 1/4 or 1/2 inch rubber wheel placed between the cusps to diagnose a tooth fracture. (REF. 46-p. 139)

566. B. The depth of a fracture pulpally is often highly difficult to determine. Thus the prognosis of any restoration for treatment of the fracture is questionable. (REF. 46-p. 142)

567. C. Carving the amalgam should be accomplished to contours desired in the finished restoration with a slight excess for subsequent finishing and polishing. The operator must never fail to carve the amalgam back to the cavity margin since failing to accomplish this will leave thin portions of material lying on the external enamel surface. (REF. 46-p. 162)

568. E. Carving the occlusal portion of the enamel may be commenced immediately following condensation while the matrix band remains in place. Sharp discoid instruments are to be recommended as carvers. The larger discoid instruments should be used first, followed by the smaller ones in regions no longer accessible to larger instruments. (REF. 46-p. 168)

569. E. Carving on the proximal surface should be at a minimum when the matrix is properly applied. Very small amounts of excess amalgam may be present at the facial and lingual margins and at the faciogingival and linguogingival. Check the gingival margin with the side of the explorer. If excess is found, remove it with amalgam knives. (REF. 46-p. 168)

570. D. Cohesive gold foil is pure gold foil or crystal gold that will weld at room temperature under pressure. Cohesive gold foil, mat gold, and Goldent are the major kinds of cohesive gold in use today for operative dentistry. (REF. 46-p. 175)

571. A. Since gold foil welds into a single mass in the annealed state, the manufacturer exposes the gold foil to ammonia gas to prevent cohesion of ropes and pellets during packaging and shipment. The original cohesiveness can be restored readily by annealing in the dental office as the gold foil is used. (REF. 46-p. 175)

572. E. Mechanical condensation can be accomplished by use of the automatic hand mallet since it releases a spring-loaded blow when pressure is applied parallel to its long axis. The pneumatic condenser provides repeated blows by compressed air as long as the condenser point is held against the gold foil with hand pressure. High frequency-low intensity Electromallet also provides repeated blows when the condenser point is held against the gold foil with hand pressure. (REF. 46-p. 177)

573. E. Restorations of cavities for Class III cavities requires the following: the area to be restored must be small or moderate in size, the incisal angle must remain strong, and esthetic requirements must be satisfied. (REF. 46-p. 178)

574. E. Goldent is the name of a new type of cohesive gold developed at the School of Dentistry, Loma Linda University, California. Goldent appears to be a core of gold dust or powdered gold enclosed in a thin layer of cohesive gold foil. (REF. 46-pp. 179, 180)

575. C. Pure gold is inherently cohesive. However, the sheets removed from the Gold Beater's Skins are considered noncohesive. The degree of cohesiveness depends upon the amount of moisture and volatile or nonvolatile substances absorbed upon the surface of the gold. (REF. 46-p. 181)

576. D. Objectives of gold foil condensation are to take advantage of the malleability of the gold and the elasticity of the dentin to produce a dense restoration that is adapted to the cavity walls and margins. Proper condensation will

result in a restoration that is wedged firmly against the walls of the cavity preparation and that presents a finished surface free of voids. (REF. 46-p. 182)

577. C. Proper gold foil condensation does not require blows of great magnitude and only slight adjustment of the condensation force is necessary within the range of condenser points recommended for most gold foil insertions. Where many adjustments must be made during an insertion, it represents an undesired obstacle for any gold foil condensation. (REF. 46-p. 182)

578. E. The gold foil restoration is finished with a gold file (Rhein trimmer) using a pull action to reduce the facial excess of gold down to the margins. These gold files reduce the gold foil as well as burnish and case harden the foil. The airbrasive technique is capable of reducing hard tooth structures without perceptible vibration, pressure, or heat by a stream of abrasive particles traveling at a high velocity. Histologic studies of pulpal reactions fail to demonstrate any significant damage. (REF. 46-p. 185)

579. E. Dental plaque accumulation is a chronic problem requiring repeated attention by the patient and dentist/hygienist. The control of dental plaque is the most important factor in the successful control of periodontal health. (REF. 92-p. 3)

580. E. It is generally taken for granted that the patient has been instructed in proper oral hygiene procedures and uses them adequately before undertaking the procedures of root planing and gingival curettage. Only in this way is the success of the periodontal procedure possible. (REF. 92-p. 36)

581. A. Root planing and subgingival curettage can be used for pocket reduction and control, to reduce inflammation prior to restorative dentistry, to reduce inflammation prior to other surgical periodontal procedures, to evaluate tissue response, as compromise therapy, and in acute periodontal disease (in a limited manner). (REF. 92-p. 51)

582. E. Not all malocclusions are detrimental. Orthodontics is utilized if the bone level is excellent and the patient has no evidence of wear or temporomandibular joint pain. The attachment apparatus of adults differs from that of the adolescent. (REF. 92-p. 76)

583. E. Comprehensive management of pathologic occlusions requires that the dentist evaluate the dentition as the dynamic system that it truly represents. The objectives remain the restoring and maintaining of the dentition in function, comfort, and health. (REF. 92-p. 84)

584. E. Dentists can achieve satisfactory results using electrosurgery for all of these effective treatments. The gingival tissues may be reshaped satisfactorily by the application of electrosurgery. (REF. 96-p. 112)

585. E. Long-term success in restorative dentistry requires that a healthy periodontium be restored around the teeth. Restorations, however, should be prepared in the presence of mucogingival problems and periodontal disease. (REF. 92-p. 122)

586. E. Mucogingival surgery is necessary for the proper preparation of the mouth for restorative dentistry. Follow-up oral examinations are necessary over the life of the patient in order to continue the adequacy of the gingival tissues supporting restorations. (REF. 92-p. 128)

587. A. The ultimate goal of osseous surgery is the retention of the dentition in a state of health and function. The proper procedures can only be performed if a correct diagnosis and treatment plan have been formulated.

588. C. Osseous resective techniques are excellent means of treating shallow one- and two-wall infrabony defects. Condemned teeth, however, should be extracted in the early stages of initial therapy in order to avoid exacerbations during the latter phases of treatment. Early removal of condemned teeth also facilitates the treatment of adjacent teeth and frequently minimizes the pockets associated with these teeth. Restorative dentistry can only be successful if placed on sound supporting structures. (REF. 92-p. 144)

589. B. The indications for osseous grafts are deep intraosseous defects, regeneration required to retain tooth, juvenile periodontosis, gain support for critical teeth, esthetics in cases of shallow intraosseous defects, anatomical limitations for other procedures, grafting other sites, root sensitivity problems, and time flexibility. The likelihood of osseous regeneration is predicated on the morphology of the defect. (REF. 92-p. 162)

590. A. Pulpal therapy eliminates the diseased pulpal tissue which is spilling inflammatory exudates and products into the periodontal ligament. Interceptive pulpal therapy is undertaken when the actuarial experience projects that a tooth with such clinical and x-ray findings will precipitate into a pulpal-periodontal problem. (REF. 92-p. 224)

591. E. It is always desirable to create a cleansable area to allow and encourage patients to keep the embrasure area relatively free of bacterial plaque. If the operator is unable to produce adequate embrasure areas during fabrication of restorations, the need for increased tooth reduction is thus evident. (REF. 92-p. 248)

592. C. Bone loss in the bifurcation or trifurcation area is the most common reason for performing root amputations. In instances where the bone loss is rather extensive, a flap is not required and the root is quickly and efficiently removed and the crown of the remaining tooth is contoured. (REF. 92-p. 298)

593. B. The increased surface area made available provides for denture base stability. The combination of tooth-to-bone support and satisfactorily recorded soft-tissue support helps to minimize the traumatic effect of excessive force on the residual ridge. (REF. 92-p. 307)

594. E. Overdentures, however, are not indicated for individuals who constantly fail to have an acceptable level of oral hygiene and do not practice plaque control. Overdentures are contraindicated for those individuals who have unrealistic expectations of the function of prosthodontic appliances. (REF. 92-p. 308)

Chapter 11 Oral Pharmacology

595. C. A drug is a substance used for the treatment or diagnosis of a disease or to modify a physiologic body process. Drugs are produced from animal, plant, or mineral sources. Some drugs are now synthesized; other drugs are extracted from plants, microorganisms, or tissues. (REF. 23-p. 11)

596. A. The essential information to put on a prescription includes the following: name and address of dentist prescriber, name and address of patient, date, preparation, form and quantity to be dispensed, instructions, and dentist's signature. The dentist should always use the official name of the drug. (REF. 23-p. 24)

597. E. Schedule 2 drugs can be prescribed by dentists. However, in practice few schedule 2 drugs are actually prescribed by the dentist. The dentist's Bureau of Narcotics and Dangerous Drugs (BNDD) number must be indicated on the prescription. (REF. 23-p. 26)

598. D. Local anesthesia is equivalent to local analgesia. Local anesthetic agents act by blocking the rapid inflow of sodium ions essential for transmission of the nerve impulse across the nerve cell membrane. Local anesthetic agents act selectively on sensory fibers because these fibers are smaller in diameter compared to motor fibers and hence more sensitive to the blocking action of drugs acting on the cell membrane. (REF. 23-p. 42)

599. D. General anesthesia is a state of unconsciousness in which the subject cannot be roused by external stimuli. The depth of anesthesia is such that pain is abolished but must be controllable in depth and must be reversible. (REF. 23-p. 43)

600. C. Examples of analgesics are aspirin, acetaminophen, mefenamic acid, phenylbutazone, indomethacin and its analogues, and ibuprofen and its analogues. The problem of analgesic dose-dependent toxicity can sometimes be overcome by combining several analgesic drugs together in small doses. However, it becomes difficult to assess the potency of the analgesic drugs when in combinations, and it is possible that the efficacy of the combination is due to the high total amount of analgesic used. (REF. 23-p. 43)

601. B. Aspirin may cause allergic reactions such as bronchospasm and urticaria. Aspirin therefore should not be given to dental patients with a history of bronchial asthma. Petechial or erythematous rashes are further side effects. However, allergy to aspirin appears to be uncommon. Large doses of aspirin cause tinnitus and temporary deafness. (REF. 23-p. 47)

602. E. Narcotic analgesics are interchangeable with major analgesics and the opiates. The narcotic analgesics include morphine, codeine and their derivatives, and synthetic morphine-like drugs. The latter are powerful analgesics, cough and respiratory depressants, and inhibitors of intestinal motility. Tolerance and dependence develop with all these drugs. Thus, the dose has to be increased, with repeated administration, to maintain the same level of effect and that addiction may accompany this procedure. (REF. 23-p. 55)

603. E. Codeine is a natural alkaloid found in the juice of the unripe seed capsule of the oriental poppy. It is a weaker analgesic compared to morphine. Large doses of codeine cause unpleasant side effects. It is not significantly addictive, but drug abuse has been reported. (REF. 23-p. 57)

604. E. Morphine diminishes the sensation of pain and the emotional response to pain is suppressed. Morphine depresses the rate and depth of respiration by decreasing the sensitivity of the respiratory center to carbon dioxide. Narcotic analgesics are dangerous in patients with lung diseases (chronic bronchitis, asthma, and pneumonia) because of the depression of the rate and depth of respiration. (REF. 23-p. 60)

605. E. Meperidine (pethidine) is a synethetic major analgesic with many of the properties of morphine. It relaxes the smooth muscles of the ureters. Respiration and cough are depressed. This drug produces dizziness and vomiting. Addiction is similar to that of morphine. (REF. 23-p. 60)

606. E. Methadone is a synthetic analgesic similar to morphine in potency and pharmacological activity. It causes smooth muscle spasm. Methadone has less addictive potential than morphine and pethidine (meperidine), but dependence can develop. (REF. 23-p. 62)

607. E. Local anesthetics may stimulate and depress the central nervous system and have toxic effects upon the heart. Local anesthetics in dentistry contain a vasoconstrictor to prevent rapid absorption and give a prolonged effect. Most preparations are safe and effective with uncommon side effects. When side effects occur they are generally due to the vasoconstrictor component. (REF. 23-p. 66)

608. E. Procaine has a short duration of action when given by local infiltration. The main toxic effect of procaine is cerebral stimulation or excitement and restlessness passing on to depression and coma. Hypersensitivity to procaine can develop among dentists who frequently administered this drug. Procaine, however, is obsolete in modern dental practice. (REF. 23-p. 69)

609. E. The purpose of adding a vasoconstrictor to dental local anesthetic agents is to reduce the local circulation at the side of injection in order to prevent the agent from diffusing rapidly. The reduced rate of absorption may minimize the toxic effects when the local anesthetic reaches the general circulation. The most toxic portion of local anesthetics used in dentistry is the vasoconstrictor. (REF. 23-p. 69)

610. B. Felypressin is a more recent vasoconstrictor. The vasoconstrictor produces a relatively bloodless field of operation for the oral surgeon. (REF. 23-p. 70)

611. C. Penicillin is the commonest cause of acute anaphylactic reactions and leads all drugs which cause fatalities in the United States. Penicillin has been so widely used over the years that it has caused many deaths. (REF. 23-p. 73)

612. E. The usefulness of topical anesthetics is highly limited. Topical (surface) anesthetics are used in the form of ointments or sprays to lessen the pain of injection of local anesthetics. Lidocaine has some topical anesthetic action with superficial effectiveness. Cocaine is a highly effective topical analgesic. Topical anesthetics have little effect when the tissues are being torn by the injected fluid. (REF. 23-p. 76)

613. E. General anesthetics mode of action is currently obscure. However, the latter produce a state of altered cerebral and nervous system function. The potency of anesthetic action is related to the degree of alveolar concentration and the factor of solubility. (REF. 23-p. 78)

614. E. The stages of anesthesia are Stage I, analgesia; Stage II, excitement; Stage III, surgical analgesia; and Stage IV, respiratory paralysis or stage of vital arrest. (REF. 23-p. 80)

615. E. Inhalation agents fall into the following categories: gases and volatile liquids. Gases (such as nitrous oxide and cyclopropane) are a heterogeneous collection of agents varying widely in their chemical structure, actions, and potency. Volatile liquids include esthers (diethyl ether and divinyl ether). (REF. 23-p. 82)

616. E. Nitrous oxide was the first anesthetic to be used and is still the safest. It is nontoxic and a weak agent so that it does not depress the medulla with the highest concentration (80% N_2O:20% O_2). When nitrous oxide is used with not less than 20% oxygen it has no adverse actions on the heart, circulation, respiratory tract, liver, or kidneys. Nitrous oxide is a strong analgesic. (REF. 23-p. 86)

617. E. Ether is a classical anesthetic agent. The irritant nature of ether allows only low concentrations to be used at first, and the slow induction may be followed by a long excitement stage. Muscular relaxation is produced in deep anesthesia and is satisfactory for abdominal surgery. It does not cause cardiac arrhythmias or increased myocardial excitability, and the depth of anesthesia can be reliably gauged by the level of reflex activity, eye signs, and depth and rhythm of respiration. (REF. 23-p. 88)

618. E. Barbiturates include thiopentone for intravenous general anesthesia. Thiopentone is widely used and is powerful, inducing unconsciousness rapidly and pleasantly without excitement. It has no analgesic effect in low dosages. Muscular relaxation is poor if the dose is insufficient to give deep anesthesia. Deep anesthesia with thiopentone produces depression of respiration and also of cardiac output. (REF. 23-p. 98)

619. E. The minor tranquilizers (anxiolytic agents) are used to alleviate anxiety, without causing drowsiness. However, there is really sharp demarcation between sedatives and tranquilizers. The most widely used minor tranquilizers are the benzodiazepines (as diazepam). The major tranquilizers are neuroleptics, such as phenothiazines, and are used to suppress psychotic overactivity in the treatment of schizophrenia. (REF. 23-p. 109)

620. E. Acute, disabling depression is a nervous breakdown. Drugs are used extensively for the treatment of depression, and psychotherapy also can be given. There are two main types of antidepressive drugs: tricyclic antidepressants (such as imipramine and amitriptyline) and monoamine oxidase inhibitors (such as nialamide, and phenelzine). (REF. 23-p. 113)

621. E. Antibiotics are substances produced by microorganisms which act in small concentrations to kill other organisms or prevent them from proliferation. The main features of antibiotics are they are substances produced by microorganisms; they act in extreme dilution, they are highly specific in their action, and the specific activity of antibiotics is against microorganisms and not against the host's cells. (REF. 23-p. 124)

622. E. Penicillin G (benzyl penicillin) is a natural penicillin that is mostly destroyed by gastric acid and thus must be given by injection in order to be reliably absorbed. It is not effective against many gram-negative bacilli. However, this is of no consequence since in the mouth these organisms are not important. The relatively narrow spectrum of activity makes super infection less likely to develop. (REF. 23-p. 131)

623. D. Tetracyclines are effective against virtually all common groups of pathogenic bacteria (gram negative and gram positive), mycoplasma, rickettsias, chlamydia, and even against tuberculosis and the malaria parasite. Tetracyclines are bacteriostatic and may be antagonistic to bactericidal drugs, particularly penicillin. The tetracyclines interfere with protein synthesis by bacteria. (REF. 23-p. 134)

624. D. Chloramphenicol is a broad spectrum antibiotic which is bacteriostatic and effective against Salmonella typhi. It is a potent inhibitor of bacterial protein synthesis. The danger of chloramphenicol is its toxic action in the bone marrow. Its use is justifiable only for severe infections when no more effective drug is available. (REF. 23-p. 138)

625. A. Allergic reactions are counteracted by antihistamines (receptor-blockers) which compete with histamine for the receptor sites. Antihistamines are useful for continued control of seasonal hay fever, urticaria, and angio-edema in patients subject to frequently recurring attacks. Antihistamines are of no value in asthma where histamine is not the important mediator of the reaction. (REF. 23-p. 156)

626. B. The main emergencies taking place in the dental office include myocardial infarction, cardiac arrest, anesthetic accidents, acute allergic (anaphylactic) reactions, circulatory collapse in patients on corticosteroid treatment, drug reactions and interactions, epilepsy, acute hypoglycemia, and hemorrhage. (REF. 23-p. 185)

627. E. Essential measures in emergencies in the dental practice are to make sure the patient can breathe, relieve pain, relieve anxiety, be aware and alert to the possibility of an emergency in the dental office. (REF. 23-p. 187)

628. E. As soon as the diagnosis of anaphylactic reaction is made the patient should be laid flat to maintain cerebral blood flow. Epinephrine (1 ml of 1:1000) should be given by intramuscular injection. Adrenaline should be followed immediately by 200 mg of hydrocortisone sodium succinate into a vein. There should be no delay in giving hydrocortisone in the hope that adrenaline alone may be effective. (REF. 23-p. 199)

629. C. Management of patients under systemic corticosteroid treatment should follow these guidelines: major oral surgery must be carried out in the hospital, and minor operations (extractions) should be carried out under local anesthesia; where a brief general anesthetic is required, a corticosteroid must be given prophylactically; for extractions under local anesthesia, 100 mg hydrocortisone

should be given intravenously and repeated if necessary; and patients should be kept under observation for 1-2 hours. (REF. 23-p. 203)

630. E. The main hazards that the dentist may have to face are: myocardial infarction, cardiac arrest, anesthetic accidents, acute allergic (anaphylactic) reactions, circulatory collapse in patients on corticosteroid treatment, drug reactions and interactions, epilepsy, acute hypoglycemia, and hemorrhage. (REF. 23-p. 207)

631. E. As soon as the diagnosis of anaphylactic reaction is made, the patient should be laid flat to maintain cerebral blood flow. Adrenalin (1 ml of 1:1000) should be injected intramuscularly, making sure to withdraw the plunger and make certain that the needle is not in a vein. Follow the adrenalin immediately with 200 mg hydrocortisone sodium succinate intravenously. Adrenalin acts rapidly but is short-lived. Hydrocortisone maintains the blood pressure for several hours, and its use is essential for such cases. (REF. 23-p. 211)

632. D. A substance (as acetylcholine) which binds to a receptor and then stimulates is an "agonist." However, a substance which binds to a receptor and then has no action (except preventing agonists from reaching the receptor) is called an "antagonist." (REF. 24-p. 31)

633. E. In Stage 1, analgesia is not complete. In Stage 2, the patient is unconscious, reflexes are intact, and there may be automatic movements. Stage 3 is divided into four planes of increasing depth, and reflex activity and muscle tone are progressively lost. Stage 4 must never be reached. It is due to overdosage and immediate resuscitative measures must be started. (REF. 24-p. 58)

634. C. Adverse effects from halothane affect the cardiovascular system (depression of blood pressure) and liver function (jaundice and postoperative hepatitis). Halothane is not proven to cause hepatitis; hepatitis, however, is likely to follow several administrations at short intervals. (REF. 24-P. 68)

635. E. Complications of thiopental anesthesia are laryngeal spasm, extra-vascular injection, intra-arterial injection, and overdose. Thiopental, however, is safe and useful in skilled hands. (REF. 23-p. 70)

636. E. Di-vinyl ether produces rapid induction, analgesia, good muscle relaxation and rapid recovery. It is only suitable for short anesthetics; however, this agent is obsolete today. (REF. 23-p. 72)

Chapter 12 Complete Denture Prosthodontics

637. C. The basis for determining when a complete denture has failed is the following: Is it compatible with the surrounding oral environment? Is there a restoration of masticatory efficiency within realistic limits? Is there harmony with the functions of speech, respiration, and deglutition; is there esthetic acceptability? Is there preservation of the supporting tissues. (REF. 25-p. 391)

638. D. Diagnosis in complete dentures is a continuous process and not accomplished in one short visit. The full evaluation in many patients may occur when the planned treatment nears completion. (REF. 25-p. 101)

639. D. Treatment for complete dentures does not terminate with the construction and delivery of the dentures, and the patient should be advised of this fact. (REF. 25-p. 101)

640. C. This bony growth is present on the lingual cortical surface of the mandible. The tori should be removed prior to denture construction, as a relief in the denture base is rarely satisfactory treatment. Generally the patient will not tolerate the denture with the torus in place. (REF. 25-p. 145)

641. A. The anterior sulcus extension begins from slightly anterior to the mental foramen to the same relative position on the opposite side of the arch. Surgical correction of the denture-bearing area is accomplished by the following: the anterior sulcus slide and the reverse anterior sulcus slide, the mucosal graft. (REF. 25-p. 158)

642. A. The anatomy of the TMJ allows some freedom of movement, but not random and freely swinging movements. The TMJ has a high degree of adjustability which varies greatly within different individuals. (REF. 25-p. 24)

643. D. The Bennett movement is the bodily lateral movement of lateral shift of the mandible resulting from the movements of the condyles along the lateral inclines of the mandibular fossae in lateral jaw movements. Bennett movement, like all other movements from the centric occlusion position, is important if teeth contact or are in gliding occlusion as they move from and to centric occlusion or if clearance is provided to avoid contact. (REF. 25-p. 24)

644. A. Occlusal harmony in complete dentures is necessary if the dentures are to be comfortable, to function efficiently, and to preserve the supporting structures. It is difficult to find occlusal discrepancies intraorally with complete dentures. (REF. 25-p. 378)

645. D. Patients are seldom aware of faulty occlusion in complete dentures. However, the patient knows when the dentist makes an improvement by correcting the faulty occlusion. The eye cannot be relied upon to observe occlusal discrepancies and the patient cannot be depended upon to diagnose faulty occlusion. (REF. 25-p. 378)

646. D. There are many intraoral methods for correcting occlusal disharmony. The intraoral methods are more accurate if the uneven contacting of the teeth has been first corrected with laboratory remount and patient remount procedures. The intraoral methods include articulating paper, central-bearing devices, occlusal wax, abrasive paste, and patient remount and selective grinding. (REF. 25-p. 379)

647. C. Rugae are raised areas of dense connective tissue radiating from the median suture in the anterior one-third of the palate. The area is a secondary bearing area, as it resists anterior displacement of the denture. (REF. 25-p. 176)

648. D. The following represent objectives for complete dentures: preservation, support, stability, esthetics, retention, atmospheric pressure, adhesions, cohesion, mechanical locks, muscle control, and patient tolerance. (REF. 25-p. 179)

649. D. The external oblique line appears as a slight groove. (REF. 25-p. 179)

650. A. The lingual tuberosity forms a light depression or fossa in the mandible. (REF. 25-p. 179)

651. A. Inflammatory fibrous hyperplasia and hypertrophy of the alveolar mucosa is the result of denture irritation and is frequently present about the anterior vestibule when the patient has natural mandibular anterior teeth opposing a complete maxillary denture. Papillomatosis is frequently present under ill-fitting maxillary complete dentures, especially those having an unnecessary relief chamber. (REF. 25-p. 148)

652. A. Centric jaw relation is the jaw relation when the condyles are in the most posterior, unstrained position in the glenoid fossa at any given degree of jaw separation from which lateral movement can be made. It is the most posterior relation of the mandible to the maxillae at the established vertical dimension. It is the relation of the mandible to the maxillae when the condyles are in their most posterior position in the glenoid fossa from which unstrained lateral movements can be made at the occluding vertical dimension normal for the individual. (REF. 25-p. 512)

653. E. A natural positioning of teeth will prevent defective speech by permitting the tongue and lips to function in a natural method during the production of linguodental and labiodental sounds. Natural positioning of artificial teeth is a vital factor in both phonetics and esthetics. (REF. 25-p. 155)

654. A. Placing artificial teeth in the position of their natural predecessors reproduces the natural appearance of both the teeth and lips. One common error is to place artificial teeth too far lingually in order to approximate the ridge because an unnatural appearance of the teeth and lips will result. (REF. 25-p. 163)

655. D. The positions of the teeth in a full denture bear a direct relationship to abuse of the denture-supporting tissues because the tooth positions have a direct effect on the stability of the denture during function. (REF. 25-p. 356)

656. B. A stable denture means minimum movement in a horizontal plane. When an imbalance in occlusion causes a denture to move in a horizontal plane, bone loss can be the result. (REF. 25-p. 99)

657. B. A balanced occlusion is important between teeth during all movements of the mandible and in every possible position to insure stability of the complete dentures. (REF. 25-p. 211)

658. B. Stability can be complemented by centralizing the forces of occlusion as close to the geometric center of the denture base as possible, (REF. 25-p. 128)

659. C. In compromising for stability it is necessary to place the predominant forces of occlusion in about the second bicuspid to first molar area. Placing only slight or no contact between the anterior teeth enhances centralization and torques that follow hypercontact between the anterior teeth. (REF. 25-p. 245)

660. A. The orientation of the plane of occlusion should be parallel to the crest of the edentulous ridge in order for the forces of occlusion to be directed at right angles to the ridge. The mandibular plane of occlusion should be slightly below the level of the tongue in order to minimize the opportunity for the tongue to lift the denture and to favor the action of the tongue in keeping food on the occlusal table. (REF. 25-p. 233)

661. E. If the patient's normal tongue position is to assume a position of retraction, then the stability and retention of the lower denture will be adversely affected. The patient should be taught tongue exercises in order to regain or establish the normal tongue position. Normally when the mouth is slightly open the tongue should fully occupy the floor of the mouth with the tip of the tongue covering the lingual surfaces of the mandibular anterior teeth with the dorsum of the tongue above the occlusal plane. (REF. 25-pp. 245, 246)

662. E. The recording of the mandibular position of centric relation for complete dentures is absolutely vital to a position opposing artificial teeth in harmonious, maximum intercuspation at centric relation and is a requirement for preservation. At centric occlusion are the initial and

terminal contact points of the masticatory cycle and the bracing point of the mandible for swallowing. (REF. 25-p. 257)

663. E. Nearly 50% of edentulous and partially edentulous patients have unsuspected lesions revealed by survey radiographs of the jaws. One-third have oral conditions requiring surgical intervention. Females are more likely to have retained roots and oral lesions compared to males. Radiographic examination is vital in the edentulous patients, but it is not necessary to purchase the panoramic radiographic equipment in order to make the diagnosis. (REF. 26-p. 79)

664. E. A ridge form may increase in dimension after initial contours are measured indicating that a process of growth and development occurs in the edentulous ridges of the maxilla and mandible. (REF. 26-p. 131)

665. C. Most complete denture problems are related to depleted bone support, which is generally accompanied by friable mucosa and altered neuromuscular control. (REF. 26-p. 339)

666. E. Stable dentures produce high pressures on the supporting tissues and transmit these pressures from region to region, varying the denture use. Nonmasticatory pressures produced under dentures are as great or greater than masticatory pressures. (REF. 26-p. 344)

667. D. Subclinical signs of mandibular dysfunction are common in young adults, but the awareness of symptoms is of less frequency. The most common manifestations of dysfunction are tenderness in the lateral pterygoid muscles plus sounds in the temporomandibular joint. (REF. 27-p. 45)

668. B. Overdentures appear to exhibit better retention than complete dentures. The tooth roots offer more discrete discriminatory input than the oral mucosa. Therefore, the periodontal ligament plays a role in the efficiency of muscular activity during chewing in patients wearing over dentures. (REF. 27-p. 143)

669. C. The use of splints increases vertical dimension and establishes a new postural position of the mandible and a new interocclusal distance. The splints reduce postural muscle activity but do not alter activity during maximal closing or swallowing. (REF. 27-p. 266)

670. B. Artificial teeth on complete dentures should be placed in the approximate positions occupied by the natural teeth. (REF. 27-p. 310)

671. A. Acrylic resin teeth wear down faster than porcelain teeth, but the total wear of resin-to-porcelain teeth is not less than resin-to-resin teeth. Porcelain-opposing porcelain teeth have the least wear. (REF. 27-p. 339)

672. B. Narrower teeth appear to be less traumatic for patients than wider teeth on complete dentures. There are no significant differences in the rates of residual ridge reduction between patients given dentures made by a complex technique involving a fully balanced occlusion and those given dentures made by a standard method. (REF. 27-p. 339)

673. E. The lower posterior teeth should be set directly over the lower ridge. They should not be placed on the part of the denture base lying over the posterior part of the mandibular ridge that curves upward to the ascending ramus. The optimum position for the lower incisors can be found by replacing the anterior segment of the record block with a moldable substance and asking the patient to speak with both upper and lower record blocks in the mouth. The upper block should be carved to restore the lips and cheeks to their prior positions before the lower incisors are set in place. (REF. 27-p. 341)

674. A. An average or smaller Bennett side shift is compatible with the use of semiadjustable articulators. The important relationship between cusp form and Bennett shift is not adequately understood by dentists and generally results in excessive occlusal adjustment. The reduction of the lower buccal cusps is useful because it diminishes options for lateral movement interferences when the Bennett shift exceeds the mean variance in shift distance. (REF. 27-p. 371)

675. E. The prognosis of a maxillofacial prosthesis will be improved by the use of a gentle resilient lining material for retention of the prostheses. A long-lasting resilient lining material is useful under clinical conditions. (REF. 50-p. 3)

676. E. Various implants, properly constructed and fitted accompanied by mature patient evaluation, can be successful for a considerable time. Most implants have been fitted by private dental practitioners and the subject of implants is highly controversial. (REF. 50-p. 20)

677. E. However, the most common defect-producing disease is oral and facial cancer. The surgical procedures required to eradicate or control cancer produces typical defects in the maxillary and mandibular arches. Congenital oral defects occur as a result of incomplete formation of a body part and exist before or at birth. (REF. 93-p. 11)

678. A. If the anatomy of the patient is restored without allowing him or her to function in society, the validity of the restoration is questionable. The causative mechanism of the patient's disease may be in part sociologic or psychologic. The patient, therefore, may well require adjunctive psychosocial assessment and assistance to help him or her to accept the problem and the maxillofacial prosthesis. (REF. 93-p. 21)

679. C. Cineradiographic films and videofluoroscopic techniques can be useful for direct visualization of the movements of the temporomandibular joints, the tongue, and the palatopharyngeal structures. Examination of the maxillofacial prosthetic patient can never be too extensive since the prognosis for rehabilitation is based upon the diagnosis. (REF. 93-p. 66)

680. B. Design of the guide-flange prosthesis is similar to the design of other types of removable prostheses. Support is the same as that of any removal prosthesis, the natural teeth and the residual alveolar ridge are the primary areas of support. Retention, however, should be distributed as widely as humanly possible to avoid considerable force being applied to the retentive structures. (REF. 93-p. 108)

681. E. Loss of extensive structure in the maxillary arch can result in oronasal or oroantral communication for which surgical or artificial closure must be considered. Surgical closure often necessitates the use of labial or buccal mucosa which obliterates the vestibule and creates a potential problem for the design of a prosthesis and the placement of artificial teeth. (REF. 93-p. 117)

682. E. All teeth that are to be used as abutments or overload must be adequately protected. Particularly in the case of the patient with a cleft palate, preservation of all maxillary teeth is extremely important for the conservation of bone tissue and the provision of support for the prosthesis. Malposed or supernumerary teeth that compromise maintenance should be considered for extraction. (REF. 93-p. 176)

683. E. A controversy has been centered on radiation sequelae produced by orthovoltage, i. e., intracavitary or interstitial therapy. The rationale for dental treatment of the patient irradiated with supervoltage or megavoltage therapy is not the same as that when external orthovoltage radiation is utilized. (REF. 93-p. 188)

684. E. Osteoradionecrosis is the major complication of irradiation to the head and neck. A significantly greater frequency of osteoradio-necrosis occurs in the mandible compared to the maxilla. The latter is due to an impaired mandibular blood supply. A controversy exists concerning the rationale for the preirradiation or postirradiation removal of the teeth to reduce the possibility of osteoradionecrosis. Another controversy concerns the postirradiation use of a removable denture prosthesis. (REF. 93-p. 193)

685. E. Splints may be designed and adapted for use in special circumstances, such as therapeutic devices for the physically handicapped. (REF. 93-p. 216)

686. B. Manipulation of the plane of orientation and cusp height is desirable to reduce interference in lateral excursion. Bilateral balanced occlusion in eccentric movements is not necessary when the natural teeth support the maxillofacial restorations. (REF. 93-p. 266)

687. E. Biocompatibility is of major importance for a prosthetic material; however, the prosthesis must also be easy and inexpensive to fabricate. The finished prosthesis should be skin-like in touch and appearance. Materials utilized must not irritate the tissues and yet should be strong enough about the periphery to endure. (REF. 93-p. 281)

688. E. Facial prostheses have been retained with mechanical devices. Most patients, however, may be served best by the use of a suitable adhesive for retention of the facial prostheses. (REF. 93-p. 305)

689. B. A removable partial denture is designed so that it can be removed conveniently from the mouth and replaced by the patient. A removable partial denture either may be entirely tooth supported or may derive its support from both the teeth and the tissues of the residual ridge. The denture base of a tooth-borne removable partial denture derives its support from abutment teeth at each end of the edentulous area. (REF. 32-p. 4)

690. D. The dentist should be responsible for the design of the partial denture framework from the beginning to the finish. The dentist is accountable for providing the technician with all of the information needed to construct the partial denture. (REF. 32-p. 5)

691. D. For the distal extension partial denture, a base made to fit the anatomic ridge form does not provide adequate support under occlusal loading. Therefore, some type of correction impression is necessary. (REF. 32-p. 6)

692. B. Kennedy's method of classification is probably the most widely accepted classification of partially edentulous arches. (REF. 32-p. 11)

693. E. The classification of a partially edentulous arch should satisfy the following: it should permit immediate visualization of the type of partially edentulous arch being considered; it should permit immediate differentiation between the tooth-borne and tooth-tissue-supported removable partial denture; and it should be universally acceptable. (REF. 32-p. 12)

694. D. Applegate provided eight rules governing the application of the Kennedy method. (REF. 32-p. 13)

695. C. A typical removable partial denture will have the following components: major connector, minor connectors, rests, direct retainers, reciprocal or stabilizing components, indirect retainers, and one or more bases, each supporting one to several replacement teeth. (REF. 32-p. 26)

696. D. The major connector should be located in a favorable relation to moving tissues and at the same time should avoid impingement of gingival tissues. It also should be located so that areas of bony and tissue prominence are not encountered during placement and removal of the denture. (REF. 32-p. 25)

697. B. The occlusal rest should be designed so that transmitted forces are directed along the long axis of the supporting tooth as nearly as possible. A rest must be placed so that it will prevent movement of the restoration in a cervical direction. (REF. 32-p. 26)

698. B. Most impression materials for removable partial dentures are rigid materials, thermoplastic materials, and elastic materials. Elastic materials include reversible and irreversible hydrocolloids, Mercaptan rubber-base impression materials, and silicone impression materials. (REF. 32-p. 37)

699. C. An impression of the partially edentulous arch must record accurately the anatomic form of the teeth and surrounding tissues. The latter is required before a partial denture may be designed to follow a definite path of placement and removal and also so that the support and retention on the abutment teeth may be precise and accurate. (REF. 32-p. 39)

700. E. Elastic materials are the only ones that can be withdrawn from tooth and tissue undercuts without permanent deformation and the only impression materials suitable for impressions of irregular contours of oral tissues. The elastic materials are most commonly used for the making of impressions for partial dentures. (REF. 32-p. 45)

701. E. A dental surveyor is an instrument used to determine the relative parallelism of two or more surfaces of the teeth or other parts of the cast of a dental arch. The surveyor is used for surveying the cast, recontouring abutment teeth on the cast, contouring wax patterns, measuring a specific depth of undercut, surveying ceramic veneer crowns, placing the intracoronal retainers, placing internal rests, machining casts restorations, and surveying and blocking out the master cast. (REF. 32-p. 98)

702. C. The path of placement is the direction in which a restoration moves from the point of initial contact of its rigid parts with the supporting teeth to the terminal resting position, with rests seated and the denture base in contact with the tissues. (REF. 32-p. 101)

703. C. The path of removal is the reverse of the path of placement, since it is the direction of restoration movement from its terminal resting position of the last contact of its rigid parts with the supporting teeth. (REF. 32-p. 101)

704. E. Esthetics should not be the primary factor in partial denture design. Replacement of missing anterior teeth should be accomplished by means of fixed restorations whenever possible, rather than permitting their replacement to influence the mechanical and functional effectiveness of the partial denture. (REF. 32-p. 104)

705. E. The partial denture must be designed so that it will not stress abutment teeth beyond their physiologic tolerance, can be easily placed and removed by the patient, will be retained against reasonable dislodging forces, and will not create an unfavorable appearance. (REF. 32-p. 105)

706. E. Failures of partial dentures, other than structural defects, can generally be attributed to poor and inadequate diagnosis, failure to properly evaluate the conditions present, and failure to prepare the patient and his mouth properly prior to construction of the master cast. (REF. 32-p. 114)

707. E. Consideration of caries susceptibility is of primary importance. The number of restored teeth present, any signs of recurrent caries, and evidence of decalcification

should be noted. During the oral examination each arch should be considered separately but also its occlusal relationship with the opposing arch. (REF. 32-p. 114)

708. E. The number of teeth remaining, the location of the edentulous areas, and the quality of the residual ridge will have a definite bearing on the proportionate amount of support that the partial denture will receive from the teeth and the edentulous ridges. (REF. 32-p. 119)

709. E. The objectives of a complete intraoral roentgenographic examination are to locate areas of infection and pathology; to reveal the presence of root fragments, foreign objects, bone spicules, and irregular ridge formations; to reveal the presence and extent of caries and the relation of the carious lesion to the pulp; to permit evaluation of existing restorations as to evidence of recurrent caries, marginal leakage, and overhanging gingival margins; to reveal the presence of root canal fillings; to evaluate periodontal conditions present and to establish the need and possibilities for treatment; and to evaluate the alveolar support of abutment teeth. (REF. 32-p. 121)

710. D. Mouth preparation must be accomplished prior to the impression procedures that will produce the master cast upon which the denture will be constructed. Oral surgical and periodontal procedures should precede abutment tooth preparations. A period of at least six weeks to three months should be provided between oral surgery and restorative dentistry procedures. (REF. 32-p. 129)

711. E. Failure to provide and maintain adequate occlusion on the partial denture is primarily due to lack of support for the denture base and the fallacy of establishing occlusion to a single static jaw relation record only. (REF. 32-p. 140)

712. A. Resin and porcelain veneer crowns are used because of cosmetic reasons on abutment teeth that would otherwise display an objectionable amount of metal. (REF. 32-p. 151)

713. D. Frequently a tooth is too weak to use by itself as an abutment for a partial denture because of its short length or tapered single root. In such cases multiple abutment and/or splinting of weak abutment teeth to the adjacent

tooth or teeth is utilized as a means of gaining multiple abutment support. Thus two single-rooted teeth may serve as a multirooted abutment. (REF. 32-p. 151)

714. C. Splinting should not be used to retain a tooth that would otherwise be condemned for periodontal reasons in the hope that the tooth may be retained. The latter is futile and unjustified. A gamble may be justified when, if successful, the need for a prosthetic restoration would be avoided. (REF. 32-p. 151)

715. D. The distal extension partial denture does not have the advantage of total tooth support, since one or more bases are extensions onto the residual ridge from the last available abutment. It is, therefore, dependent on the residual ridge for a portion of its support. (REF. 32-p. 159)

716. E. Support from the residual ridge becomes greater as the distance from the last abutment increases and will depend on several factors: quality of residual ridge, extent of residual ridge coverage by the denture base, type and accuracy of the impression registration, accuracy of the denture base, design of the partial framework, and total occlusal load applied. (REF. 32-p. 161)

717. A. In the case of the tooth-supported base which is secured at either end by the action of a direct retainer and supported at either end by a rest, this degree of support and direct retention are lacking in the distal extension restoration. For this reason, a distal abutment should be preserved whenever possible. (REF. 32-p. 160)

718. D. The broader the residual ridge coverage by the denture base, the greater is the distribution of the load, thereby resulting in less load per unit area. A denture base should cover as much of the residual ridge as possible and be extended the maximum amount within the physiologic tolerance of the limiting border structures or tissues. (REF. 32-p. 165)

719. D. An occlusal rest should be designed so that the transmitted forces are directed along the long axis of the supporting tooth as nearly as possible. A rest must be placed so that it will prevent movement of the restoration in a cervical direction. (REF. 32-p. 171)

720. E. It is through the rigidity of the major connector that all other component parts of the partial denture may be effective. The major connectors must be located in favorable relation to moving tissues and must avoid impingement of gingival tissues. (REF. 32-p.174)

721. D. Relief of free gingival margins must be provided for any component of the framework, plus the denture bases. The lingual bar should be used for mandibular removable dentures where sufficient space exists between the elevated alveolar lingual sulcus and the lingual gingival tissues to place a rigid bar. (REF. 32-p. 177)

722. E. True adjustment is impossible with most cast clasps. Despite this disadvantage, the cast circumferential clasp arm may be used effectively, and many of these disadvantages may be minimized by proper design. Adequate preparations will permit its point of origin to be far below the occlusal surfaces to avoid bad esthetics and increased tooth dimension. (REF. 32-p. 187)

723. C. Stress breakers (stress equalizers) or articulated prosthesis is applied to a broken-stress partial denture. The subject of stress breakers is a controversial one today. It is only the improperly designed or ineffectively fabricated rigid restoration that has proved to be harmful to abutment teeth. Some form of mechanical stress breaker is preferable to a poorly designed and ineffectively fabricated rigid restoration. (REF. 34-pp. 7, 109)

724. E. Indications for removable partial dentures include: distal extension situations as the use of a cantilevered fixed restoration and replacement of missing posterior teeth without the assistance of a posterior abutment; after recent extractions; in cases of a long span; when esthetics is desired in the anterior region; where there is excessive loss of bone (residual), where there is unusually sound abutment teeth; and for economic considerations. (REF. 34-pp. 8, 12, 186)

725. E. The following data should be on record as the result of the oral examination and diagnosis: the patient's present and predictable future health status, periodontal conditions that are present throughout the mouth, oral hygiene habits, caries activity, the need for surgery or extractions, the need for fixed restorations for toothbounded spaces, the need for occlusal correction, the need for

periodontal consultation and treatment, the need for orthodontic treatment of malposed and disarranged teeth, the need for restorations elsewhere in either arch, and the selection of the type of mandibular major connector. (REF. 34-pp. 161-166)

726. E. Failures of removable partial dentures are due to structural defects, inadequate diagnosis, failure to properly evaluate the conditions present, and failure to prepare the patient and his or her mouth properly prior to construction of the master cast. (REF. 34-pp. 2, 422)

727. E. A partial denture made from a one-piece impression places the masticatory load only on the abutment teeth and that part of the bone that underlies the distal end of the extension base. The balance of the bony ridge will not function in carrying the load. The result will be a traumatic load to the bone underlying the distal end of the base and to the abutment tooth, which will result in bone loss and loosening of the abutment tooth. (REF. 34-pp. 273-412)

728 E. Denture bases should be designed and fabricated so that they will provide the greatest possible retention to the partial denture. Retention of denture bases is the result of the following types of forces: adhesion, cohesion, atmospheric pressure, the plastic molding of the tissues around the polished surfaces of the denture, and the effect of gravity on the mandibular denture. (REF. 34-pp. 118, 119)

729. E. The requirements for the ideal denture base include the following: accuracy of adaptation to the tissues, with low volume change; dense, nonirritating surface that is capable of receiving and maintaining a good finish; thermal conductivity; low specific gravity; lightness in the mouth; sufficient strength; resistance to fracture or distortion; self-cleansing factor or easily kept clean; esthetic acceptability; potential for future relining; and low interest cost. (REF. 34-pp. 101, 261)

730. E. In the final analysis, it is bone tissue which provides the support for a removable restoration. Alveolar bone provides the support for partial dentures. When potentially destructive forces are minimal, then the physiologic tolerances of the supporting structures need not be

tested. The forces accruing through a partial denture are widely distributed and can readily be minimized by design and location of component parts, together with a harmonious occlusion. (REF. 34-pp. 125-130)

731. E. A linguoplate (continuous bar retainer) does not in itself act as an indirect retainer. Rather the linguoplate serves more as an orthodontic appliance on inclined tooth surfaces than as the support for the removable partial denture. When the linguoplate is utilized in a partial denture, terminal rests should always be provided at either end to stabilize the denture and to prevent orthodontic movement of the teeth contacted. (REF. 34-pp. 189, 190)

732. E. Full palatal coverage major connectors are indicated for use as follows: in most cases where only some or all anterior teeth remain, Class II arch with a posterior modification space and some missing anterior teeth in distal extension edentulous area, Class I arch with 1-4 premolars and some or all anterior teeth remaining, abutment support is poor and cannot otherwise be enhanced, and in the absence of a pedunculated torus. (REF. 34-pp. 25-33)

733. B. All partial dentures have the following in common: they must be supported by oral tissues; they must be retained against reasonable dislodging forces; the best possible support must be obtained; the method of direct retention must be taken into account; and the partial denture having one or more distal extension denture bases must be designed so movement of the unsupported end away from the tissues will be prevented. (REF. 34-pp. 36, 37)

734. B. Internal occlusal rests (not an internal attachment or a retainer) are utilized for both occlusal support and horizontal stabilization. The abutment crowns contain the internal rests. Occlusal support is derived from the floor of the rest and an additional occlusal bevel when the latter is provided. (REF. 34-pp. 40, 41)

735. A. Occlusal rests in sound enamel should be made with diamond points equal in size to Nos. 6 and 8 round burs. Whenever a small enamel defect is encountered in the preparation of an occlusal rest, it is usually better judgement to ignore it until the rest preparation has been completed. Then prepare the remaining defect with small burs to receive a small gold foil restoration. (REF. 34-p. 227)

736. E. Two basic types of sprues are multiple or single sprues. Multiple spruing includes the following points: use a few sprues of larger diameter, keep all sprues as short and direct as possible, avoid abrupt changes in direction, avoid T-shaped junctions as much as possible, and reinforce in all junctions with additional wax to avoid constrictions in the sprue channel and to avoid V-shaped sections of investment that might break away and be carried into the casting. (REF. 34-pp. 354-357)

737. E. The sprue channel is the opening leading from the crucible to the cavity in which the appliance framework is to be cast. Sprues have the purpose of leading the molten gold from the crucible into the mold cavity. Therefore, the sprue should be large enough to accommodate the entering stream and of the proper shape to lead it into the mold cavity as quickly as possible with minimal turbulence. (REF. 34-pp. 355, 356)

738. E. All methods of casting vary; however, they all use force to inject quickly the molten metal into the mold cavity. This force may be either centrifugal or air pressure. Either too much or too little force is very undesirable. (REF. 34-p. 364)

739. E. It is essential that the time of burn-out be sufficient to entirely eliminate the moisture from the investment. If moisture remains, its presence results in a porous casting due to the continued emission of steam by the investment. It is best to err on the side of too long a burnout period than on too short a period of time. (REF. 34-p. 362)

740. E. Sprues should not be removed from the casting until the majority of the polishing and finishing is completed. Reasonable care, however, should be exercised to avoid any distortion when the sprue must be removed because it is not practical to leave it. Avoid careless handling of castings during finishing. (REF. 34-p. 364)

741. E. Heat hardening by allowing the casting to completely cool in the investment is not recommended for gold alloys. The latter method of heat hardening is not only uneven but shrinkage also is nonuniform, resulting in an inaccurate casting. Under no conditions should the casting be heated and plunged into a pickling solution. (REF. 34-pp. 364, 365)

742. E. Porcelain or plastic tube or grooved teeth may be attached to a metal base by cementation or, with the use of resin teeth, attached with acrylic resin under pressure, i.e., the pressed-on method of attaching resin teeth to a metal base. (REF. 34-pp. 380, 381)

743. E. The interdental papilla must end near the labial face of the tooth and never slope inward to terminate toward the lingual portion of the interproximal surface. The correctly formed interdental papilla should be so produced that it will be self-cleansing. (REF. 34-pp. 391, 392)

Chapter 14 Crown and Bridge Prosthodontics

744. B. There are three requirements for bridge construction: an appreciation of forces developed by the oral mechanism and of the capability of the tooth and its supporting structures to resist them; modification of normal tooth form that are designed to reduce forces or increase resistance to them; and establishing and maintaining normal tissue tone. (REF. 29-p. 2)

745. B. A bridge is contraindicated when the space to be filled is of such length that the additional load generated from the occlusion of the pontics will impair the health of the tissues around the teeth (as abutments). (REF. 29-p. 3)

746. B. Splints and long bridges have been utilized for the stabilization of teeth in the patient with advanced periodontal disease. Too many dental practitioners avoid the use of splints while a few enthusiasts overestimate the efficacy of these procedures. As a result, patients may be misled. Therefore, sound restorative judgment should be followed. (REF. 29 p. 7)

747. E. Failures are minimized when the following steps are taken: a comprehensive study of existing conditions; an evaluation of the potential of the remaining teeth and supporting structures; a discriminating assessment of the relationship of one arch to the other, with the optimal load-bearing ability of the bridge structure; an eventual selection of a method of restoration that gives consideration to the esthetic requirements imposed by the patient as well as his caries index; oral hygiene; and a plan of treatment that will accomplish this satisfactorily. (REF. 29-p. 9)

748. E. The existing vertical dimension and maxillo-mandibular relationship are accepted and maintained and the most conservative approach is always utilized. Conservative approach means conservation of tooth structure and of the surface enamel. A fixed partial denture is a mechanical repair, a treatment for a local disease, and a prophylactic against a systemic disease. (REF. 29-p. 10)

749. A. In certain instances, the position of an abutment tooth can often be improved by orthodontics. Minor or uncomplicated orthodontic treatment can often be undertaken by the dental practitioner. If the case is complicated the patient should be referred to an orthodontist to upright the abutment tooth. (REF. 29-p. 10)

750. E. When carving an inlay pattern directly, the operator uses a circular matrix band fitted loosely around the tooth, the band being trimmed both occlusally and cervically to accommodate the opposing cusps and avoid cutting the soft tissues. (REF. 29-p. 13)

751. B. Gross carving can be done with a Wagner or Ash instrument, a No. 12 Crenshaw scaler, or some other suitable and convenient instrument. Proximal carving is best done with the No. 23 explorer. The occlusal surface is carved with the instrument of choice (as the flat end of a Wagner instrument or No. 5 explorer). There can be no overextended margins, occlusally, proximally, or cervically. (REF. 29-p. 13)

752. E. Study casts are essential in the planning of a bridge. The casts enable the dentist to evaluate the forces that will act against the bridge, to decide whether any grinding or rebuilding of teeth will be necessary so an improved opposing occlusal plane can be formed; to use the surveyor to locate the path of insertion and outline the reduction necessary to make abutment preparations parallel; to visualize the directions in which forces will be applied to the finished restoration; to select, contour, and position the facings and to use them as guides in preparing abutments. (REF. 29-p. 76)

753. E. Traumatic centric occlusion may involve the anterior teeth. If the anterior teeth have a good incising relationship, the premature contact is removed by grinding the lingual aspect of the maxillary tooth because shortening the mandibular tooth would take the teeth out of occlusion

in protrusive movement. If both centric and protrusive relationships are traumatic, the lower incisal edge is altered. If removal of the faulty centric contact fails to eradicate the protrusive interference, the incisal edge of the maxillary tooth is also ground. (REF. 29-p. 80)

754. B. If a cusp loses its centric stop following the removal of cusp interference, the opposing sulcus or marginal ridge will have to be built up by means of a restoration. There is support for a tooth arrangement having an anterior guidance that permits little contact of posterior teeth away from centric occlusion. (REF. 29-p. 81)

755. E. Any lack of skill and absence of comprehension of the potential of a crown and bridge can preclude achievement of the results expected. (REF. 29-p. 85)

756. D. After a thorough analysis of the patient's problem, the form of the appliance is considered. The appliance must correct the problem. The analytical process should show the directions and the distance sought in any tooth movements. The limiting factors include those inherent in the appliance, the patient, and the operator. (REF. 29-p. 86)

757. E. With a fixed partial prosthesis, it is possible to stabilize a tooth, minimize or eliminate shock from occlusion, and improve the health of the supporting structure in every way, especially if the involved tooth can be made an intermediate abutment. (REF. 29-p. 89)

758. E. The inlay may be used as a bridge retainer in the following circumstances: the span must be short, no wider than one tooth; the mouth must be caries free; the clinical crown must be of average length; and in functional occlusion, must not be subjected to undue leverage. The tooth should be vital, with dentin lining all of the cavity walls.

759. E. The inlay retainer is contraindicated for the tooth that is rotated, extensively carious, short, extruded, or pulpless or one that has a large cervical restoration. A cavity prepared in a rotated tooth will give substantial retention only when supplemented by two or more pinholes. Even then an inlay may not offer an area receptive to the solder joint. (REF. 29-p. 93)

760. E. The partial veneer, three-quarter crown is utilized as a bridge retainer but is also used in combination with resin or silicate cement in the form of a single unit restoration for a fractured tooth. The partial veneer crown covers the proximal, lingual, and occlusal surfaces or incisal edge of the tooth, with the labial or buccal surface untouched except for the labioincisal or bucco-occlusal margin. (REF. 29-p. 93)

761. E. The partial veneer crowns should not be placed on the following teeth: short teeth with extensive caries and teeth that have a poor long-axis relationship with the path of insertion; upper cuspids with long incisal arms, contact areas at the gingival margin, and very short mesial and distal surfaces; teeth too small or too thin for accurate positioning and cutting of the proximal grooves; or teeth with extensive cervical caries; and in mouths with a high caries index. (REF. 29-p. 93)

762. E. The partial veneer crown is indicated on maxillary centrals, cuspids, and bicuspids, and also on mandibular second bicuspids which are of medium length. This retainer placed in maxillary bicuspids can support posterior bridges supplying one, two, or three teeth and anterior bridges replacing the cuspid or the cuspid and lateral. (REF. 29-p. 94)

763. E. The posterior tooth partial-veneer crown may be placed on rotated or tipped bicuspids if the latter is not too pronounced. It may also be used on the upper first molar when the mouth is caries-free, when the crown is long occlusocervically, and when the mesiobuccal area of the tooth is exposed as the patient talks or smiles. (REF. 29-p. 94)

764. A. Splinting is a rigid or semirigid attachment of one tooth to another, or the comparative immobilization or support of a series of teeth by either a removable or fixed appliance. Teeth are splinted in the construction of fixed partial prostheses, in preparing mouths to support and retain removable partial prostheses, and for mutual or individual support in periodontally affected mouths. (REF. 29-p. 95)

765. E. Splinting is indicated in fixed partial construction when the space is long or when an individual abutment tooth at one or both ends of the space will yield to the torque from the lever arm of the prosthesis. Because of counterbalancing, two splinted teeth will provide support, and resistance to forces, in excess of the sum of the support or the resistance of the individual teeth. (REF. 29-p. 97)

766. B. The full veneer crown may be placed on any tooth that cannot be returned by alternate methods to an effective working capacity and contour. It should be used as a bridge abutment when the caries index, torque, leverage, or load contraindicates the partial veneer crown, the pin-ledge, or the inlay. (REF. 29-p. 98)

767. E. There are five types of finishing lines or cervical margins. (1) The feathered edge is to be avoided since it is indefinite and makes difficult exactness in carving patterns or finishing castings. (2) The chisel edge is satisfactory and is produced very often in lingual and proximal reduction. (3) The bevel is used where shallow caries has made it necessary to cut deeper. (4) The chamber is the ideal finishing line to be developed when routine preparation does not produce a chisel edge. (5) The shoulder is used for areas to be veneered and for jacket crowns. The shoulder can be beveled. Circumferential shoulders require excessive removal of tooth structure. (REF. 29-p. 100)

768. E. When forming the cervical margin, one of the principal points of the axial reduction is to achieve a prepared form that will make the cervical margin of the preparation the largest diameter of the prepared portion of the clinical crown, without undercuts and without the tooth being too tapered for maximum retention. (REF. 29-p. 101)

769. E. Inlays may be used to support the free end of a broken-stress bridge because little or no stress will be transferred from the bridge. An inlay should not be utilized to build up one section of the occlusal surface of a tilted abutment tooth because the leverage from the casting may be greater than the stability of the inlay. (REF. 29-p. 105)

770. C. In the preparation of a mandibular bicuspid, retention may be increased by a bevel 1.0 mm wide on the buccal surface along the distobuccal margin. Because the latter is not parallel to the path of insertion, it should go as far cervically as the convexity of the tooth can tolerate. Partial veneer crowns on lower bicuspids are satisfactory when splinted to each other or to a retainer on the cuspid. (REF. 29-p. 107)

771. E. With ultrahigh-speed rotary cutting, most crown and bridge preparations are completed in less time with less effort and trauma. However, when rapid cutting has taken place a larger percentage of teeth exhibit sensitivity following cementation of bridges, and an increase occurs in the number of candidates for endodontic therapy. Ultrahigh speed has virtues, but it is not a panacea. (REF. 29-p. 122)

772. E. Ultrahigh-speed cutting should be done in a wet field. While some visibility is affected adversely by water, this is not to a degree that instrumentation is impossible. Finishing and refinement of all preparations should be done at slower speeds with hand instruments. (REF. 29-p. 122)

773. B. The type of occlusion that is ideal for most patients is highly controversial. A completely balanced occlusion has been advocated. A tooth arrangement recommended is one having an anterior guidance that permits little contact of posterior teeth away from centric occlusion. Most natural dentitions are of the latter type. (REF. 29-p. 149)

774. E. Bonded porcelain veneer crowns are accepted in all respects by most patients and dentists. However, they are frustrating, ineptly utilized, and badly constructed by some dentists and dental technicians. With modern techniques, building and bonding or fracture of the porcelain veneer are no longer problems. (REF. 29-p. 162)

775. E. All aspects of construction of a veneered crown or bridge can be done in the dental office laboratory. The equipment required is not excessive. Clasps of a removable partial denture may be supported by the bonded porcelain veneer. (REF. 29-p. 163)

776. A. Fused porcelain is recognized as a restorative material that is compatible with oral soft tissues plus it has superior esthetic qualities. With the use of albuminous porcelains the strength has been increased and the incidence of porcelain fractures has been reduced greater. Crowns constructed of aluminous porcelain cores or occluding surfaces are incapable of replacing veneered crowns in advanced situations. (REF. 29-p. 172)

777. A. Facings made of resin are on the market, but they should be recommended only for temporary replacements not permanent facings. (REF. 29-p. 174)

778. C. Hue is that quality of sensation through which an observer is aware that one color is green and another color is red. Brilliance or brightness is represented at its extreme by white and black and is indicative of the amount of light reflected from a matte-colored surface. Saturation is the property that makes one sample of a pair of the same hue appear more intense or pure. (REF. 29-p. 174)

779. E. The porcelain facings commonly used are the following: pin, flatback with a slot, Trupontic, Sanitarypontic, porcelain biting-edge, and the reverse-pin. (REF. 29-p. 176)

780. B. Facings may be shaped and positioned on the working cast by grinding to mesiodistal width, adjusting to occluso cervical or incisocervical length, with adaptation of the facing to the ridge; forming the mesiodistal convexities and occlusocervical contour, and adjusting the long-axis inclination. (REF. 29-p. 184)

781. E. The broken-stress joint or nonrigid connector is used in bridge construction only where the span is short and the supporting alveolus is not extensively reduced or actively receding. The need for this type of connector is very limited. Thus it should be bypassed in favor of the solder or rigid connector. (REF. 29-p. 187)

782. E. The semirigid connector (subocclusal rest) is used when two inlays act as retainers for a bridge. A solder joint will attach the pontic to the retainer in the stronger abutment (posterior abutment), and the subocclusal rest will be placed in the other inlay. (REF. 29-p. 191)

783. A. The second nonrigid connector is the dovetail occlusal rest. This connector is an extension of the pontic casting fitted into a dovetail-shaped rest seat prepared in the occlusal surface of the retainer. The isthmus must not be less than 1.5 mm wide and 2.0 mm deep, and the rest at its extremity should measure 2.5 cm at the widest point. A groove can be cut, 1.5 mm wide, 1.0 mm deep, and 2.5 mm long, on the proximal surface of the retainer to receive a cast strut as a part of the rest. (REF. 29-p. 191)

784. E. The casting should be seated on the tooth with a mallet and orangewood stick. If it does not seat, the inside must be scrutinized for irregularities, which should have a shiny, burnished appearance. If a plus-contact obstructs seating, it should be polished further until the casting can be seated. (REF. 29-p. 194)

785. B. Although discomfort from cementation is very short, some patients desire anesthesia for this purpose. The cement serves merely as a luting material to fill the small space that exists between the tooth and the restoration. (REF. 29-p. 195)

786. E. Oral hygiene should be stressed and preventive therapy should be practiced when bridge retainers are used that do not cover all surfaces of the crown. (REF. 29-p. 197)

787. E. Failures in bridge construction includes the following: discomfort, looseness of bridges, recurrence of caries, recession of supporting structure, degneration of the pulp, fractures of bridge components, loss of veneers, loss of function, loss of tissue tone or form, and failure to seat. (REF. 29-p. 199)

788. E. In tooth reduction for abutment preparations, especially those involving stones or accelerated speeds, sufficient consideration for the pulp must be emphasized. One of the greatest pulpal irritants can be heat generated by the high-speed cutting tools used in modern cavity preparation. If the preparation on the abutment is deep, the heat must be controlled and dissipated or a severe pulpal reaction may develop. Lubrication and cooling are essential. (REF. 29-p. 209)

789. A. A bridge is a fixed partial denture, rigidly attached to one or more abutment teeth, replacing one or more lost or missing teeth. (REF. 30-p. 3)

790. E. The intangibles may be defined as an appreciation of the following: forces developed by the oral mechanism, the capability of the tooth and its supporting structures to resist them, modifications of a normal tooth form that are designed to reduce forces or increase resistance to them, and establishing and maintaining normal tissue tone. (REF. 30-pp. 9, 10)

791. E. Bridge construction exacts a superior level of technical proficiency and concern in the following: the removal of caries from the abutment or from any associated tooth, the loss of which might affect the design or life of the bridge; the sterilization or cleansing of the tooth surface; the protection of the pulp during preparation of the tooth and construction of the bridge; the restoration of the tooth surface so the tooth will function normally and comfortably and not abuse the supporting structures; and the restoration of multiple areas of occlusion, and a comprehensive and applicable knowledge of tooth form and esthetic tooth alignment. (REF. 30-p. 9)

792. C. A bridge is indicated whenever there are properly distributed and healthy teeth to serve as abutments. The abutment teeth must have suitable crown-root ratios and are capable of sustaining an additional load. Criteria for suitable abutments are proper distribution, crown-root ratio or periodontal support, radiographic studies, and oral examination. (REF. 30-pp. 10-14)

793. E. A bridge is contraindicated when it cannot be constructed so as to restore arch form and occlusion. When the proposed abutments have exposed root areas that are sensitive and cannot be covered by bridge retainers, the construction of a bridge is contraindicated. (REF. 30-pp. 14-18)

794. A. Diagnostic casts help the dentist to evaluate the forces that act against the bridge, to decide whether grinding or rebuilding of teeth will be obligatory so that a suitable or improved opposing occlusal plane can be formed, to use the surveyor to locate the path of insertion and outline the reduction necessary to make the preparation of abut-

ment preparations parallel and esthetical, and to visualize the directions in which force will be applied to the final restoration. (REF. 30-pp. 10, 13)

795. D. Short teeth may be used when the preparations are altered to develop resistance to displacements. Frail teeth also may be used as abutments provided the spaces to be restored are also narrow and the opposing forces are small or relative. (REF. 30-p. 68)

796. B. Shoulders are outlined grossly with high-speed cutting, given definitive form with lesser speeds, and then honed and smoothed with hand instruments. Shoulders invariably must be smoothed with hand instruments. (REF. 48-p. 103)

797. E. The full veneer crown may be utilized as a single-unit restoration or as a retainer for a bridge. Function, comfort, and improvement of the environment must be introduced or continued with the seating of the full veneer crown. (REF. 48-p. 210)

798. E. The basic dental investment for gold alloys include dental stone, a form of silica, reducing agents, accelerators, and retarders. Quartz or cristobalite types of silica are present in dental investment. (REF. 33-p. 420)

799. B. Casting failure may be due to investment fracture. The fracture in the investment is caused from burning out too rapidly, overheating the gold, or too thin a mix of investment. (REF. 48-p. 427)

800. E. A bridge that becomes loose and must be removed because a retainer casting did not fit should never have been cemented in place in the first instance. Only one retainer may move on its abutment so that the dentist must recall the patient periodically to check for this situation. (REF. 48-p. 466)

801. E. Human chewing movement pathways are made by the teeth and condyles and their relationship to border movements, occlusal forces, mandibular dysfunction, and growth and development. (REF. 94-p. 45)

802. E. Alteration of the occlusion by the occlusal splint therapy followed by complete occlusal rehabilitation clearly affects muscle palpation and nocturnal EMG activity. (REF. 94-p. 49)

803. A. The closing strokes of mastication and other jaw closures are influenced by the anterior teeth (anterior guidance). Anterior guidance is the incisal and cuspal guidance. (REF. 94-p. 51)

804. B. Centric relation is any place along the arc of closure where the condyles are bilaterally in their most superior position and in intimate contact with the meniscus in the glenoid fossae when no lateral forces are applied. (REF. 94-p. 54)

805. E. The wearing down of teeth by primitive people associated with little or no dysfunction of the TMJ or of periodontal disease may prove that nature intends for the teeth to wear that identical way in other races. (REF. 94-p. 58)

806. D. Bruxism is aggravated if not caused by occlusal disharmonies. Emotional stress also is a common denominator. Some kind of occlusal interference can be found in the patient with bruxism. The dentist must improve his or her knowledge and skills in order to eliminate the occlusal disharmonies responsible for bruxism. (REF. 94-p. 61)

807. B. In patients where it is not feasible to do orthodontics, orthognathic surgery should at least be explored to determine if it is possible to better the relationship of the anterior teeth. It is frequently necessary to undertake orthodontics, orthognathic surgery and restorative procedures to solve the occlusion problems. (REF. 94-p. 65)

808. C. There is, however, a tendency to produce more horizontal chewing cycles, and, therefore, wear on the teeth usually continues. To derive benefits from occlusal equilibration, the anterior teeth as well as the posterior teeth should make simultaneous contact with the opposing teeth when the condyles are in centric position. (REF. 94-p. 67)

809. C. Articulators, however, do not have a central nervous system, muscles, ligaments, or nerves. They cannot show mobility of teeth and possess no ability to learn. The most common error in rehabilitative dentistry is treating the teeth before the TMJ complex has become stable. In any study of occlusion, the muscles must be given consideration. (REF. 94-p. 77)

810. D. Any management of the occlusal system can influence the function and shape of the TMJ to greater extent than was previously thought. Extensive remodeling of the TMJ takes place through adult life leading to marked changes in condylar shape. (REF. 94-p. 102)

811. E. Other symptoms of jaw dysfunction are the need for treatment, problem with sleeping, inability to work, and seriousness of the dysfunction. (REF. 94-p. 116)

812. E. The treatment also must be compatible with the patient's financial and time constraints without jeopardizing their health. (REF. 94-p. 119)

813. E. The conservative therapy measures recommended for symptoms of jaw pain and dysfunction, begin with the prescription of a nonnarcotic, anti-inflammatory analgesic. It is important to avoid biomechanically stressful forces because of the accompanying temporomandibular joint symptoms. (REF. 94-p. 120)

814. E. To alleviate harmful oral habits the dentist should suggest that patients repeatedly say to themselves, "Teeth apart and jaw relaxed." Since longstanding stress is one of the primary factors of musculoskeletal pain, there are alternative stress control methods that should be considered. (REF. 94-p. 121)

815. B. Referral to a psychologist for relaxation training may be necessary if physical therapy produces little or transient improvement after two to three visits. Usually a form of cognitive behavioral counseling will be combined with electromyographic biofeedback and progressive relaxation. (REF. 94-p. 125)

816. E. One or more of the latter dysfunctions may produce the symptoms of the TMJ pain-dysfunction syndrome. They may be eliminated using bite stent therapy or occlusal adjustment. (REF. 94-p. 127)

817. B. Bite stents generally eliminate nocturnal clenching and bruxing in the chronic bruxer. Some of these patients are stimulated to bruxing and clenching by interceptive occlusal contacts. Therefore, the latter patient requires occlusal adjustment. (REF. 94-p. 130)

818. B. The lesions of occlusal traumatism range from necrosis on the pressure side to dilated blood vessels and elongated periodontal fiber bundles on the tension side. (REF. 94-p. 143)

819. E. The severity of the sequelae of partial edentulism is dependent on the duration of the edentulism, the patient's age, and the neuromuscular adaptation to the state. All of the latter sequelae are the result of a break in the integrity of the occlusal surface of one or both arches. The objective of prosthodontic treatment, therefore, is tc restore the integrity of the occlusal surfaces. (REF. 94-p. 161)

820. E. However, the harmonious functioning masticatory system is not dependent upon specific morphologic tooth-to-tooth relation and to intercuspation. A highly rigid adherence to one occlusal concept is short-sighted. Epidemiological and clinical data show increased frequency of dysfunction signs and symptoms in individuals with loss of teeth and unbalanced tooth loss. (REF. 94-p. 162)

821. E. The long term integrity of the occlusal surface is a function of the integrity of the supporting tissues and the integrity of the occlusal surface. (REF. 94-p. 165)

822. C. The term vertical dimension should have an adjective describing the position of the mandible at the time of measurement, i. e., rest vertical dimension or occlusal vertical dimension or postural vertical dimension. REF. 94-p. 168)

823. C. A wide range of instruments are currently available for measurement of vertical jaw position. The choice is dependent upon the accuracy, cost and degree to which they disrupt the individuals normal behavior. (REF. 94-p. 179)

824. E. The dentist should recognize those factors that affect wear. The selection of materials and the development of treatment planning to establish occlusal conditions should be based upon minimizing tooth wear. (REF. 94-p. 184)

825. A. A discrepancy in the size or relationship of the jaws as unusually large permanent teeth, tongue thrusting or thumb sucking, developmental anomalies, frenal invagination, cleft lip and palate, and endocrine disorders (acromegaly) are contributing factors to tooth malposition. In adults, the following factors produce tooth malposition: large interproximal fillings, loss of teeth, bruxism, loss of periodontal support, and primary and secondary occlusal traumatism. (REF. 94-p. 191)

826. E. In the absence of inflammation the signs of occlusal traumatism are reversible. The periodontal alterations are, however, inflammation and a lack of the attachment apparatus. The teeth, therefore, are unable to withstand the forces of occlusion. (REF. 94-p. 192)

827. E. Therapeutic occlusion is one produced by the dentist which conforms to the physiologic needs of the patient. A therapeutic occlusion is a well balanced and stable occlusion but is not an ideal occlusion. (REF. 94-p. 193)

828. D. The purpose of the biteguard is to alter the patient's occlusion. The occlusion of the biteguard should be developed with care and exactness. The insertion of the biteguard can be made at the same appointment at which the impression is taken. (REF. 94-p. 221)

829. E. The major disadvantage of preparing the biteguard is that the dentist must have a vacuum adapter available for his use. However, after the initial investment the instrument's value will outweigh any costs.

Chapter 15 Oral Surgery

830. B. Mixed tumor of the salivary gland (pleomorphic adenoma) is treated by surgical excision. However, the exact surgical procedure is controversial. Intraoral lesions of the pleomorphic adenoma are generally treated by conservative extracapsular excision. Some oral surgeons prefer to remove the entire lobe of the salivary gland that

contains the mixed tumor. When the capsule is invaded by tumor cells a wider excision with removal of a margin of normal tissue is sufficient to prevent a recurrence of this neoplasm. The use of x-ray radiation is useless in treating the mixed tumor of salivary glands. (REF. 35-p. 723)

831. A. Treatment of osteomyelitis demands that drainage be established and continued and that the infection of bone tissue and bone marrow be treated with antibiotics to prevent further spread and undue complications, as pathologic jaw fracture. If a large sequestrum forms, it should be removed surgically. Without prompt treatment, acute suppurative osteomyelitis may proceed to the development of periostitis, abscess, or cellulitis. (REF. 35-p. 788)

832. B. Odontoma is any tumor of odontogenic origin. However, it has come to mean a growth composed of both epithelial and mesenchymal cells exhibiting complete differentiation, with formation of enamel and dentin. Treatment of the odontoma consists of surgical excision with no expectancy of recurrence following surgery. All odontomas that are surgically excised should be sent to the oral pathologist for histopathologic examination. The latter is necessary since the ameloblastic odontoma appears similar to the common odontoma on radiographic examination. (REF. 35-pp. 858, 1030)

833. C. There is still a great deal of controversy about the preferred method of treatment of the ameloblastoma. Oral surgeons agree, however, that complete removal of this odontogenic neoplasm, regardless of how it is accomplished will result in resolution of the mass. Treatment consists of radical and conservative surgical excision, currettage, chemical and electrocautery, radiation therapy, or a combination of surgery and irradiation. Some form of surgical resection is preferred because the recurrence rate following surgery is considerably less than with the other available treatments. (REF. 35-pp. 993, 996)

834. B. The oral surgeon or dentist plans the extraction conservatively in the following manner: using elevator and/or forceps delivery of the tooth; sectioning the tooth; re-

moving only bone that will regenerate during healing; and removing cortical bone to facilitate extraction of the tooth or root. (REF. 36-p. 10)

835. E. The first measure in oral surgery is early diagnosis and extraction before extensive bone destruction takes place. For instance, if an indication for third molar extraction exists, it should be accomplished prior to 25 years of age. The oral surgeon should plan and execute procedures to create minimal periodontal problems, conserve bone, remove pathologic tissues and osseous irregularities, and cause minimal distortion to the soft tissues to compromise the vestibule. (REF. 36-p. 1)

836. A. The surgeon should perform necessary treatment with the least amount of trauma and eradicate associated pathologic areas causing minimal distortion of the soft tissues. (REF. 36-p. 2)

837. E. Before extractions the dental clinician should observe clues relating to mechanical factors that will enable him to determine whether the extraction can be accomplished relatively easily or with difficulty. Factors indicating difficult extractions include the following: old age, short crown and long root, functional wear, heavy alveolar plates, dense supporting bone, atrophic periodontal membrane, high bony socket, hypercementosis, broken down crowns, crowded tooth alignment, endodontically treated teeth, and tortuous roots. (REF. 36-p. 6)

838. E. The clinician should not place too much emphasis on the radiograph. Radiographs are an essential aid in exodontia. However, they are limited in the amount of clinical information that they impart to the dentist. (REF. 36-p. 125)

839. E. When the dentist sits down to extract teeth, he finds that certain forceps are more effective than others. When extracting mandibular teeth, the most comfortable forceps would be the anterior and posterior Ash forceps rather than the no. 23 and 151 instruments. Generally, fewer mistakes and complications occur during surgery when the dentist is sitting because he has a relaxed position, ability to use controlled force, and the restraining of the impulse to hurry the extraction. (REF. 36-p. 99)

840. E. There are instances when broken roots are difficult to visualize, especially when the root tip is in the maxillary or mandibular third molar regions. Third molar roots are small and very fragile and may fracture at the apex, leaving a root tip a few millimeters long. Common sense indicates that if the dentist cannot clearly see the root tip, he or she should explain the situation to the patient and note the event on the patient's record. If a retained small root tip becomes symptomatic, it is best to consult promptly with an oral surgeon. (REF. 36-p. 18)

841. E. The dentist should follow a practical diagnostic sequence as follows: evaluate the patient from the overall management standpoint, carefully examine the site of surgery and weigh factors that will dictate whether it will be a forceps extraction or a surgical removal, and then study the radiograph. (REF. 36-p. 16)

842. E. Breakage of root tips during an extraction may not be the result of poor technique, especially when the roots are tortuous. The root tips can generally be removed at the time of extraction when they can be clearly visualized and the proper instrument technique is employed. (REF. 36-p. 16)

843. E. A common case of unnecessary extraction is the removal of unerupted third molars in teenagers without evidence of existing pathology. It is generally agreed that the recommended treatment is to remove teeth that have not erupted and which probably will not assume proper position and function. (REF. 36-p. 16)

844. E. The extraction of a lower third molar with a pericoronitis should not be considered as poor judgment, if the pericoronitis is chronic and the third molar presents favorable factors for extraction. When the pericoronitis is subacute or acute and the third molar shows evidence of unfavorable factors for extraction, then to attempt to remove the tooth would be a mistake of judgment. (REF. 36-p. 226)

845. E. Extraction of teeth may lead to hemorrhage either during the extraction or postoperatively. Hemorrhage during the extraction can be handled better since the tissues are anesthesized, thus the operator counts on good assistance. The operator should determine if the hemor-

rhage is from soft tissue or bone. For bony hemorrhage, sterile bonewax is an excellent agent to arrest hemorrhage. (REF. 36-p. 224)

846. E. The use of uncontrolled force by either an elevator or a forceps during extraction is a major factor in unnecessary complications. An example is the forceful removal of an upper molar with forceps alone. Excess force applied to a second molar causes fracture and loss of the maxillary tuberosity. (REF. 36-p. 226)

847. B. The prophylactic removal of third molars for periodontal reasons should be considered if the teeth appear to remain impacted. Partially erupted third molars should be treated similarly. The rationale for the prophylactic extraction of third molars for periodontal reasons should be based upon experience and sound judgment. (REF. 36-p. 178)

848. E. The dentist may fail to identify nervous or unmanageable patients. All patients should be profiled as manageable with local anesthesia or as unmanageable. Unmangeable patients should be referred to an oral surgeon who will administer nitrous oxide. (REF. 36-p. 171)

849. E. Most infections of dental origin respond quickly to a combination of antibiotics and other supportive care. However, many serious complications are currently possible. The selection of the proper antibiotic theoretically should be preceded by a Gram stain as well as a culture and sensitivity test, both aerobic and anaerobic. (REF. 36-p. 317)

850. E. An antibiotic may be broad spectrum, related to microbiology, and may include many organisms that are rarely pathogens within the oral cavity. A broad-spectrum drug effective against Salmonella, Shigella, E. coli, Proteus, and Hemophilus should not be considered as broad-spectrum for dental use when it is not effective against staphylococci and streptococci. (REF. 36-p. 311)

851. B. There is a need for reliable and effective methods for alveoplasty. Clinical studies are needed to improve, refine, and innovate methods and thereby assure excellent results. (REF. 36-p. 311)

852. B. Submucous vestibuloplasty preserves the integrity of the oral mucosa. It is generally used only on the maxillary arch and is dependent on having adequate healthy covering mucosa without submucosal fibrosis or scarring. Vestibuloplasty is ridge extension or sulcus extension. (REF. 36-p. 270)

853. E. Preprosthetic oral surgery includes the following procedures: surgical repositioning, segmental osteotomy, orthognathic surgery, submucous vestibuloplasty, vestibuloplasty with secondary epithelialization, vestibuloplasty with mucosal or skin grafts, bone graft to the ridge crest, palatal osteotomy, and visor osteotomy. (REF. 36-p. 253)

854. E. The dental clinician should consider the following 4 types of postextraction pain: intense pain with no apparent cause, pain from a traumatic extraction (molar), pain from a foreign body, and pain from localized osteitis (dry socket). (REF. 36-p. 244)

855. E. The dental practitioner should not continue to treat an oral infection that is not responding to antibiotic therapy. If no improvement takes place in the oral infection in 2 or 3 days, the general practitioner should refer the patient to the oral surgeon for evaluation. The oral surgeon has the option of changing antibiotics, performing an incision and drainage for culture purposes, admitting the patient to the hospital for intravenous antibiotic administration and if necessary an exploratory incision and drainage performed under general anesthesia. The patient is in the hands of an oral surgeon qualified to follow any treatment plan and manage the complication. (REF. 36-p. 226)

856. E. Some degree of postextraction hemorrhage or oozing of blood is normal and varies from one subject to the other. However, the leakage of blood stops within an hour if the patient bites on a 2 x 2 inch gauze with pressure. For cases of secondary hemorrhage, the following therapy is recommended: reanesthetize the extraction site and have the patient bite on a fresh 2 x 2 inch gauze for 20 minutes. Remove all debris from the alveolus if bleeding has not ceased in 20 minutes. Place the surgicel in the alveolus if bleeding occurs from soft tissues. Use a hemostat to clamp the end of a bleeding vessel. Oxidized regenerated cellulose (surgicel) is also excellent for arresting bony hemorrhage. (REF. 36-p. 336)

857. E. Everything possible should be done to decrease the patient's apprehension. The following represent some helpful procedures: improve communication, assurance of adequate sedation and complete anesthesia, avoidance of physical trauma, and planning the oral surgery in order to complete the operation efficiently and in a reasonable time. (REF. 36-p. 329)

858. G. A too common solution to the problem of shock is to let someone else shoulder the responsibility and narrow the scope of understanding and activity to a tooth or teeth as if they were unrelated to the patient. Obviously, the dentist's obligation is to be familiar with the prevention and treatment of shock in dental patients. (REF. 36-p. 319)

859. B. The past history and review of systems provides the dentist with a systematic appraisal of the aspects of health which place dental patients as candidates for syncope. Syncope may be due to administration of quinidine and any positional changes should be made cautiously with patients taking antihypertension medications since they are subject to orthostatic hypotension. (REF. 36-p. 638)

860. F. Most drugs prescribed for the treatment of cardiovascular disease also can adversely affect systemic health. To prevent cardiac arrest, the dentist should know the patient through physical evaluation, know the nature of the medications the patient is taking, and to know himself by being aware of his own capabilities and limitations. (REF. 36-p. 637)

861. E. Drugs may lead to angioneurotic edema; therefore, a detailed history should be taken. The patient's medications should never be considered apart from the patient's health and physical condition. Concurrent with the obligation is the impossibility of being familiar with all of the drugs on the market today. (REF. 36-p. 639)

862. C. The patient with cardiac infarction should be viewed as a threat to life during dental treatment. Myocardial infarction is more likely to develop in the presence of congestive heart disease. The dentist should have a competent evaluation of the heart patient. (REF. 36-p. 640)

863. A. Complications must be expected during the practice of oral surgery. A careful past medical history is essential for all patients. Physical evaluation is of importance and is the determination of a particular patient's physical and emotional ability to withstand a specific dental procedure. Many of the limitations of therapy are necessitated by a disease rather than by the drugs with which the dental patient is being treated. (REF. 36-p. 638)

864. E. A program of in-office evaluation of the oral surgery patient is necessary for the prevention of emergencies and will upgrade emergency preparedness and will also serve the doctor as a deterrent to malpractice claims. (REF. 36-p. 637)

865. E. Serious morbidity may be related only randomly to dental therapy (as heart attack or stroke) or may be directly related to the stress of therapy. About 20% of all nonaccidental deaths (400, 000) are sudden and unexpected without prior history or diagnosis of a systemic disease. (REF. 51-p. 4)

866. C. For diabetics on a stabilized dosage of oral hypoglycemics, the most common problem develops when dental treatment interrupts the established caloric intake. Without a sufficient supply of blood glucose, hyperinsulinism can occur and acute hypoglycemia results. (REF. 51-p. 5)

867. E. Patients who are prone to the intravascular coagulation phenomena (as from intimal irregularities, prosthetic heart valves, narrowed coronary vessels, low flow or turbulent condition of venous channels, and history of repeated pulmonary emboli) may be taking medications that interfere with the production of vitamin K-dependent coagulation factors produced by the liver. (REF. 51-p. 9)

868. E. An example of drug interaction occurs in the administration of drugs which decrease the prothrombin time in patients already taking coumadin (as antacids, barbiturates, corticosteroids, glutethimide, meprobamate, and oral contraceptives). (REF. 51-p. 12)

869. E. Everything possible should be done to diminish apprehension in the oral surgery patient, including the following: improved communication, assurance of adequate sedation

and complete anesthesia, avoidance of physical trauma, planning the surgery in a strategic approach to complete the operation efficiently and within a reasonable time period, and management of rapport, building confidence, and providing the patient with understanding. (REF. 51-p. 13)

870. E. Oral-facial pain may result from the following: intense pain from no apparent cause, pain from a traumatic extraction (as a molar), pain from a sharp healing alveolar ridge, pain from tight sutures, pain from a foreign body, and pain from a localized osteitis (dry socket). REF. 51-p. 16)

871. E. Little mistakes common in the diagnosis of oral-facial pain may lead to complications, dissatisfied patients, and frustration for the dentist. (REF. 51-p. 26)

872. E. Removal of third molars may be required for preventive periodontal measures (as removal of malpositioned and impacted teeth, teeth with potential for replacement of diseased or compromised adjacent teeth, and teeth which can be brought into position orthodontically). There is a periodontal rationale for the prophylactic removal of third molars. (REF. 51-p. 34)

873. E. If the practitioner provides care without the patient's affirmative consent, except in a few emergency situations, the doctor not only will be subject to problems arising from failure to obtain informed consent but also may well be subject to civil charges of assault and/or battery. (REF 51-p. 44)

874. E. Express consent, either written or verbal, is the preferred method of obtaining patient acquiescence to extraction of teeth.

875. C. Drugs commonly encountered in the treatment of cardiovascular disease may predispose patients to systemic complications of dental treatment and therefore require modification of the treatment plan. Digitalis, methyldopa, quinidine, coumadin, and heparin have similar untoward reactions with implications on dental treatment. (REF. 51-p. 44)

876. A. In preventive aspects of oral surgery, numerous problems are encountered ranging from prevention of errors in diagnosis to prevention of death from malignant neoplasms. Severe mutilation may occur when oral surgery follows errors in diagnosis. Mandibles have been resected when cysts have been mistaken for serious pathology. (REF. 51-p. 46)

877. A. Treatment in oral surgery should be predicated on an accurate diagnosis. The oral surgeon should obtain all possible information about the patient and the patient's disease before instigating treatment. Consultation with allied specialists in dentistry and medicine may be indicated. (REF. 51-p. 46)

878. B. A preoperative evaluation is vital in order to prevent operative and postoperative complications. The preoperative evaluation should include a careful history of blood pressure and heart disease, a thorough examination, indicated laboratory procedures, and necessary consultations. Oral surgery should not be undertaken until it is determined that the patient is capable of withstanding the stress the procedure will produce. (REF. 51-p. 46)

879. E. Timely, sound, and conservative surgical procedures are indicated in multiple extractions in order to prevent untoward results, unnecessary hemorrhages and other complications, and needless mutilation in the eradication of diseased teeth. (REF. 51-p. 47)

880. D. No oral surgical procedure should be performed on the teeth or their hard and soft supporting structures until adequate radiographs are available. Radiographs may reveal hidden pathology, operative complications, and involvement of contingent structures. Radiographs assist the oral surgeon in determining a surgical approach to the oral problem. Procedures carried out without radiographs may result in fractured roots, fractured bones, involvement of the maxillary sinus, nerve injuries, and other injuries, many of which could be prevented by the intelligent use of good radiographs. (REF. 51-p. 50)

881. A. Complications will be minimized if a well-regulated oral surgical plan is formulated prior to starting any oral procedure. The surgical plan should include a step-by-step procedure that will facilitate the operation and yet be

flexible enough to allow the management of any unanticipated problem or emergency that may develop. (REF. 51-p. 50)

882. D. Procedures carried out (as extractions) without radiographs lead to complications that could readily have been avoided. (REF. 51-p. 57)

883. E. The dentist or oral surgeon must be able to evaluate the magnitude and difficulty of the oral surgical procedure and determine when suturing is required. Not all procedures require suturing because they are not of the same magnitude. (REF. 51-p. 59)

884. B. It is recommended that radiographs be taken at the time of eruption of the third molars, at approximately 18 to 21 years of age. If this survey reveals the teeth to be hopelessly impacted, they should be removed as soon as practicable. At this age, removal of impacted third molars is generally a relatively simple procedure accompanied by minimal postoperative complications. If the tooth is allowed to remain, a cyst, ameloblastoma or other complication may arise. (REF. 51-p. 60)

885. A. The early prophylactic removal of malposed third molars that have no chance of erupting into the dental arch is preventive dentistry. These malposed teeth cannot possibly aid the patient and are capable of producing complications. (REF. 51-p. 62)

886. C. Removal of the follicle and its epithelial remnants at any early age prevents development of a cyst and ameloblastoma from the unerupted tooth. (REF. 51-p. 63)

887. E. The fractured maxillary tuberosity generally results from failure to adhere to sound oral surgical principles. (REF. 51-p. 63)

888. E. The majority of postoperative bleeding problems are local in nature and may be effectively managed by the dentist. Systemic causes of postoperative hemorrhage are occasionally encountered. It is important for the oral surgeon to recognize these patients with hemorrhagic disease preoperatively so that correct therapy can be instigated to prevent serious bleeding when surgery is necessary. (REF. 51-p. 78)

889. C. Extractions may produce a beneficial result in jaw and facial deformities requiring orthodontic treatment. The extractions improve function and cosmetic appearance but also frequently improve the patient's overriding psychological problem that may be present. (REF. 51-p. 86)

890. E. Many postoperative complications are unpredictable and unavoidable. However, others are undoubtedly self-generated and result from negligence, inadequately planned oral surgical procedures, or ignorance on the part of the operator. The best way to treat a complication in the dental office is to prevent its occurrence. (REF. 51-p. 88)

891. E. The following sound oral surgical principles will prevent postoperative hemorrhage in the oral cavity: asepsis, complete and profound anesthesia; adequate access to the operative field; hemostasis; use of controlled force; conservative manipulation of the oral tissues; adequate cleansing and closure of the wound; and a well-regulated post operative regimen. (REF. 51-p. 99)

892. E. Acute infections of the oral cavity have the potential of developing into a serious, life-endangering space infection. However, if the dental infection is properly treated early in its development, serious complications are generally avoided. (REF. 51-p. 106)

893. E. Delayed treatment of the acute infection of the oral cavity is not tenable. Immediate extraction of an infected tooth, regardless of the length of time the infectious process has been developing or the amount of soft tissue swelling that is present, is the treatment of choice. The latter is possible because of the use of antibiotics, improved anesthetic agents, and refined surgical techniques. (REF. 51-p. 112)

894. E. When an acutely infected tooth is extracted, it should be accomplished by a simple atraumatic procedure. However, if the extraction requires a complicated procedure, with removal of bone tissue and tooth sectioning, extraction should be postponed until the infectious process has been resolved. (REF. 51-p. 121)

895. E. When the use of an antibiotic is indicated it should be prescribed in an intelligent manner, depending, whenever possible, on positive bacteriological findings to determine

the antibiotic of choice. The antibiotic should be administered in sufficient quantity and for sufficient time to control the infection and to prevent the emergence of resistant strains of the organisms. (REF. 51-p. 130)

896. E. The following signs and symptoms, if present in the oral cavity should make the dentist suspicious of a malignant neoplasm: local lesion (insidious in onset, chronic and progressive, indurated, ulcerated and fixed to its base, or does not respond to recognized treatments), pain, asymmetry of the face, regional adenopathy, loose teeth, radiographic evidence of bone changes, paresthesia, trismus (altered mobility of the tongue and difficulty in swallowing), and increased salivation with bad breath and hemorrhage. (REF. 51-p. 131)

897. E. Bone grafting materials of autogenous and allogenic origin have been used with increased frequency during the past decade in the surgical specialty areas of dentistry. Allogenic banked bone is considered as a second-rate graft material when compared to autogenous bone. Cryogenically preserved bone allografts have been used for some time in the oral surgical treatment of many types of minor defects of the facial bones, in some patients as substitutes for autogenous grafts, and in patients for whom the second operation to obtain the autogenous bone is contraindicated. (REF. 51-p. 221)

898. E. Autogenous bone marrow has been used in periodontal therapy by the placement of grafts in intrabony pockets. The technique is that of taking a small amount of the highly osteogenic graft material from the iliac crest in order to obtain a maximum osteogenic graft by a technique that is minimally traumatic and inconvenient to the donor. (REF. 51-p. 248)

899. E. Both allogenic and autogenous bone grafts are used in clinical dentistry to produce osseous repair in the treatment of cystic bone cavities, in periodontal therapy, in the treatment of maxillary clefts, in the treatment of the edentulous atrophic alveolar ridge, and in the recontouring of facial bones. (REF. 51-p. 250)

900. B. Facial evaluation for surgical orthodontics begins with a systematic three-dimensional assessment of the frontal and profile views in the vertical, transverse, and

horizontal planes. During the esthetic examination it is essential that the patient's lips and facial soft tissues be relaxed, not strained. In assessing frontal esthetics the surgeon and orthodontist should analyze asymmetry and vertical disproportion to describe abnormalities in the vertical and transverse (facial width) planes. (REF. 51-p. 250)

901. E. An assessment is made of functional occlusion which includes an analysis of the mandibular position in centric relation, opening and closing movements of the lower jaw, excursive movements of the mandible, orofacial musculature, and TMJ articulation. An altered mandibular position is frequently found coexisting with dentofacial deformities. (REF. 51-p. 270)

902. D. When the entire mandible is to be repositioned, the vertical oblique ramus osteotomy is performed through an incision in the posterior mandibular vestible. An osteotomy is performed obliquely from the sigmoid notch to the angle of the mandible. The mandible is then repositioned posteriorly. When the mandible is to be moved posteriorly more than 6-8 mm, the coronoid process is sectioned to prevent adverse traction from the temporal muscle. (REF. 51-p. 270)

903. D. Mandibular advancement is indicated for the correction of mandibular retrognathism (horizontally deficient mandible). The sagittal ramus osteotomy is the operation preferred by a number of oral surgeons. The latter procedure is performed in the body and ramus of the mandible. and allows the mandible to be advanced without bone grafts. Morbidity to the inferior alveolar nerve is very minimal. (REF. 51-p. 287)

904. A. Maxillary surgery is currently possible to correct a horizontal facial disproportion (maxillary deficiency). Maxillary deficiency can occur as part of a cleft lip and palate disorder as well as in patients with craniofacial syndromes. A modified high LeFort I maxillary osteotomyis performed to correct the maxillary deficiency. The bilateral sagittal ramus osteotomy is performed and the mandible is set back and asymmetry corrected. (REF. 51-p. 291)

Chapter 16 Anesthesia

905. E. Major oral surgery makes regional analgesia unfeasible. Infection rules out the use of regional anesthesia. (REF. 36-p. 7)

906. E. Before premedication, the dentist should make an evaluation of the patient. The evaluation will determine the following: patient's general physical and psychological condition, need for medical consultation, history of unpleasant drug experience, drug sensitivities of the patient, and true need for premedication. A complete history sheet should be attached to the patient's treatment chart to become a part of the permanent record. (REF. 36-p. 9)

907. A. Pain is difficult to control by regional anesthesia when inflammation exists in part (as in the dental pulp). Through the use of various conscious-sedative-analgesic techniques the dentist may manage the inflamed part (dental pulp) without resorting to general anesthesia and loss of consciousness. (REF. 41-p. 90)

908. B. Pain perception is localized within the cortex of the brain. However, it also is dependent to some degree on other anatomical structures such as free nerve endings, or pain receptors, and afferent sensory fibers for conducting the impulses from the site of the original stimulus. (REF. 37-p. 1)

909. B. Psychogenic pain is that unpleasant sensation which has no organic basis. The pain originates wholly within the mind but is fixed on some portion of the anatomy. The pain may represent a symptom of a deep underlying neurosis of which the patient is unaware. (REF. 37-p. 14)

910. C. Analgesia is the absence of all pain without the loss of consciousness. Hypoalgesia is a synonym of analgesia. It depicts the lessened pain reaction caused by elevating the pain threshold. (REF. 37-p. 71)

911. B. Nerve block is that method of securing regional analgesia (anesthesia) by depositing a local anesthetic solution within close proximity to a main nerve trunk, thus preventing afferent impulses from traveling centrally beyond that point. (REF. 37-pp. 61, 63)

912. A. In performing a paraperiosteal injection, the dentist inserts the needle in contact with the periosteum and deposits the anesthetic solution so that it will diffuse through the periosteum and cancellous bony plate. The solution is always deposited beside the periosteum. (REF. 37-pp. 61, 64)

913. E. The advantages of regional anesthesia are that the patient remains awake and cooperative; there is little distortion of normal physiology; there is low incidence of morbidity; the patient may leave the dental office unescorted; no additional trained personnel are needed; the technique is not difficult to master; the percentage of failure is small; there is no additional expense to the patient; and there is no need to omit a previous meal. (REF. 37-p. 63)

914. A. The mental nerve block uses the following anatomical landmarks: bicuspid teeth, lower edge of body of mandible, supraorbital notch, infraorbital notch, and pupil of the eye. The mental and incisive nerves are anesthetized. (REF. 37-p. 119)

915. E. The lingual nerve block is indicated for surgical procedures of the anterior two-thirds of the tongue, floor of the oral cavity, and mucous membrane on the lingual side of the mandible. The technique used for this nerve block is the same as that for the inferior alveolar nerve. Tingling and numbness develops in the anterior two-thirds of the tongue. (REF. 37-p. 112)

916. E. The inferior alveolar nerve block anesthetizes the inferior alveolar nerve and its subdivisions, mental nerve, incisive nerve, and on occasions the lingual nerve and buccinator nerve, both branches of the mandibular nerve. (REF. 37-p. 105)

917. E. The maxillary nerve block is indicated when anesthesia of the entire distribution of the maxillary nerve is required for extensive surgery, to block all the subdivisions of the maxillary nerve with one needle insertion, when local infection and trauma make blocks of the terminal branches difficult or impossible. (REF. 37-pp. 27, 61)

918. C. The infraorbital block anesthetizes the infraorbital nerves, inferior palpebral, lateral nasal and superior labial nerves, anterior and middle superior alveolar nerves, and sometimes the posterior superior alveolar nerve. This nerve block should be carried out under aseptic conditions (surgical scrub, sterile gloves, surgically prepared field). (REF. 37-p. 61)

919. B. Epinephrine is a levorotatory alkaloid secreted by the adrenal medulla. Epinephrine is administered as a hydrochloride salt and acts by vasoconstriction in the local area caused by its arteriolar effect. Epinephrine is the most potent and efficient of the vasoconstricting drugs used in dental anesthetic solutions. Concentrations of 1:50, 000-1:250, 000 are commonly administered (1:200, 000 appears to be the optimal concentration). (REF. 37-pp. 198-199)

920. E. No local anesthetic in use in modern dentistry fulfills all of these requirements especially the duration of action. Systemic toxicity is directly related to anesthetic potency (difficult to measure). (REF. 37-pp. 65, 132)

921. A. The potency of a local anesthetic depends solely on its chemical structure and the duration of action can be altered by the addition of a vasoconstrictor drug. Local anesthetic activity is related to a variety of structural configurations other than those of the local anesthetic agent. (REF. 37-p. 126)

922. E. True toxicity (overdose) is due to the following: sufficiently high blood stream level to affect vital centers by inadvertent intravascular injection, too large a volume, too great a percentage strength, and rapid absorption into the blood stream. Symptoms are early central nervous system stimulation followed by a proportionate degree of
Occasionally, central nervous system de-
ay appear as the first sign of toxicity. (REF.

mary cause of allergic reactions is a specific
body reaction in a patient previously sensi-
cal a[illegible]thetic agent. Symptoms of allergic
rticaria, angioneurotic edema,
on (rhinitis, asthmatic symp-

toms). The symptoms of toxic overdose to vasoconstrictor drugs are palpitation, tachycardia, hypertension, and headache. (REF. 37-p. 165)

924. E. Mepivacaine (Carbocaine) is a nonester local anesthetic agent which produces anesthesia of moderately long duration (2-4 hours). The maximum safe dosage is approximately 300 mg (15 ml of a 2% solution). REF. 37-pp. 127, 145)

925. A. Lidocaine (Xylocaine) is the first nonester anilide derivative to be used in dentistry. In toxic doses it first produces stimulation and then depression of the central nervous system. Lidocaine administered intravenously is capable of producing a degree of analgesia and even general anesthesia. Respiratory arrest (apnea) is the most common cause of death due to the overdose of lidocaine or any local anesthetic agent. (REF. 37-pp. 127, 143)

926. C. Tetracaine (Pontocaine) can be combined with epinephrine, procaine, and norepinephrine. Procaine in combination with tetracaine solutions do not potentiate each other but rather act as separate drugs in a physical, not chemical combination. Tetracaine is a potent, toxic, local anesthetic agent (10 times more potent and toxic compared to procaine). (REF. 37-pp. 126, 136)

927. A. Syncope (fainting) is a frequent complication following the administration of local anesthetics in dentistry. It is caused by cerebral ischemia secondary to a vasodilatation or increase in the peripheral vascular bed with a corresponding drop in blood pressure. The dentist should treat syncope in its early phases before the patient has lost consciousness. Elevate the patient's legs slightly so the patient is in a semireclining position. (REF. 37-pp. 210-211)

928. C. Muscle trismus may follow blocks of the inferior alveolar nerve. Any muscle soreness or limitation of motion is termed trismus. Trismus is due to trauma to a muscle during the insertion of a needle. Trismus may be prevented by using sharp, sterile needles in order to prevent trauma and low-grade infections. (REF. 37-p. 173)

929. E. The dentist can consistently and effectively be informed of his patients' physical conditions by physically evaluating all patients. Physical evaluation means that the dentist is attempting to evaluate the status of any existing systemic condition. History taking includes the following: to ask clear, concise questions; to listen attentively; to observe; and to integrate. A good listener will get much more information from the patient's answers. (REF. 43-p. 19)

930. E. Light anesthesia produces the following signs: slow breathing, prolonged inspiration, purposeful movement or rigid muscles, facial expression of pain or semiconsciousness, large pupils, eyelids resist opening, accelerated pulse rate, normal blood pressure, and pink color to skin. The objectives of anesthesia for all forms of surgery are the control of pain, muscular relaxation, and reduction of hemorrhage. (REF. 44-p. 3)

931. E. The preliminary safeguards for administration of volatile anesthetics are a case history, a physical examination, no food, and an empty bladder. (REF. 44-p. 35)

932. B. Cardiac arrest and the essential treatment of cardiac asystole are highly important problems facing the dentist. The treatment consists of maintaining cardiac compression plus the injection of 5-10 ml of 1% calcium chloride given intravenously every 4 minutes. If calcium chloride is ineffective, adrenaline should be administered (5 ml of 1:10,000) intravenously. A direct intracardiac injection may be given if venipuncture is impossible. (REF. 44-p. 173)

933. D. The chemical grouping of local anesthetics are the following: para-aminobenzoic acid esters and the anilides or amide derivatives. There is actually little to choose between the modern local anesthetic solutions with reference to onset of anesthesia. If the dentist has difficulty in achieving satisfactory local anesthesia with one drug, a substitute anesthetic solution of different chemical structure may well be successful. (REF. 44-p. 194)

934. B. The anaphylactic reaction (shock) may develop within minutes or seconds of the administration of the drug and demands immediate or emergency treatment. Lay the dental patient flat and administer oxygen or mouth-to-

mouth resuscitation and intramuscular adrenalin (0.5 ml of 1:1000 solution). In the absence of an immediate response, administer 100 mg hydrocortisone hemisuccinate intravenously. (REF. 44-p. 200)

935. B. Topical anesthetics have a place in dentistry, since with a sharp needle the topical anesthetics make injections painless. Topical anesthetics in use include the following: 5% lidocaine, 1 or 2% tetracaine, ethyl aminobenzoate (benzocaine), benzyl alcohol, and combinations of the latter with vehicles or flavoring agents. (REF. 44-p. 196)

936. C. Local anesthetic solutions are eventually absorbed into the general circulation and thus have the potential for toxic manifestations. The dental practitioner therefore should choose the local anesthetic with consideration and basic rules of good technique should always be followed during their use. (REF. 44-p. 195)

937. C. The doses utilized for local anesthetic drugs should be on the conservative side in order to afford the dentist a wide margin of safety. It must be remembered that dental patients are ambulatory and these individuals expect to have no side effects or reactions from the anesthetic. Likewise, the vasoconstrictor dosage automatically increases as the local anesthetic volume is increased. (REF. 45-p. 96)

938. C. The duration of action further depends upon the chemical nature of the drug, the concentration of the drug administered, the rate of diffusion of both the anesthetic salt and the free base, and the addition of vasoconstrictors, which influence the time during which the free base remains in contact with the nerve. (REF. 45-p. 136)

939. C. The injectable local anesthetics undergo biotransformation according to their basic ester or amide linkage in the intermediate chain. Local anesthetics of the ester group are inactivated by hydrolysis. Local anesthetics of the amide group primarily undergo biotransformation in the liver by microsomal enzymes. Degradation of the compound leads to a hydrolysis or splitting of the amide and the presumed hydroxylation of the aromatic ring. (REF. 45-p. 219)

940. B. Nitrous oxide has a definite analgesic action in small concentrations (as 10-20%). In this dosage range the ability to concentrate is decreased, as is the ability to interpret painful stimuli. A rise in the pain reaction threshold is associated with a decrease in psychomotor performance. No known chemical reaction involving nitrous oxide occurs when this gas is inhaled. (REF. 40-p. 35)

941. C. The air we breathe contains 80% nitrogen and 20% oxygen. The blood takes up only 1.7% by volume of nitrogen. It has been demonstrated that blood serum dissolves 26% by volume of nitrous oxide. Solubility of nitrous oxide in blood is about fifteen times that of nitrogen. Thus a mixture of 80% or 90% nitrous oxide and 10% or 20% oxygen can produce anesthesia. (REF. 25-p. 40)

942. E. Nitrous oxide is eliminated through the lungs primarily. As a general anesthetic nitrous oxide suppresses the cough reflex only to a moderate degree. Nitrous oxide does not cause any change in heart rate or cardiac output or a change in arterial or venous pressure. The sensitivity of the nasolaryngotracheal area is markedly reduced and the sense of smell is diminished. Nitrous oxide does not appear to stimulate nor depress metabolism (oxygen uptake). (REF. 47-p. 41)

943. B. Relative analgesia does not put a patient completely to sleep. During relative analgesia the respiration is normal, there are no movements of muscles, nausea is rare, pupils are normal and contract normally to light, eyelids do not resist opening, normal pulse rate, normal blood pressure, and normal skin color. Relative analgesia is not as good as local anesthesia. (REF. 47-p. 42)

944. B. Relative analgesia was never meant to be a substitute for local anesthesia. Analgesia alone may suffice in man cases in which local anesthesia is currently used. Relative analgesia permits a greater freedom of action in many cases. Analgesia may be used in synergistic combination with analgesia which permits an ideal psychosomatic solution to the problem. (REF. 47-p. 48)

945. B. Relative analgesia (nitrous oxide and oxygen) is useful in the following situations: differential diagnosis in cardiac conditions, patients with hypertension, psycho-

analysis and psychiatric care, venipuncture, postoperative analgesic, cystoscopy, changing and removing of dressings, incisions, suturing and removing sutures, removing foreign bodies, irrigations, insertion and removal of drains, injections, placing and removal of casts, painful or uncomfortable examination procedures, esophageal dilation, gastroscopy, and proctoscopy. (REF. 47-p. 49)

946. B. Nitrous oxide inhalation makes the surface veins more prominent and thus more accessible for venipuncture. (REF. 47-p. 98)

947. A. The arguments against conscious sedation include the premise that those who administer a general anesthetic (and nitrous oxide if given in sufficient dosage will produce general anesthesia) should be able to perform all the necessary technical procedures required for those who administer general anesthesia. Anesthesiologists believe that all who administer conscious sedation should be able to perform endotracheal intubation. However, conscious sedation techniques do not require general anesthetic training provided the baseline concept of Jorgensen is maintained. (REF. 95-p. 5)

948. E. The fact that premedication is not necessary is of great value since the administration of a drug out of the dentist's purview is a serious medicolegal hazard and should always be avoided. (REF. 95-p. 7)

949. E. The dentist is not always aware of early pregnancy. The majority of drugs should be avoided in early pregnancy because of possible teratogenic effects induced by medication. The drug manufacturers place inserts into their products which disclaim responsibility for teratogenic effects induced by medication. (REF. 95-p. 8)

950. B. Minimum anesthetic concentration is an experimental tool and is not for clinical use by the dentist. The minimum anesthetic concentration for nitrous oxide is 101%. Anesthesia ensued at between 80% to 140% nitrous oxide. It would be difficult to produce general anesthesia in any patient with less than 80% nitrous oxide. (REF. 95-p. 12)

951. E. Benefits of hypnosis range from full analgesia, requiring no adjunctive agents, t. decreased anxiety and tension permitting easier patient management with lower

dosages of local anesthetics or inhalation agents. Reducing the total drug exposure may decrease untoward reactions. (REF. 95-p. 23)

952. E. Narcotics will produce good relief of anxiety. Their disadvantage is the tendency to produce emesis. Meperidine is a narcotic that will frequently produce hypotension and cardiac arrhythmias. (REF. 95-p. 31)

953. A. Premedications which act for long periods after the oral procedure are definitely unsatisfactory for the dental patient. The purpose of the premedication is primarily to allay anxiety. (REF. 95-p. 31)

954. E. Ketamine (intramuscularly) is not satisfactory for use in dentistry because of the prolonged action of the drug militates against outpatient use. The incidence of hallucinations in adults is very high and it is contraindicated in teenagers and younger children. However, it can be used in uncooperative children. (REF. 95-p. 33)

955. B. When the tube is removed a sore throat occurs in 100% of patients. Laryngeal edema may occur followed by ulceration and laryngeal granuloma and 45% of patients have some degree of respiratory infection postoperatively. (REF. 95-p. 38)

956. E. The most successful anesthetics have balanced lipophilic and hydrophilic properties so that the anesthetic can arrive at the nerve at a sufficient concentration to effect local anesthesia. The drugs most commonly used in dentistry are lidocaine, mepivacaine, and prilocaine. (REF. 95-p. 46)

957. B. The concentration of the particular drug used does not necessarily alter the systemic toxicity or the actual blood level attained. An increased concentration of local anesthetic may increase the local tissue damage, however, it cannot alter systemic toxicity. (REF. 95-p. 51)

958. A. The Gow -Gates technique requires only one needle insertion rather than the usual two. The anesthetic solution is deposited via the intraoral approach at the neck of the translated condyle. It appears to be a reliable substitute for the standard inferior alveolar block in cases where adequate anesthesia is not achieved. (REF. 95-p. 63)

959. A. Aspiration prior to injecting vasoconstrictor plus local anesthetic will minimize the risk of intravascular deposition of vasoconstrictor. The common vasoconstrictors used with local anesthetics are epinephrine, norepinephrine, and nordefrin. Vasoconstrictors definitely have a place in dentistry. (REF. 95-p. 65)

960. E. There is quite a large number of drugs that react with monoamine oxidase inhibitors. This indicates their rather widespread activity. (REF. 95-p. 83)

961. E. An important feature for the dentist who uses conscious sedation in his practice is a review of all equipment and facilities before the operation at the beginning of each day. The latter is true of conscious sedation but also to routine dental practice. (REF. 95-p. 111)

962. E. Two specific reference points are utilized to evaluate the level of sedation, i. e., the first cortical sign and Verril's sign. Verril's sign is generally the end point of drug administration for conscious sedation. (REF. 95-p. 154)

963. C. Conscious sedation is not for every dental patient, every dental office and every dentist. However, when properly used it provides more efficient dental care and control of the apprehensive patients. (REF. 95-p. 160)

964. E. There may be some controversy among dentists concerning the type of patient who is really suitable for conscious sedation. (REF. 95-p. 165)

965. E. The latter signs are major in character. Physiologic signs indicate alterations in cardiovascular parameters. (REF. 95-p. 174)

966. E. Some patients are unable to cooperate, others are psychotic. (REF. 95-p. 176)

967. E. Minor complications in some patients may turn out to be major complications in certain dental patients. (REF. 95-p. 200)

Chapter 17 Community Dentistry

968. E. To enhance the health of the community, the dentist should direct efforts toward: maximum use of preventive procedures, provisions of the highest quality of dental service to the most people, the promotion of the total health of the community, and the organization and support of specific effects to improve oral health. (REF. 47-p. 6)

969. E. Health insurance applicable to dentistry has grown in demand over the past 20 years. The public is likely to continue to broaden its health insurance including dental care. There is an increasing demand for prepaid health coverage. The lessons learned from medical and hospital insurance programs can be useful in planning dental prepayment plans. (REF. 49-p. 9)

970. E. The modern dental practice must be organized to utilize all available preventive procedures if the dentist is to render the highest caliber of professional service to his patient. The latter includes a recall system, provisions for patient education, the use of topical applications of fluorides and dietary fluoride supplements, routine oral prophylaxes, use of radiographic procedures, and sterilization techniques. (REF. 49-p. 45)

971. E. The Oral Hygiene Index provides a systematic assessment of debris and calculus and has been useful in studying the relation between periodontal disease and oral cleanliness. (REF. 49-p. 83)

972. E. Hospitals, important health resources in any community, provide significant opportunities for the dentist. Unfortunately, the dental profession has not capitalized on the opportunities in this area. The dentist is not integrated into the hospital, the center of the delivery of health care. (REF. 49-p. 94)

973. A. The need for dental service often is confused with the demand for care. One can be aware of a need and not demand care for it. The unqualified desire for dental care is defined as potential demand whereas the desire plus the ability to obtain dental service is defined as effective demand. (REF. 57-p. 101)

974. E. Group private practice (joint dental practice) is classified as open panel and closed panel. An open panel is characterized by the following: a licensed dentist may elect to participate; beneficiary has his choice of a licensed dentist; and dentists may accept or refuse any beneficiary. In the closed panel, beneficiaries may go only to those dentists who agree to provide the prepayment plan. Dentists must accept any beneficiary as a patient.. (REF. 49-p. 105)

975. E. Group practice is nothing more than the conduct of a dental practice by two or more dentists who share the staff, facilities, and services. The dentists work together and consult with each other. The dental profession has viewed the growth of closed panel group practice as a threat to the private practice of dentistry. (REF. 55-p. 116)

976. E. Fluoridation has proved itself fully in practice after 20 years of experience. No hazard to health has resulted. However, despite the favorable experience, opposition to fluoridation has not ended. Fluoridation, despite its overwhelming advantages must not be considered a cure-all. (REF. 49-p. 123)

977. E. The new graduate should build a preventive dental practice. It is a better choice for several reasons. Once the objective has been attained and the majority of patients are returning for examination, prophylaxis, and routine maintenance service, the practice will be less taxing for the dentist. Second, rarely will it be necessary to perform major reconstructive procedures which are very difficult and demanding for the dentist and patient to accept. (REF. 49-p. 143)

Chapter 18 Dental Practice Administration

978. A. Work simplification requires studies of operations in motion, a critical analysis of floor plans, traffic flow, instruments, equipment, furnishings, business management, the relative functions of the operator, staff, the patient, and of the psychological attitudes as well as the physical movements that are part of a dental practice. (REF. 52-p. XVI)

979. C. Many individuals, including some dentists, regard work simplification as a series of statistics and formulas. Industry and dentistry, however, are adopting time and motion studies to increase efficiency by methods of motion economy. (REF. 52-p. 1)

980. E. The Class V motion is extremely fatiguing, and it should be eliminated. A Class V motion is the movement from the oral cavity to the working tray, attached to the unit, and back to the oral cavity. The latter demands the arm movement and movement from the center of the body. (REF. 52-p. 70)

981. E. In a comparison of time factors for eight operators, the following observations were made: most cavity preparation times were the same but one operator took four times longer than average; injection time varied from 10 seconds to 1 minute, 45 seconds; operators using high velocity suction did not require time for rinsing; and one operator spent over one-third of the total working time for carving the restoration. (REF. 52-p. 30)

982. E. The dentist will find that equipment needs, the number of personnel using the treatment room, the general arrangement, and the size of the room will vary from year to year with progress. However, the broad, basic concepts will not alter. (REF. 52-p. 84)

983. E. There is an arrangement that fits under the chair base and permits the chair to be pushed nearer the fixed unit. Sufficient space must be available in front of the chair to take advantage of these mechanisms. (REF. 52-p. 135)

984. D. There is evidence that large quantities of water do not actually cool as much as was originally believed. The high speed of a cutting tool creates a vortex, which can throw water away from the desired location. (REF. 52-p. 185)

985. E. Lighting inside the oral cavity should be supplied from a luminaire easily adjustable to exclude high brightness in the patient's eyes and at the same time provide lighting that is needed by the dentist to see fine details over long periods of time. (REF. 52-p. 190)

986. C. The preprepared tray is a link in a chain of prepared areas. To gain maximum efficiency from the system the staging or make-ready area must be well defined. All materials should be coded and indexed. (REF. 52-p. 206)

987. E. No stereotyped tray arrangement can substitute for the dentist's own thinking and planning. For a system to be effective, the dentist, together with his assistant, should determine what instruments are to be used, in what order, and with what frequencies. (REF. 52-p. 219)

988. E. Many dentists have a tendency to instruct the new assistant as something comes to their mind. With this kind of instruction, the assistant may not understand the purpose, the why, or the philosophy of the dental practice. Before beginning training, the dentist should be prepared to help the assistant understand something of his philosophy of practice. (REF. 53-p. 236)

989. E. The idea is to make the child patient feel important by some little attention. Overtalkative patients are the biggest time and money wasters in any dental practice. The dental assistant can break into a conversation by telling the doctor he is wanted on the phone or the next patient is waiting and in a hurry. Terminate the conversation, but do not offend the talkative patient. (REF. 54-p. 311)

Chapter 19 Pedodontics

990. E. Caries control is an essential part of preventive pedodontics. Research has reinforced the past observations about the role of sugars, particularly sucrose, in the production of carious lesions. The use of fluorides represents the most promising approach to caries control when incorporated in a program that also includes sugar restriction and oral hygiene. (REF. 58-p. 548)

991. E. The utmost effort should be made to educate parents and children on the need for children to curtail their consumption of foods with high sugar content (such as cookies, candies, jams, jellies, adhesives, and carbohydrates). There is a need to utilize more than one approach to the problem of caries prevention. (REF. 58-pp. 11-13)

992. C. Children in the mixed dentition period (ages 6 to 12) are generally easier to manage and more amenable to reason than their younger counterparts. Less problems are encountered in their behavior pattern and management. Reinforcement of acceptable behavior is a desirable approach, especially if complicated procedures are anticipated. (REF. 58, pp. 15-21)

993. A. Tranquilizers are frequently of benefit if children are unduly apprehensive and fearful. Where fear of an injection is the major problem to be surmounted, alternative procedures can be suggested. Proceed in some children with treatment with the local anesthetic or in others use nitrous oxide-oxygen analgesia as an alternative. (REF. 58-p. 20)

994. E. The fundamental principles of behavior modification successful with young children should be utilized with the adolescent as well. Reinforcement of good behavior, step by step procedural acquaintance and courtesy, all help in creating a favorable dentist-patient relationship. (REF. 58-p. 35)

995. E. A good examination includes evaluation of all aspects of a child's appearance and behavior before arriving at any conclusions about the oral cavity. (REF. 58-p. 73)

996. E. A health questionnaire or past medical and dental history should be completed in writing by the parent prior to the child's introduction to the dentist. Adequate health questionnaires should provide basic information as the child's name, nickname, age, weight, birthplace, chief complaint, and past medical and dental history. (REF. 58-pp. 334, 528, 529)

997. E. The oral examination of the child patient should consist of a detailed inspection of the soft and hard tissues of the mouth and a radiological survey. It may be necessary to perform special tests, diet surveys, medical reports, or consultation with specialists. A good order is to inspect the lips, externally and internally, the buccal mucosa and mucobuccal fold, the hard palate, the sublingual area, the tongue, and the gingivae. (REF. 58-pp. 73, 79)

998. E. The radiographic examination should involve a technique that is practical in regard to useful information gained by the dentist, the safety and comfort of the patient,

and the time required to perform such a survey. The radiograph is a tool in diagnosis that should be employed judiciously. (REF. 58-p. 104)

999. E. Every effort should be undertaken to reduce the amount of radiation exposure to the minimum. Precautions for the child's safety include the following: use of shielded equipment that is in good working order, have patient wear a lead apron, and use film that produces the least possible exposure. The largest film that fits the child's mouth is the most desirable one. (REF. 58-p. 101, 111)

1000. E. There are occasions when it is helpful to employ drugs as adjuncts to reduce the anxiety level of the child patient prior to operative procedures. Sedatives and hypnotics have been suggested to aid in relieving tension and emotional stress. One safe and effective sedating agent for children is a combination of hydroxyzine hydrochloride and chloral hydrate. The appropriate dosage must be given orally about 45 minutes before the dental appointment. (REF. 58-p. 130)

1001. B. Operative procedures for the child can be accomplished that are equal to those of the adult. Full coverage steel crowns have been a major breakthrough in economically solving the problem of restoring the badly broken down tooth in the primary and mixed dentition. (REF. 58-p. 164)

1002. D. The number of handicapped children is small, and pedodontists are called upon to treat relatively few. Handicapped patients require extra time, energy, preparation, and thought as compared to normal children. The dental problems of the handicapped are usually the same as those affecting normal children. Mangement is more difficult and dental care is frequently neglected. (REF. 58-p. 584)

1003. E. The use of the rubber dam in pedodontics provides many advantages, most important of which is the high degree of patient control during operative procedures. If it is not used with some children, the area of operation becomes contaminated with saliva despite all efforts of the dentist to keep it dry. (REF. 58-p. 143)

1004. E. The primary tooth is smaller and the pulp chamber relatively large. It is necessary to scale down the usual cavity preparation as well as to change it in certain aspects. A shallower pulpal floor is indicated. Since the contact areas of the primary molars are flat, the extension of the interproximal cavity should be wider to attain a selfcleansing area. No bevel is needed on the gingival since the enamel rods on primary teeth incline occlusally in the gingival third. (REF. 58-p. 45)

1005. C. Marginal defects are the greatest failure occurring in Class II amalgam restorations in both primary and permanent teeth. There is a need to eliminate traumatic cuspal occlusion and the desirability of a conservative occlusal outline to minimize marginal defects. Modifications such as grooving, rounding of floors, and gingival reverse bevels all improve resistance to bulk proximal fracture in vivo. (REF. 58-p. 168)

1006. E. The development of the full coverage steel crowns has been a major breakthrough in economically solving the problem of restoring the badly broken down tooth in both the primary and mixed dentition. Operative procedures in the child patient will gradually become less necessary due to fluorides and caries control agents. Thus a shift will be seen in the direction of greater emphasis on preventive orthodontics, habit control, and treatment of the handicapped. (REF. 58-p. 247)

1007. E. Carving and polishing of amalgam restorations in primary teeth should be carried out with the same care as in permanent teeth. It is not desirable to carve deep central and secondary grooves when restoring primary molars. It is necessary to check the occlusion a second time with articulating paper after final carving and removal of the rubber dam. Finai polishing of all amalgam restorations is necessary because it reduces corrosion and marginal deterioration and results in more comfort for the pedodontic patient. (REF. 61-p. 168)

1008. B. Use of good condensing force and properly shaped trapezoidal condensers is necessary to secure adaptation of amalgam. Corrosion and marginal deterioration are held to a minimum if amalgam is properly finished. The opposing cusps should always be checked for traumatic interdigitation and ground off if necessary. (REF. 58-p. 174)

1009. B. The cavity design should be prepared to minimize accidental pulp exposure and reduce the incidence of marginal breakdown of silicate cement. Other factors are responsible for failure regardless of the cavity preparation. These factors include lack of removal of caries, improper silicate cement manipulation and faulty placement and condensation of the silicate cement. (REF. 58-p. 180)

1010. E. Zinc oxide and eugenol may be used in indirect pulp capping. This preparation is sealed in teeth with deep carious lesions approaching the pulp, especially in young permanent teeth with incompletely formed root ends. (REF. 58-p. 187)

1011. E. Calcium hydroxide paste is widely utilized for indirect pulp capping following accidental operative exposures or for small carious exposures of 1 mm or less. Capping of the pulp exposure has never been a consistently successful approach to pulp management and should be employed sparingly. Calcium hydroxide appears radiolucent in a radiograph. (REF. 58-p. 169)

1012. C. The operator may undertake partial removal of caries and placement of calcium hydroxide under a temporary amalgam restoration when the permanent first molar has incomplete root apices. Continued development of root ends takes place. (REF. 58-p. 208)

1013. C. For the inferior alveolar injection the index finger or thumb is moved along the anterior border of the ramus until the greatest concavity is palpated (the coronoid notch). The finger is moved lingually to the internal oblique ridge. The needle is inserted from the opposite side of the mouth to bisect the fingernail and the soft tissue is penetrated. The needle continues its penetration until it gently touches bone and anesthetic solution is slowly injected after aspiration reveals no blood. (REF. 58-pp. 386-391)

1014. D. Indirect pulp capping is the sealing in of a suitable drug over partially excavated carious dentin. This pulp capping should arrest the existing caries process and stimulate sclerosis and hardening in the remaining vital dentin. Small surgical exposures may be capped with a paste of calcium hydroxide. (REF. 58-p. 201)

1015. B. In the case of a large carious exposure in a primary second molar, a formocresol pulpotomy is the treatment of choice. This type of pulpotomy is done on primary teeth only. (REF. 58-p. 236)

1016. B. Contraindications for the formocresol pulpotomy are history of spontaneous pain, pain from percussion, suppurative, calcified globules in the pulp, internal resorption, pathologic bifurcation radiolucency, and pathologic periapical radiolucency. (REF. 58-p. 212)

1017. C. The following are important points to remember when pulpectomy is performed on primary teeth: do not penetrate past the apical ends of the tooth; use a resorbable compound as zinc oxide and eugenol as the filling material; introduce filling material into canal with light pressure; and do not perform an apicoectomy except when the permanent tooth is absent. (REF. 58-p. 235)

1018 D. The maxillary primary molar roots contain flat shaped root canals. (REF. 58-pp. 45-70)

1019. E. The technique for endodontics on primary teeth may consist of filing out the root canals as thoroughly as possible at the first appointment and flushing with sodium hypochloride. A paper point containing camphorated monochlorophenol or formocresol should be sealed in each root canal. At the second appointment the paper points are removed and root canals are filled with resorbable material (zinc oxide and eugenol or Oxpara paste). (REF. 58-pp. 218, 219)

1020. D. Accidents to primary teeth are most common at 1-1/2 to 2-1/2 years of age. Fracture of teeth may involve the following: enamel fracture of primary maxillary incisor, dentin fracture of primary maxillary incisor, and fractures involving the pulp in a primary maxillary incisor. (REF. 60-p. 19)

1021. D. When a primary incisor tooth has a horizontal and vertical fracture of the crown, it is so severely mutilated that extraction is generally the treatment of choice. (REF. 60-p. 18)

1022. E. Severe intrusion of maxillary primary incisors may frequently lead to devitalization following the injury. These should be treated endodontically or extracted to prevent abscess formation adjacent to permanent tooth buds or developing permanent teeth. It is however possible for re-eruption to occur in intruded primary teeth 5-6 months following the intrusion. (REF. 60-p. 30)

1023. E. Overprotection produces a shy, anxious child. Overindulgence results in an aggressive, demanding, and spoiled child. Underaffection produces a well-behaved child which may be unable to cooperate; may be shy, and may cry easily. Rejection produces an aggressive, overactive and disobedient child. Authoritarianism produces an evasive and dawdling child. (REF. 96-p. 16)

1024. E. There is also an emotionally immature child patient. They are very young children who cannot rationalize the need for dental treatment. (REF. 96-p. 75)

1025. E. With children who exhibit disruptive behavior, the dentist must use procedures to allow them to receive dental treatment plus condition the child to accept dental treatment psychologically. (REF. 96-p. 76)

1026. E. When inhalation sedation with nitrous oxide-oxygen is not desired or indicated there is general agreement that the intravenous route is the method of choice. (REF. 96-p. 175)

1027. D. The most accurate and effective premedication for the conscious patient is produced by titrating a sedative directly into a vein. (REF. 96-p. 176)

1028. E. Palpation of the injection site before the placement of the tourniquet, a thorough knowledge of the anatomy of the venipuncture techniques by the dentist will prevent the latter problems. (REF. 96-p. 185)

1029. E. An adequate health questionnaire is essential since it provides information that is helpful to the dentist's diagnosis of a child's immediate and long-range problems. (REF. 97-p. 18)

1030. E. The objectives of treatment are to eliminate infection; repair and retain all primary teeth until exfoliation; correct any variation from normal in the developmental pattern of permanent teeth; prevent and intercept incipient malocclusion; educate families to control and prevent dental disease; and condition the child to be a good dental patient. (REF. 97-p. 30)

1031. E. The toxic effects of lidocaine include depression without the preliminary stage of stimulation. (REF. 97-p. 69)

1032. E. The eruption process is frequently associated with excessive irritability, refusal to sleep or eat, excess drooling, fever, vomiting, and dermatitis. Fever and systemic disturbances are not related to the teething process but rather to infections, loss of maternal antibodies, and development of immunologic responses. (REF. 97-p. 94)

1033. A. The latter four characteristics must depend on the interaction of technical factors primarily under the control of the dentist. Panoramic radiology has enhanced the diagnostic capability of the pedodontists. (REF. 97-p. 119)

1034. E. Radiation hygiene is of importance in children because of their high biological susceptibility to x-rays. The risk of damage is proportional to the dose administered, therefore, avoid any amount of unnecessary radiation. However, radiographs are essential in pedodontics and they should be used whenever necessary. (REF. 97-p. 127)

1035. E. The technique involves the application of a phosphoric acid solution to the enamel prisms, which alters the tooth surface. An acrylic resin is applied and bonds to the enamel surface. Failures of the bond may take place partially or entirely within the resin rather than at the resin-enamel interface. Failure may also occur within the enamel. (REF. 97-p. 148)

1036. A. Injuries during the adolescent years are primarily due to contact sports. Children with protruding anterior teeth with lack of lip coverage are predisposed to fractured teeth during contact sports. (REF. 97-p. 207)

1037. B. The dental practitioner should determine space needs carefully in relation to the restoration of defective teeth (crowns and roots). The child with partial or complete anodontia will no doubt require space analysis and treatment planning which provides the most in functional and esthetic occlusion. (REF. 97-p. 246)

1038. E. Vertical problems in orthodontics are due to environmental factors and abnormal growth. Their treatment is highly complex. (REF. 97-p. 226)

1039. E. Dentists who treat handicapped children will experience the gratitude of patients who never have been able to find a dentist to perform dental treatment. The reward to the dentist is a sense of high accomplishment, pride, and foremost a feeling of satisfaction. (REF. 97-p. 392)

1040. A. No ideal preventive dentistry program exists but there are successful preventive programs that every dentist should revise or augment to suit his personal needs and desires. Preventive care is a long-term relationship between the dentist and staff and patients. The patient must comply with the dentist's treatment to ensure long-term success. (REF. 98-p. 37)

1041. E. Water fluoridation should be our goal in every community with a central water supply in the United States. The fluoridated communities in the United States have reduced the incidence of dental caries by 50-60%. Patients who live in nonfluoridated communities require topical fluoride treatments semiannually. Children should receive a fluoride supplement at 6 months of age (except those breast-fed when fluoride drops should be given starting at birth). (REF. 98-p. 69)

1042. C. All evidence indicates that physical and chemical barriers applied to caries-susceptible teeth plus oral hygiene and restriction of sucrose, are the most effective therapy for prevention and control of dental caries. (REF. 98-p. 100)

1043. E. Emphasis in the young is on the use of systemic fluoride and diet control by early elimination of the nursing bottle and parent awareness of the importance of early dental care. The child should progress over the years from being the object of the preventive dental program to providing his own program. (REF. 98-p. 174)

1044. E. The maximum benefit from fluoridation comes from lifelong residence in a fluoridated area. Fluoridation is probably the most investigated preventive dentistry measure. There is substantial evidence of efficacy and the dental and economic benefits are tremendous. (REF. 98-p. 274)

Chapter 20 Orthodontics

1045. C. There is a large degree of variation among individuals in the sequence or the timing of calcification and crown formation. (REF. 59-pp. 168, 169)

1046. A. The rule is that a tooth contact proximally is different in the deciduous dentition following the establishment of a continuous dental arch (3 -7 years). Except for the deciduous molars, no other teeth are in proximal contact. Spacing of teeth is not abnormal in the latter situation. Normal occlusion is not a rigid relationship of the teeth. What is normal interdigitation in the deciduous and mixed dentition is abnormal in the permanent dentition. (REF. 59-pp. 196-198)

1047. C. It has been demonstrated by experimental studies that it is possible with orthopedic forces to increase the transverse dimensions of the maxillae, along with the alveolar processes and dental arches. Orthopedic forces also produce secondary effects, i. e., remodeling adjustments at the circummaxillary sutures and broadening of the nasal cavity. (REF. 59-pp. 196-198)

1048. A. The overbit of incisors is the amount of labial vertical overlap of the maxillary incisors over the mandibular ones. It usually corresponds to one-third the mandibular incisor crown height. Normal variation in the overbite ranges from zero to 3 to 4 mm. (REF. 59-pp. 584, 585)

1049. E. Normal occlusion is a requisite for facial esthetics. The canines have been selected as representing the keys to occlusion. The canines can further be related to facial skeletal landmarks (as the orbitale and Frankfort horizontal). Malocclusion can thus be defined in anteroposterior and transverse directions. (REF. 59-p. 205)

1050. B. The purposes of orthodontic treatment are esthetics, interception of imbalanced forces, preprosthetics, preventive periodontics, prevention of pathosis, correction of speech defects, and facilitation of surgery. (REF. 99-p. 1)

1051. E. The latter six prerequisites should be fulfilled in order to warrant an attempt at minor tooth movement. Minor tooth movement techniques should be considered if the jaws are in correct relationship, if the malpositions are limited to relatively few teeth, and if the desired movement is not more than a few millimeters. If the mandible and maxilla are in an incorrect relationship to the skull or to each other, specialized training in orthodontics is required. (REF. 99-p. 6)

1052. E. An individual tooth can be in several different versions at the same time. The tooth may be in labio-, mesio-supra-, and torsiversion all at the same time. (REF. 99-p. 18)

1053. A. A negative overjet occurs when the maxillary incisor teeth are positioned posterior to the mandibular anterior teeth.

1054. B. Certain skeletal or environmental abnormalities may cause a supraeruption of posterior teeth or an infraeruption of the incisors. In the latter case the incisor teeth do not approximate in occlusion and the patient has an anterior open bite. (REF. 99-p. 19)

1055. E. According to Angle, the key to occlusion is the maxillary first permanent molar. A Class I occlusion is an ideal occlusion in a well balanced muscle system. The mesiobuccal cusp of the maxillary first permanent molar occludes in the buccal groove of the mandibular first permanent molar. The lips and soft tissue are in a harmonious relationship. (REF. 99-p. 22)

1056. C. The most common removable appliance is the acry lic and wire appliances. The appliance consists of the acrylic baseplate that covers the palate. the retentive clasps around molars and premolars, and the active force. (REF. 99-p. 93)

1057. D. In planning the design of the auxiliary springs (labial wire spring, free-ended spring, and accessory spring), it is necessary to design these springs so that they will exert suitable pressure over an adequate distance. (REF. 99-p. 102)

1058. C. In orthodontic therapy, the physical properties desired are generally those of a long spring. However, the latter may not be possible because of the limited space available. This disadvantage is overcome by disposing of some of the surplus length in the form of a coil. (REF. 99-p. 106)

1059. E. It is generally of great value for the dental practitioner who desires to undertake minor tooth movements for his patients to consult with an orthodontist. This is particularly true in those borderline cases in which a question exists as to whether or not the orthodontic problem can be successfully treated with minor tooth movements. (REF. 99-p. 106)

1060. E. Proper instrumentation is important in the construction of orthodontic appliances. The basic pliers and orthodontic instruments should be included in the armamentarium of every dental office. (REF. 99-p. 116)

1061. E. Maxillary and mandibular Hawley appliances will close the anterior diastemas and produce a satisfactory occlusion. (REF. 99-p. 117)

1062. D. It is important to construct the anterior labial wire with great attention to detail. The palatal portion of the Hawley wire is embedded into acrylic for retention. The occlusal portion of the anterior labial wire should be contoured above the contact area and close to the premolar in order to prevent occlusal interferences. (REF. 99-p. 122)

1063. E. The mattress spring is utilized to produce a labial or buccal tooth movement. (REF. 99-p. 132)

1064. B. The purpose of the maxillary acrylic biteplate is to increase the vertical dimension in cases of deep overbite. By causing the eruption of the posterior teeth, the mandible will assume a resting position with relaxation of the muscles of mastication. The tense muscles of mastication cause problems in the temporomandibular joint. (REF. 99-p. 139)

1065. C. Preformed, pre-welded orthodontic bands are available from manufacturers. They must be crimped and adapted to improve the fit. (REF. 99-p. 152)

1066. E. The attachment or bracket is the most important part of the band and serves to attach the arch wires and devices for force application. The bracket is used for the insertion of the labial arch wires. (REF. 99-p. 155)

1067. B. This type of therapy should be performed by an orthodontist because imprudent use of orthopedic forces can produce unwanted results. (REF. 99-p. 167)

1068. C. Thumbsucking creates unilateral and bilateral crossbites. With abnormal forces applied to the maxilla by the buccinator muscle during sucking, it is possible to prevent the proper growth in the width of the maxilla. Thus, there is a difference in the width of the maxillary and mandibular dentitions. The narrow maxillary arch causes the patient to shift the mandible to the left or to the right in order to create a functional occlusion. A bilateral problem results. (REF. 99-p. 202)

1069. E. A removable appliance utilizing elastic traction may be used to close anterior diastemas. Since every force produces an equal and opposite force, it is necessary to have an anchoring mechanism for the removable appliance. One retention device is the ball clasp. A Hawley type of appliance with a labial arch wire may also be used to close a diastema. (REF. 99-p. 216)

1070. B. If resorption of the frenum fails to occur after 3-4 weeks the frenectomy is then performed while retaining the orthodontic result produced prior to surgery. (REF. 99-p. 232)

1071. A. Individual anterior cross-bites are due to ectopic eruption, misplaced tooth bud, arch length discrepancy, or other factors that produce individual malposition (as anterior teeth in linguoversion). (REF. 99-p. 243)

1072. E. The tooth bud of the third molar is located in a superficial position at an early age. Therefore, it may be easier to remove the impacted third molar at the early stage of development than at a later stage when the tooth is present in a deeper location within the bony mandible. (REF. 99-p. 265)

1073. E. The following are indications for the use of minor tooth movement appliances (teeth are to be moved short distances and the number of teeth is small): esthetics and prosthetics. In modern times, adult dental patients are seeking orthodontic therapy as they desire increasingly comprehensive dental care. The dental pracitioner thus should be better educated in the principles and techniques of providing limited orthodontic treatment. (REF. 99-p. 277)

Chapter 21 Oral Pathology

1074. B. In congenital syphilis the infection is transmitted to the newborn by the mother at birth or prior to delivery. The infection may take place through the placenta beginning at the fifth month of pregnancy. Congenital syphilis is generally not responsible for abortion during the early months of the infection. There is always the possibility that an uninfected living newborn may be delivered from a syphilitic pregnant woman. The child with congenital syphilis may be born prematurely. Spoon-shaped hutchinsonian incisor and the mulberry molar are characteristic of congenital syphilis. (REF. 70-p. 149)

1075. D. Oral lesions of tuberculosis are rare. However, they may occur on the tongue, palate and lips. The lesions of tuberculosis vary but are generally flat, with ulcerations on the tongue simulating traumatic ulcerations. They may be granulomatous or take the form of an indurated mass suggestive of malignancy of the tongue. (REF. 64-p. 104)

1076 D. Osteoporosis produces a decreased density with weakness of the bones of the jaws. The decreased density is the result of an inadequate or depressed matrix formation with an impediment to formation of new bone.

The balance between bone formation and bone resorption is upset by a decrease in the bone formation rate. (REF. 88-p. 322)

1077. D. Primary (congenital) and secondary (acquired) macroglossia may be recognized. Overdevelopment of tongue musculature is the primary type, and the acquired type results from relaxation of the tongue musculature, regardless of etiology. (REF. 88-p. 93)

1078. B. Malignant oral neoplasms vary from very large easily recognized lesions to small lesions with minimal or no features of cancer thus no clinical diagnosis is possible. A biopsy is essential in establishing the diagnosis or in confirming the clinical impression. Malignant oral neoplasm is diagnosed only after obtaining positive histopathologic evidence. Basically, the clinical, historical, and histopathologic approaches must be emphasized in the diagnosis of oral malignancy. (REF. 69-p. 786)

1079. C. Hodgkin's disease may be a chronic inflammatory process of viral or bacterial origin. Its behavior pattern is indicative of malignant neoplasia similar to other lymphomas. Three distinct histopathologic entities comprise Hodgkin's disease, i.e., paragranuloma (least malignant variety), Hodgkin's granuloma, and the sarcoma (most malignant variety). All three types have the binucleate giant cell (Reed-Sternberg cell), which is pathognomonic for Hodgkin's disease. (REF. 83-p. 252)

1080. B, C. Keratotic lesions (keratoses) of the mouth may be precancerous. Leukoplakia is an example of a precancerous oral disease. It is histopathologically different from other keratotic diseases because it is characterized by dyskeratosis and thus precancerous. Hyperkeratosis is not a precancerous disease. Leukoplakia appears as a grayish-white or whitish adherent patch of any size and shape occurring on any region of the oral cavity. (REF. 67-p. 85)

1081. D. Ankylosis is a chronic limitation of motion in a joint. It may be partial or complete, fibrous or bony, true or intra-articular, false or extra-articular, and unilateral or bilateral. Combinations of the latter also may take place. (REF. 71-p. 294)

1082. C. Lymphosarcoma may arise from mature lymphocytes or lymphoblasts. The clinical behavior pattern is more benign than the reticulum cell sarcoma. Lymphosarcoma occurs in males after 40 years of age, with the development of nontender enlargement of the deep cervical lymph nodes. The lymph nodes are firm, discrete, and mobile during the early stages of the neoplasm. (REF. 88-pp. 261, 326)

1083. C. Leukemia is a malignant neoplasm involving the blood-forming cells with an abnormal proliferation of white blood cells and their precursors. Metastasis of the abnormal white blood cells takes place to the spleen, liver, lymph nodes, and infiltration occurs in the bone marrow. Marrow function is inhibited with development of anemia and thrombocytopenia. Leukemic infiltration produces hypertrophic gingivae. (REF. 64-p. 284)

1084. D. Infectious mononucleosis is an acute disease with an obscure etiology. However, it may be a hypersensitivity reaction or is caused by a virus. The acute disease occurs primarily in children and young adults but no age is immune. Lymph node enlargement, sore throat, and stomatitis, gingivitis, or ulcerations are present in the oral cavity along with petechiae. (REF. 88-pp. 26, 76, 155)

1085. D. Oversecretion of the pituitary growth hormone subsequent to dental development and epiphyseal closure produces acromegaly. There is bossing of the frontal bones, enlarged nose, lips are protuberant, mandible is enlarged (mandibular prognathism), flattened palatal vault, normal size and shape of the teeth, large interdental spaces in the mandible, migration of teeth leading to periodontal disease and malocclusion. (REF. 68-p. 22).

1086. C. The teeth are pigmented with a bluish color due to the deposition of blood pigment in the dentin and enamel of developing teeth. The pigment does not involve the portions of the teeth that develop after birth or after blood hemolysis has ceased. Only the deciduous teeth of children are affected. There is excessive attrition of the deciduous teeth, rounded teeth, thin occlusal enamel, and blue-green or brown pigmentation in deciduous teeth. The deciduous teeth have a groove encircling the crown called the Rh hump. The groove represents the cessation of the growth of enamel at birth. (REF. 72-p. 74)

1087. D. Xerostomia is present in Sjogren's syndrome with or without salivary gland swellings. Decreased salivation leads to complaints of dryness and burning of the mouth. When teeth are present, rampant dental caries reminiscent of radiation caries may be present. The edentulous patient finds it difficult to tolerate dentures due to dry and inflamed oral mucosa. (REF. 88-p. 36, 100)

1088. A. Amelogenesis imperfecta is a developmental disturbance of enamel formation that affects all teeth (deciduous and permanent). The dentin is normal since mesodermal tissues of the tooth are not involved. The disease appears to be of genetic origin and probably transmitted as a simple dominant medelian characteristic. (REF. 68-p. 46)

1089. C. The incidence of cleft palate in Caucasians is 1:2500. The cleft occurs more frequently in females than males. The cleft palate may be complete in a number of syndromes and diseases. The cleft appears as a defect of varying length in the midline of the palate, exposing the nasal cavity to the oral fluids. The cleft palate patient may have impaired hearing and labyrinthitis. (REF. 68-p. 15)

1090. A. The torus palatinus is an exostosis located in the midline of the palatal vault. It results from the overlapping of the medial surfaces of each palatal process forming a single protuberance. About 25% of adults exhibit some bony enlargement of the palatal vault (REF. 68-p. 135)

1091. D. Paget's disease produces various radiographic bone patterns in the periapical regions of the jaws, i. e., a granular pattern, a "Cotton-ball" pattern, a stippled pattern, and a striated pattern. Paget's disease of bone is a chronic bone disease characterized by connective tissue proliferation which disturbs the bone architecture. New bone formation is prominent leading to enlarged and deformed bones. The skull is involved in 15% to 20% of patients and one or both jaws are generally affected (maxilla more commonly affected than mandible). The etiology of this bone disease is obscure. (REF. 88-p. 198)

1092. B. Monostotic fibrous dysplasia involves only a single bone (maxilla, mandible, skeletal bone). Polyostotic fibrous dysplasia involves more than one bone but no other abnormalities exist. Albright's syndrome is a form of polyostotic fibrous dysplasia plus associated endocrine disturbances (abnormal skin pigmentation, precocious growth with early epiphyseal closure, precocious sexual development, and on occasion hyperthyroidism or diabetes mellitus). (REF. 80-p. 296)

1093. D. Periapical granulomas are common in the jaws. They are located at the root apex and arises due to bacterial infection of an involved pulp which spreads to the periapical tissues. Chemical products of necrotic pulps lead to periapical granulomas. (REF. 68-p. 38)

1094. C. Mottled enamel (fluorosis) is a form of enamel hypoplasia. Hypocalcification results from the ingestion of fluorides during tooth formation. Mottling of enamel occurs when the fluoride level significantly increases above 1 part/million. No mottling of enamel occurs when the fluoride level is below 1 part/million parts of water. Fluorosis may be classified into the following: mild fluorosis, moderate fluorosis, and severe fluorosis. (REF. 68-p. 53)

1095. E. Pulpitis is applied to all types of inflammatory and infective changes that occur in the pulp of teeth. It is difficult to produce a differential diagnosis of pulpitis. Clinical investigation should consist of exploration, thermal applications, percussion, palpation, excavation, electric pulp testing, and radiographic examination. (REF. 72-p. 332)

1096. D. Clinically, salivary gland tumors are unilateral, with recurrent neoplasms becoming multicentric. The salivary gland benign neoplasm may be an asymptomatic, mobile, enlargement. The benign neoplasm is slow growing with an intermittent or rapid growth period. Pain is associated with malignant neoplasms but not with the benign growth. Benign mixed tumors demonstrate a bosselated configuration clinically. (REF. 23-pp. 46, 94, 506)

1097. C. Mucocele (mucous cyst) may occur at any age in both sexes which arises from an obstruction of the duct of the mucous gland or from traumatic severance (as biting the lips). A collection of fluid accumulates within the tissue spaces leading to a mucous retention phenomenon rather than a retention cyst. The mucocele occurs in any location in the oral cavity but is common in the lower labial mucosae. (REF. 68-p. 453)

1098. C. The ranula is a true cyst, arising from the retention of salivary fluid in the ducts or body of the submaxillary or sublingual gland. It is the result of obstruction. (REF. 68-p. 456)

1099. B. Paget's disease of bone (osteitis deformans) is a chronic bone disease affecting the sacrum, femur, spine, skull, and in 15 to 20% of patients one or both jaws are involved. Paget's disease of bone has a positive family history. (REF. 68-p. 571)

1100. C. Oral lichen planus frequently precedes lichen planus of the skin. About 50% of patients with lichen planus have oral lesions. This oral disease differs from hyperkeratosis and leukoplakia (common keratotic diseases) because it occurs equally in males and females and appears from 20 to 40 years of age and as frequently as in older individuals. The etiology is obscure but is related to emotional factors (fear, depression, trauma). (REF. 88-pp. 37, 50)

1101. D. Allergic stomatitis is a simple inflammatory reaction that may occur superficially and involves most or all of the peripheral tissues of the oral cavity. Clinically, the tissues are intense red color, moderately swollen, and is smooth and glistening. Moderate dryness with burning, tenderness, itching, and pain are frequent. (REF. 88-p. 154)

1102. C. The ameloblastoma arises from epithelium derived from the ectodermal component of the odontogenic tissues (dental lamina, enamel organ, rests of Malassez, Hertwig's root sheath). Thirty percent of ameloblastomas arise from epithelial rests in the walls of odontogenic cysts (primordial and dentigerous cysts). Many varieties of ameloblastoma exist (six epithelial and four mixed varieties). (REF. 68-p. 210)

1103. C. The malignant melanoma is a rare oral neoplasm but is one of the most rapidly spreading and fatal skin neoplasms. Its most frequent oral location is in the gingival and palatal tissues. The oral tissues show increasing melanin pigmentation leading to formation of a dark-colored patch. The lesion spreads in all direction with a dark abnormal mass of tissue. This neoplasm is dense, borders are indurated, and ulceration plus meta static lymphadenopathy are present. (REF. 68-p. 96)

1104. C. The tongue, gingivae, and buccal mucosae are commonly involved in amyloidosis. The tongue is a site for a single oral lesion of amyloid. Single or multiple firm nodules of varying sizes, pale or gray in color, develop in the tongue. (REF. 68-p. 521)

1105. E. The basal cell carcinoma of the face rarely (less than 1% of cases) metastasizes. It infiltrates and invades the surrounding tissues. Its clinical appearance is varied since it develops as a fungating, infiltrative or verrucous patterns. (REF. 68-p. 100)

1106. D. Tuberculosis of the oral cavity is rare. Lesions can occur in the tongue, palate and lips and appear as flat, persistent ulcerations that simulate those of traumatic origin. The lesions may be granulomatous or inflammatory, and form a firm, indurated mass. A biopsy is indicated to make a definitive diagnosis. Calcified bodies may develop in the submandibular lymph nodes during tuberculosis. (REF. 68-p. 262)

1107. D. Actinomycosis develops as a cervicofacial cellulitis with purple nodules in the cheek and face. Actinomyces bovis is the common cause. A conclusive diagnosis cannot be made without laboratory studies confirming the clinical findings. Smear cultures should be made and/or biopsy performed of the oral lesions. The exudate serves as an excellent culture specimen. (REF. 64-p. 144)

1108. B. Focal infection is that infection in which pathogenic microorganisms and/or their toxins located in a one localized area spread by way of the lymphatics, blood stream, nerve channels, or by direct passage to other parts of the body. The latter gives rise to or exacerbates numerous systemic diseases. (REF. 68-p. 421)

1109. E. The dentist must distinguish between an oral neoplasm or whether the disease is inflammatory, cystic, or an abnormality. The tissues of the oral cavity may give rise to a variety of neoplasms with a varied clinical appearance. There is no single clinical appearance common to oral neoplasms or cysts. Oral biopsy examination most often provides the necessary data for making a conclusive diagnosis. (REF. 68-p. 200)

1110. C. The gingival tissues may undergo the following changes: epulis, alveolar inflammatory hyperplasia, and giant cell granuloma. (REF. 68-p. 664)

Chapter 22 Oral Roentgenology

1111. C. A tissue or a part which permits relatively greater transmission of x-rays is termed radiolucent. Such an area produces darker shadows on the film because of the more ready passage of the rays and their greater effect on the silver salts in the emulsion. Substances or tissues which absorb more rays than others are considered more opaque and are termed radiopaque. (REF 74-p. 11)

1112. B. The bone adjacent to the periodontal ligament is denser (like all cortical bone) and is termed the lamina dura. It appears as a thin white line in the radiograph. (REF. 74-p. 2)

1113. D. The thin white line (lamina dura) is highly important in radiographic interpretation. (REF. 74-p. 298)

1114. B. Radiography plays an important role in the diagnosis, study and treatment of periodontal disease. However, it does have very serious limitations. Periodontal disease may be present without any radiographic indication of abnormality. Radiographic evidence may lead to error. (REF. 76-p. 83)

1115. B. Any consideration of the level of the alveolar crest or the depth of a bone pocket has to take notice of the length of the root. With naturally short teeth certain degree of bone loss is of greater significance than the same amount with a long root. Thus the length of the roots plays an important part in the progress of periodontal disease. (REF. 89-p. 399)

1116. B. There is a great tendency to cease study of the oral radiograph when one abnormality has been seen in a film. Neglect will eventually lead to error. The recognition of a second lesion in the same radiograph is often of utmost significance in arriving at the correct interpretation. (REF. 74-p. 390)

1117. B. The medullary or cancellous bone surrounding the tooth socket is made up of thin strands, or trabeculae, which cross one another in an irregular manner. Separating the trabeculae, in radiographs, are dark spaces which contain bone marrow. (REF. 89-p. 298)

1118. B. The nasal fossae is a cavity which appears as a dark shadow in the radiograph. The fossae contains air, therefore, the shadows are usually very dark, but not of uniform density. (REF. 89-p. 224)

1119. C. The incisive foramen varies widely in shape and the foramen transmits the nasopalatine nerves and vessels. It is an important structure in radiographic interpretation because it is very often mistaken for a cyst or pathologic process. (REF. 89-p. 265)

1120. A. Radiographic evidence of fracture consists of a wide and radiolucent area in the midline suture, often with the roots of the incisor teeth projected through some part of the area. (REF. 74-p. 350)

1121. A. There are dentists who attempt to make radiographic interpretations of antral infections from intraoral radiographs. The procedure is open to too many fallacies to make it justifiable. (REF. 89-pp. 224, 245)

1122. A. The relationship of the apices of the teeth and the antral cavity has been shown to be variable, and in many instances it is not possible to accurately determine the thickness of bone interposed between root and antrum. (REF. 89-p. 229)

1123. A. Nutrient canals (vascular canals) in the maxilla are less frequently seen outside of the shadow of the antrum. They are noted mostly in the bicuspid region and only rarely in the incisor area. (REF. 75-p. 387)

1124. A. The radiographic appearance of the mental foramen is that of an area of radiolucency. The shadow may be oval, rounded, oblong, or irregular in shape or there may be no shadow at all. The position of the mental foramen is also variable, the commonest sites being at of just below the apex of the second bicuspid or a little mesial to and below the latter apex. (REF. 74-p. 8)

1125. B. The occlusal radiograph can also be used to view the mental foramen. Occlusal projections reveal the buccal-lingual or labial-lingual location of teeth or other structures in the jaws. (REF. 89-pp. 120-123)

1126. C. Radiographic evidence of incisive canal cysts, including the nasopalatine and anterior palatine varieties, is an area of radiolucency situated in the midline, often with the roots of the incisor teeth projected through some part of the area. (REF. 89-p. 360)

1127. B. Mandibular third molars may fail to erupt completely, if at all. The impacted third molar may appear as a vertical impaction, mesioangular impaction, distoangular impaction, and a horizontal impaction. The third molar may become impacted against the distal aspect of the second molar or into the bone of the ascending ramus. (REF. 75-p. 437)

1128. B. The following cysts develop in the midline of the maxilla: anterior palatine foramen cyst, incisive foramen cyst, median cyst, nasopalatine cyst, and vestigial cyst. The latter cysts primarily arise either from the nasopalatine duct or the buccal epithelium. They may contain ciliated epithelium and squamous epithelium (most common), and mucous cells may be present. (REF. 89-p. 359)

1129. D. Serial radiographs, made at periods of time, may reveal extension of decalcification into the depths of the alveolus while the surface of the crest is being destroyed. Generally, loss of the alveolar crest takes place imperceptibly and without previous decalcification in the trabeculae. (REF. 89-pp. 300, 302)

1130. B. External resorption may occur in the roots of teeth which lie in contact with cysts of the jaw (such as apical cysts). Resorption (root) is more common in the presence of neoplasms than with a cyst. Rarely a clinical dental cyst may be present; however, there is no radiographic evidence of the presence of the cyst. (REF. 75-p. 274)

1131. B. The granuloma varies in size radiographically and may be very small to an inch in diameter. The full extent of the granuloma cannot be determined from radiographic studies, for they reveal only the vertical and lateral dimension and not the anteroposterior, or coronal, dimension in the lesions on the posterior teeth. (REF. 89-p. 387)

1132. A. To diagnose nutrient canals the radiograph should have a good contrast, i.e., the percentage of difference between the white and black shadows is high. (REF. 77-p. 6)

1133. C. Only foreign bodies that are radiopaque may be demonstrated by radiographic methods such as fragments of metallic filling materials, broken hypodermic needles. broken instruments, pellets from shotguns, fragments of shells or bombs, and glass particles from broken windshields. Fragments of wood, toothbrush bristles, and fish bones may become impacted in soft tissues; however, they are not visible in radiographs. (REF. 89-p. 356)

1134. D. Bone changes in the jaws occur with certain metabolic disturbances and may be revealed in dental radiographs. Substantial alterations must occur in the calcified portions of the jaws before any radiographic change appears. Failure to demonstrate disease by means of the radiograph is not proof of its absence. (REF. 89-p. 398)

1135. C. The acute alveolar abscess may develop at the apex of either permanent or deciduous teeth. Organisms appear at the apex of the root and lead to an intense inflammatory reaction in the periodontal ligament and adjacent bone. Liquefaction of cells occurs, pus is formed and burrows through bone to the surface. The radiographic changes in the early abscess are very difficult to see. The abscess occurs in an area of radiolucency of ill-defined extent, within which bone trabeculae are visible but of lessened width and density. (REF. 74-p. 9)

1136. A. Multiple myeloma occurs in the skull and skeleton. A few small radiolucent areas may be all that is present even in a fatal case. In the jaws, the maxilla rarely reveals the rounded areas of radiolucency, even when the skull shows numerous lesions. The presence of multiple small areas of bone destruction in the jaws is likely either multiple myeloma or secondary cancer (both are rare). (REF. 89-p. 378)

1137. B. It is vital to understand that the mere presence of bone pockets in radiographs may not have the significance that they appear to have. It is possible for bone destruction to persist following successful treatment, without there being any actual space between the tooth and the bone. Where bone is grossly lost so that the alveolar crest is far from its original site, the surface may be flat, which is all that the radiograph may indicate. (REF. 74-p. 105)

1138. E. Therefore, it is imperative that patient exposure or system speed, as well as other safety features, be considerations that are not overlooked by the dental practitioner. (REF. 100-p. 3)

1139. B. The single phase generators are used with a variety of films as the image receptors. All films require postexposure manual processing in wet chemicals. The use of panoramic x-ray equipment has been rather common; however, there is some evidence that suggests that this modality may not be understood by its users. A growing tendency exists toward the use of machine processing of films rather than wet tanks or manual development. (REF. 100-p. 4)

1140. E. Other factors of concern in the evaluation of a film include its resolution or its relative ability to distinguish closely approximated structures from one another, its consistency from one batch of film to another, and its packaging. Dental film also has a finite shelf life. (REF. 100-p. 8)

1141. E. The great increase in speed present with the rare earth film-screen combinations is an important factor. Reducing the exposure time lessens motion distortion. The life of the x-ray tube is increased because of the reduction in work load and the exposure of the patient can be dramatically reduced. (REF. 100-p. 11)

1142. E. By producing appropriate matches among all components of a dental x-ray system, gains are possible in image quality plus the reduction to radiation exposure. (REF. 100-p. 15)

1143. A. All modern x-ray equipment also have light fields that correspond with x-ray fields, thus the positioning of the patient and the adjustment of the x-ray field size can be readily accomplished. (REF. 100-p. 16)

1144. E. The choice of processing of x-rays is between the machine and tank. The choice is based primarily on economics and volume. Either method when used correctly and with care will produce a good radiograph. With either system, a quality assurance program should be instituted for regular testing. (REF. 100-p. 18)

1145. E. In microfocus radiography theoretical advantages are present; however, detailed technical specifications, focal spot sizes, duty cycles, and other information have not been readily available when compared with their traditional counterparts. (REF. 100-p. 24)

1146. C. It may be possible to distinguish between a carious lesion and the cavity preparation based on the quality of the hard tissue margins, it is impossible to determine radiographically whether a cavity preparation has been adequately filled with a plastic or resin material unless the material is opacified. (REF. 100-p. 50)

1147. E. Xeroradiography has been used for cepahometric analysis, for evaluation of bone lesions of the mandible, for sialography, and for the study of a variety of dental as well as nondental structures. It is of particular value in tomography of the temporomandibular joint. The advantages of xeroradiography in dentistry include an intraoral image receptor, fine detail, wide latitude, high image contrast, and relatively low exposure requirements. (REF. 100-p. 55)

1148. E. Computer tomographic scanning has proven valuable in examining the salivary glands after an injection of contrast agents. It is possible to identify tissue masses that are located adjacent to the parotid glands which cannot be recognized during routine sialography. (REF. 100-p. 70)

1149. A. When properly used, the nuclear medicine procedures with radiopharmaceuticals circulating and concentrating to varying degrees in different organs and tissues can be of considerable value in the diagnosis and treatment of dental, osseous, and salivary gland pathology. (REF. 100-p. 110)

1150. E. Lack of image sharpness in the original radiograph cannot be overcome by photographic copying. Instead, it will increase as the copy of an inferior original is enlarged for viewing or photographic printing. (REF. 105-p. 113)

1151. E. It should, therefore, be apparent to the dentist and dental student that the characterization of pathology by precise and specific radiographic criteria is impossible. In fact, radiographic interpretation by pattern recognition can lead to serious mistakes. It is impossible to arrive at definitive diagnosis as the result of image analysis. However, radiographic data can be used effectively in the development of a differential diagnosis and to provide important supporting evidence to validate a clinical diagnosis. (REF. 100-p. 142)

Chapter 23 Periodontics

1152. B. Heavy calculus deposits upon the teeth during uncontrolled diabetes mellitus. The calculus appears with a cartilaginous consistency and is easily removed. The irritation produced by the calculus causes a loss of tissue vitality and tone. (REF. 62-p. 54)

1153. A. Forty percent of pregnant women may have gingivitis probably due to hormonal imbalances. The gingivitis increases in severity from the second month of gestation until the eighth month and then decreases. Pregnancy appears to act as a modifying influence on the gingival response to local irritants. (REF. 81-p. 97)

1154. C. Gingivitis occurs with or without gingival enlargement and may be acute or chronic. The local etiologic factors in gingivitis are: plaque, bacteria and bacterial products, calculus, irritating restorations, food impactation, infections, and other causes. Other etiologic factors are drug allergy, hormonal, systemic, and idiopathic causes. (REF. 83-p. 23)

1155. D. The periodontal pocket is a diseased gingival attachment. The pocket exists only because of the pathology present in the gingival tissues, initiated for the most part by local etiologic factors. Diagnosis of a pocket is made by measuring the space between the tooth and the gingiva but also takes into account the condition of the gingival tissue. (REF. 81-p. 121)

1156. D. The importance of occlusal trauma as an etiologic factor in periodontal disease must be emphasized. Habits of clenching, bruxism, etc., are agents in producing traumatic forces. The force of the musculature of the lips and cheeks against the teeth as well as the force of the tongue from within the oral cavity also must be recognized in producing occlusal traumatism. (REF. 81-p. 170)

1157. C. There is a direct relationship between the amount of bacteria in plaque, oral debris, and calculus and the severity of periodontal disease. A direct cause-and-effect relationship exists between dental plaque and gingivitis. A cause-and-effect relationship between bacterial plaque and alveolar bone loss in man has not been documented. However, it has been demonstrated that the loss of alveolar bone increases with poor oral hygiene. (REF. 81-p. 331)

1158. B. Gingivectomy is not an outmoded surgical procedure; however, it is not a replacement for scaling and curettage or to mucogingival surgical procedures. It is a surgical procedure that fulfills specified objective. It can easily and simply produce optimum gingival morphology. (REF. 81-p. 616)

1159. D. Malocclusion is a contributing factor to periodontal disease. The time to utilize tooth movement procedures is after the reduction of the dental inflammation. Orthodontic treatment generally precedes retention, stabilization, occlusal adjustment, pocket elimination, and restorative dentistry. (REF. 81-p. 538)

1160. C. Calculus deposits are responsible for a marked inflammatory reaction in the gingival tissues. Calculus deposits result in edema of the interdental tissues on the lingual aspects of the mandibular incisors. Slight mobility of the teeth is present. Calculus forms as subgingival calculus and supragingival calculus. (REF. 81-p. 125, 128)

1161. C. Curettage is the procedure of scraping or debriding a tissue. Gingival curretage is the use of an instrument against the gingival side of the pocket in order to scrape and debride the soft tissue. It is intended to remove the chronically inflamed wound surface elements. (REF. 81-p. 171)

1162. B. Osteoplasty is the plastic contouring of the alveolar process to achieve physiologic contours in the bone and gingival tissues. Ostectomy has the same objectives as osteoplasty, but involves sacrifice of supporting bone as well as the periodontal ligament to produce the required contours. (REF. 81-p. 774)

1163. C. Gingival involvement is localized to the marginal area and is the incipient evidence of a progressive gingival hyperplasia, a condition concomitant with gingival inflammation. Gingival hyperplasia and recession are signs of periodontal disease. Inflammatory gingival hyperplasia is associated with heavy calculus deposits. (REF. 83-p. 138)

1164. B. Gingival involvement and hyperplasia may be of systemic background, such as the hyperplasia of Dilantin therapy. This gingival involvement may not be specifically diagnostic from the clinical picture but are diagnosed after careful evaluation of data obtained from clinical examination, history, and laboratory examination. (REF. 79-p. 269)

1165. D. Gingival changes are associated with vitamin C deficiency. They are commonly seen in children under 2 years of age. Gingival lesions may be the first manifestation of vitamin C deficiency in children. The gingivitis is characterized by a marked tendency toward spontaneous hemorrhage and by very painful, swollen, bluish, purple gingivae plus ulcerations. (REF. 79-p. 90)

1166. B. Migration of teeth is one of the characteristics of periodontal diseases. Tooth migration is associated with various factors, i.e., pocket formation, food impaction, occlusal traumatism, and various habits. Migration also occurs during periodontosis but it is not specific for this disease. (REF. 81-pp. 78, 80)

1167. B. The objectives of the gingivectomy are elimination of the gingival pockets and creation of physiologic gingival morphology. Morphology of the gingiva postoperatively is closely related to health and prevention of future periodontal disease. The underlying alveolar bone must be free from any deformity. (REF. 81-p. 616)

1168. B. In pregnancy there is probably some other factor introduced which, together with local bacteria, may be responsible for the gingivitis of pregnancy. Pregnancy appears to act as a modifying influence on the gingival response to local irritants. (REF. 81-p. 90)

1169. C. Gingivosis begins insidiously as a low-grade edema of interdental papilla that spreads to the marginal and attached gingiva. The second stage (acute stage) is engorgement of affected gingiva, which hemorrhage spontaneously and profusely. The chronic stage results in necrosis of the gingiva with recession and denudation of the root. (REF. 81-p. 257)

1170. D. Clinical features of the periodontal pocket are: discoloration (pink to bluish red), loss of stippling, retraction of gingival tissue, bleeding, exudate (can be expressed from pocket by pressure), and loss of architectural form. Histologic findings are: discoloration, loss of stippling, retraction, bleeding, exudation in pockets, and hyperplasia of gingiva. (REF. 81-pp. 211, 1381)

1171. B. Etiology of periodontal disease involves local environmental factors, severity, frequency of injury and duration of disease process modified by resistance and repair factors. The inflammation of the gingival units is caused by local factors, i.e., microbial, mechanical, chemical, thermal, and radiant factors. (REF. 81-p. 499)

1172. D. The depth of the pocket should be ascertained with a probe bearing a millimeter rule. Not only is the pocket depth important, but also the topography of the pocket. Pockets vary in depth around the involved tooth. (REF. 81-p. 117)

1173 D. Periodontosis affects young patients. It is a degenerative form of periodontal disease with noninflammatory destruction of the periodontium. All cases have varying degrees of gingival inflammation in spite of the latter noninflammatory definition. There is loosening and migration of the teeth in the absence of accountable local factors. (REF. 81-p. 866)

1174. A. Gingival curettage is utilized in the treatment of marginal gingivitis. Marginal gingivitis may be characterized by inflammatory hyperplasia with heavy calculus deposits. Subgingival calculus deposits are adherent to all surfaces of all teeth. (REF. 79-p. 209)

1175. C. The mobility of teeth in disease may be classified into four groups: in some subjects only single teeth are affected, whereas in others all teeth are involved; increased mobility and wandering may be the only sign of disease; teeth with restorations which are slightly high may show increased mobility for a short time and then become firm; and teeth that can be depressed in the socket show a markedly increased width of the periodontal ligament and loss of alveolar bone. (REF. 81-p. 953)

1176. D. A periodontal abscess may form in pockets above the bone crest in the gingival corium or in infrabony pockets. The abscess may point through the bone or form in the periodontal ligament not near the gingiva. The interradicular area of multirooted teeth is also a site for periodontal abscess formation. (REF. 81-p. 116, 117)

1177. C. Recognizable lesions of occlusal traumatism are the result of the magnitude, severity, and frequency of the applied force modified by the repair ability of the host. The attachment apparatus and teeth are considered to be related to the general body biology and exposed not only to local influences. (REF. 81-p. 156)

1178. C. In some situations the gingival morphology predisposes the area to plaque accumulation. The gingival margins create soft tissue craters that act as harbors for the bacterial invaders. (REF. 81-p. 259)

1179. A. Etiologic factors include both local and systemic causes of hyperplastic gingivitis. Oral debris, bacterial plaques, calculus, and gingival pathology are present. The removal of the latter plus improvement of local hygiene may lead to resolution of gingival inflammation.

Once accretions are established they contribute to further injury to the gingival tissues. (REF. 79-pp. 206, 209)

1180. B. Gingival tissue showing fibrous hyperplasia should be resected by gingivectomy and include gingivoplasty so that the fibrous tissue does not interfere with mastication or induce oral disfigurement. (REF. 79-p. 209)

1181. A. Acute necrotizing ulcerative gingivitis is a distinct, recurrable periodontal pathology having a rather complex etiology, with some factors still obscure. It is distinguishable clinically from marginal gingivitis or periodontitis and responds to therapy. (REF. 81-p. 333)

1182. B. Immediate subgingival curettage in acute necrotizing ulcerating gingivitis has only a salutary effect on the gingiva. Subgingival debridement and curettage are carefully performed as completely as possible in the affected zones, although the coronal scaling is done without completeness. (REF. 78-pp. 623, 631)

1183. B. During an oral examination one should review not only the severity of the calculus deposit but also the control by the patient (attempt and accomplishment). The better the control of calculus and oral hygiene, the less the occurrence of periodontal disease. (REF. 78-pp. 301-309)

1184. C. Pockets are classified as suprabony or infrabony. Infrabony pockets are subdivided into pockets with three osseous walls, pockets with two osseous walls, pockets with one osseous wall, and combinations of the latter three types. Suprabony pockets are classified as gingival pockets and periodontal pockets. (REF. 78-pp. 188, 189)

1185. D. The function of a temporary splint includes the following: protect the mobile tooth by stabilizing them, distribute occlusal forces to prevent teeth with lost periodontal support from trauma, retain teeth in the position to which moved by orthodontics, prevent pathologic migration, protect mobile teeth during periodontal procedures, and aid in determining if borderline teeth will respond to therapy. (REF. 79-p. 657)

1186. B. Thorough curretage may be effective. However, if the latter plus oral hygiene fail and in more advanced cases oral penicillin (1 million units daily for 4 days) may be administered, provided of course there is no previous history of sensitivity to penicillin. (REF. 81-pp. 167, 168)

1187. B. In instances where the second molar (mandibular) has been lost the third molar drifts forward to take its place. There is no contact between the first and third molars. Interdental resorptive lesion develops assuming a vertical character in relation to the third molar. This lesion is caused by food impaction resulting in marginal periodontitis and creation of an infrabony pocket. (REF. 79-p. 147)

1188. C. The indications for tooth movement for periodontics include the following: reduction of deep overbite or locked bite resulting in occlusal trauma, correction of crowded teeth detrimental to good gingival health, closure of open contacts prone to food impaction, correction of occlusal discrepancy in the presence of occlusal trauma, improvement of landmark positioning (cusp tip to central fossa line) for occlusal equilibration, and modification of elimination of gingival and osseous defects. (REF. 81-p. 514)

Chapter 24 Endodontics

1189. C. Pulp exposure may originate from the following etiologic factors: bacterial (coronal ingress), traumatic (fracture), iatrogenic (cavity preparation), chemical (filling materials, disinfectants), and idiopathic. An alarming amount of pulp involvement is caused by the treatment (as high speed technology) designed to repair the caries. (REF. 85-p. 295)

1190. C. Hyperemia of the pulp is a hyperreactive alteration characterized by increased blood flow to the dental pulp under a variety of conditions. The following stimuli give rise to hyperemia: thermal change of hot or cold or acidic or touch stimulation through exposed dentin. Hyperemia of the pulp is the midlest alteration, and it is generally transitory in nature. (REF. 85-p. 296)

1191. C. Acute pulpitis or inflammation of the pulp is generally accompanied by histopathology of chronic inflammation rather than of acute inflammation. Neutrophils are present in incipient (acute) pulpitis. Microabscesses of the pulp do develop at areas of caries exposure extended through reparative dentin. (REF. 85-p. 297)

1192. B. The acute apical abscess is resolved by either spontaneous or therapeutic drainage. Positive diagnosis of this abscess rests on clinical signs and symptoms rather than roentgenographic findings.

1193. B. Successfully capped pulp exposures have a dentin bridge formed beneath the calcium hydroxide layer. An intense cellular activity is present below the dentin bridge. Pulp capping is not recommended in instances of traumatic pulp exposure in the anterior teeth. (REF. 85-p. 305)

1194. B. Pulpotomy is more desirable than pulp capping because gross bacterial contamination occurs in traumatic pulp exposure, it is difficult to restore a pulp capped tooth, it is often difficult to obtain retention in restoring a pulp capped tooth, and success of pulpotomy compares favorably with success of pulp capping. (REF. 85-p. 305)

1195. B. Pulp capping is contraindicated after a traumatic accident where microorganisms have gained entrance into the pulp. Impact injury frequently results in devitalization of the pulp. Enormous root canal and open apex of the tooth indicate early devitalization of the pulp following a traumatic accident. (REF. 85-p. 309)

1196. B. There is some evidence that prior to the obturation of canals, greater success is achieved in cases with negative cultures than in cases with positive cultures. Antibiotic management in therapy can be better suited to the individual if antibiotic sensitivity testing is done for organisms in the root canal. Culturing is useful as a yardstick to determine if canal debridement is complete. (REF. 85-p. 310)

1197. A. Endodontic surgery is indicated when the tooth cannot be saved without surgery. Concern over apical cysts is reduced since most apical cysts will heal following root canal filling and without surgery. Indications are necessity for drainage, failure of nonsurgical therapy, predictable failure with nonsurgical therapy, impracticality of nonsurgical therapy, and procedural accidents. (REF. 85-p. 318)

1198. D. The first objective of sanitation of the root canal is achieved by skillful instrumentation coupled with liberal irrigation. Disinfection and preferrably sterilization occurs by the use of intracanal medicaments which complete the sanitation. (REF. 63-p. 487)

1199. D. The causes of endodontic failures include the following: incomplete obturation, root perforation, external root resorption, periodontal-periapical lesion, canal grossly overfilled, canal unfilled, developing apical cyst, adjacent pulpless tooth, silver point inadvertently removed, broken instrument, accessory canal unfilled, constant trauma, and perforation of nasal floor. (REF. 86-pp. 34, 167)

1200. B. External resorption produces ragged margins in the resorbed bone. Differentiating external resorption from internal resorption is based upon the following: the walls are ragged and irregular. The resorption appears on the side of the tooth or centered. The pulp always appears to pass through the lesion unaltered, maintaining its size and shape all the way to the apex. The radiolucent lesion appears to be superimposed over the pulp canal. External apical resorption results in a shortened, blunted, or square tooth. (REF. 86-pp. 29, 48, 334)

1201. B. Concomitant periapical and periodontal lesions may cause the dentist to extract the involved tooth. However, concurrent endodontic and periodontic therapy may be successful and save otherwise hopeless teeth. The primary source of the communicating lesion should be located since the origin of the lesion determines the prognosis. The periodontal-endodontal defects have been classified into five types of lesions. (REF. 86-pp. 34, 64)

1202. B. No aspect of endodontics is as important as the roentgenographic examination. It can also be extremely misleading to the dentist. The roentgen image is only a shadow which has elusive characteristics. The roentgenogram is a two-dimensional picture of a three-dimensional situation. The roentgenogram may be too short or too long and too light or too dark. Two exposures are necessary to check out detail from more than one horizontal angle. The film must be properly placed, exposed, and processed. (REF. 86-pp. 445, 471)

1203. E. The rubber dam can be placed for endodontic therapy in 1 minute. The rubber dam concept is not time-consuming, frustrating, and discouraging when applied to endodontics. There are advantages to using the thin weight rubber dam on mandibular anterior teeth as well as on partially erupted posterior teeth. (REF. 86-p. 91)

1204. B. The outline form of the endodontic cavity must be correctly shaped and positioned in order to provide complete access for instrumentation. External outline form is established during preparation by mechanically projecting the internal anatomy of the pulp onto the external surface. (REF. 86-pp. 104, 166)

1205. B. Most reamers for endodontics are manufactured by pulling and twisting a triangular wire into a sharpened tapered instrument of gradual spirals. Most files are made by twisting square wire into a tapered pointed instrument of much tighter spirals than the reamer. Files can be used for both reaming and filing. However, reamers can be used only for reaming. (REF. 86-pp. 170, 172)

1206. B. Prior to and at frequent intervals during instrumentation, the root canals should be irrigated with a solution capable of disinfecting and dissolving organic matter. The specimen for bacteriologic culture must be taken before irrigation. Irrigation reduces the microbial flora in the root canals and facilitates instrumentation by lubricating canal walls and by removing dentin filings from root canals. (REF. 86-pp. 173, 17[illegible])

1207. B. Bacteria may be effectively controlled or eliminated from diseased canals by debridement and proper irrigation while cleansing and shaping the canal and by intracanal medication. Proper cleansing of the root canal, with irrigation, is the most effective method for removing and killing bacteria. (REF. 86-p. 580)

1208. E. A highly critical act in assuring the success of treatment is the accurate determination of the length of the tooth prior to radicular preparation. The length of the tooth procedure establishes the apical extent of instrumentation and the ultimate apical level of root canal filling. Increased failure, prolonged healing, apical perforation, and overfilling may result from failure to accurately determine the length of the involved tooth. (REF. 86-pp. 179, 210)

1209. B. After a traumatic accident, if the pulp responses are negative and root development is complete, immediate pulpectomy and root canal filling are the indicated treatment. (REF. 86-pp. 222, 596)

1210. E. Avoid the use of toxic-filling materials. Toxic-filling materials play a noxious role in pulp inflammation Use a proper protective base, one covering all the walls of exposed dentin within the cavity. Dry the dentin carefully before placement of the base. Cavity liners themselves may be toxic. Prevent insult and injury to the dental pulp. (REF. 65-pp. 222, 596)

1211. E. The cements with American acceptance are primarily zinc oxide-eugenol cements, the polyketones, and epoxy. The pastes currently used are chlorapercha and eucapercha, and iodoform pastes (rapidly and slowly absorbable types). (REF. 66-p. 222)

1212. C. Electric pulp testing shows validity for the quantified results. Adequate controls are necessary for the electric pulp testing and a normal, uninvolved tooth (comparable tooth in oposite arch) should serve as an adequate control. However, it is necessary to test teeth adjacent to or near the suspected tooth, especially if trauma is an etiologic factor. (REF. 86-p. 478)

1213. D. Chronic pulpalgia produces discomfort with mild pain lasting for months to years. The pain is diffuse and it is difficult to locate the source of the pain. This discomfort causes mild referred pain. (REF. 86-pp. 504, 507)

Chapter 25 Dental Materials

1214. C. Approximately 70-80% of all dental services involve the use of dental materials. The dental materials are intended to restore both function and esthetics. (REF. 87-p. 2)

1215. B. One should understand the physical and biological properties of dental materials as well as the manipulative effects of these properties. Materials restore function and esthetics and arrest further tissue destruction, and materials conserve the nation's critical dental manpower. (REF. 87-p. 29)

1216. B. Plaster of Paris is a gypsum product to which modifiers have been added to regulate the setting time and control the setting expansion. It is used in making impressions. Plaster of Paris is generally used in an individualized tray made of modeling composition or acrylic resin as a refining wash. When border refining is not required the plaster is used in a stock tray. (REF. 87-p. 56)

1217. A. White plaster has its setting time adjusted by the addition of special accelerators. Starch is added to make the finished cast easier to separate. The added accelerator has an ionic strength that reduces expansion to a minimum. Impression plaster is not used today because of its cast separation difficulties. (REF. 87-p. 56)

1218. B. Potato starch is added to make the plaster more soluble. (REF. 87-p. 75)

1219. D. Experimentation has been undertaken with zinc fluoride and zinc sulfate treatment baths in an effort to improve the quality of gypsum casts. The latter have been successful. (REF. 87-p. 78)

1220. B. Never immerse the setting gypsum cast in water because the expansion of either plaster or stone or die stone will double or triple its size through the phenomenon of hygroscopic expansion. The cast should be separated one hour after pouring to prevent damage to the cast's surface. (REF. 87-p. 178)

1221. A. Reversible hydrocolloid (agar) is the first dental material that makes accurate one-piece impressions of undercut surfaces. When heated, this hydrocolloid converts from a solid gel into a liquid sol state suitable for dental impressions. (REF. 87-p. 110)

1222. E. Making the impression influences the preventive characteristics of a prosthesis. The design of the impression tray for the final impression and the choice of materials should provide an equitable distribution of pressure over tissue areas that are both hard and soft, thick and thin, and rigid and displaceable. (REF. 87-p. 110)

1223. C. Modeling impression compound is a thermoplastic material used as an impression material. The stick form is used as an impression material and the cake form is primarily used as a tray (impression) material. (REF. 87-pp. 83, 91)

1224. E. The thermal conductivity of modeling compound is very low. The outside of the compound softens first; the inside softens last. When the material hardens, the tissue side is the last to be affected. (REF. 87-p. 83)

1225. C. The lower the temperature of the compound at the time the impression is made the less the error from the linear thermal coefficient of expansion. The American Dental Association specifications for the compounds for impression making allow a flow of 6% at mouth temperatures. (REF. 87-p. 89)

1226. E. Prolonged heating of modeling compound makes the compound more brittle and grainy. When a flame is used to soften compound, care should be taken not to overheat, boil, or ignite the compound since these result in a change in the properties owing to the loss of important constitutents. (REF. 87-p. 89)

1227. D. A typical commercial zinc oxide-eugenol powder is composed of 70% zinc oxide, 29% rosin, and small amounts of zinc acetate and/or zinc sterate. The rosin improves the mixing properties, and the zinc salts are accelerators. The liquid is composed of 85% eugenol and 15% olive oil. The olive oil aids mixing and reduces any burning sensation caused by eugenol. (REF. 87-pp. 192, 100)

1228. C. The zinc oxide and eugenol react chemically to form a chelate compound, zinc eugenolate crystals. These crystals then form a matrix to which untreated eugenol is absorbed, while the unreacted zinc oxide is dispersed throughout the mass as a filler. A smaller particle size also tends to reduce solubility and disintegration. (REF. 87-p. 92)

1229. E. Plasticizers, fillers, and other additives are incorporated into zinc oxide-eugenol paste to alter certain properties such as smoothness of mix, adhesiveness, hardness when set, and setting time. (REF. 87-pp. 92, 100)

1230. A. Zinc oxide and eugenol pastes have no significant dimensional change subsequent to hardening. The impression can be preserved indefinitely without a change in shape from relaxation or other causes of warpage. However, it is best to pour casts as soon as practical. (REF. 87-p. 95)

1231. E. The setting time of zinc oxide-eugenol paste is not easily controlled by inexperienced operators. The temperature and humidity influence the setting time. However, the paste does not absorb the secretions in the palate, since when the secretions are profuse, distortion results. The paste is untidy to handle and difficult to control at the borders, and may distort when removed from undercuts. (REF. 87-p. 96)

1232. C. Minimal tissue distortion results when the paste is allowed to flow under the application of minimal pressure. The advantage of the paste is its ready flow and the material is not washed out by saliva. (REF. 87-p. 98)

1233. C. Compressive strengths in excess of 5000 pounds per square inch have been reported for zinc oxide-eugenol mixed at a high powder-liquid ratio. (REF. 87-p. 97)

1234. A. Hydrocolloid sols possess the property of changing to gels under certain conditions. The application of heat to a reversible colloidal gel returns the gel to the sol conditions. When the sol is cooled, it returns to the gel. (REF. 87-p. 112)

1235. A. A disadvantage of reversible hydrocolloid is that gels are subject to changes in dimension by syneresis and imbibition. Therefore, the impression must be poured in stone immediately upon removal from the mouth. (REF. 87-p. 107)

1236. C. The accuracy in reproducing detail of hard objects is not necessarily true when reproducing soft tissues. Any material that must be seated with positive pressure and held rigidly until the material hardens or gels is capable of displacing soft tissue. (REF. 87-p. 107)

1237. C. Wrapping an impression in a moist towel is acceptable for the trip to the laboratory; however, it is no substitute for pouring within the time specified. The poured cast should be covered with wet paper and stored in a humidor for one hour. This minimizes distortion of alginate during the setting period. The cast should be separated one hour after pouring to prevent damage to the cast's surface. (REF. 87-p. 109)

1238. D. A rapid cooling of hydrocolloid may cause a concentration of stress near the tray during gelation. Releasing of this stress after removal from the mouth results in distortion. Distortion may also result from varying thickness of material during gelation. (REF. 87-p. 110)

1239. C. Alginate hydrocolloid has been modified over the years to allow its use in removable partial denture fabrication. It is, however, unsatisfactory for use in fixed prosthodontics, as far as master casts and dies are concerned. Poor detail registration by the alginate and the alginate-gypsum interaction prevent casts made from these materials from showing clearly defined planes, angles, and finish lines. (REF. 87-p. 117)

1240. C. The alginates deteriorate rapidly at elevated temperatures. Material stored for a month at 60°C or over is unsuitable for dental use. (REF. 87-p. 117)

1241. A. The composition of the alginate radically affects its gel strength. (REF. 87-p. 114)

1242. E. The reaction rate of the alginate impression materials can be controlled by varying the temperature of the mixing, or gauging water. (REF. 87-p. 114)

1243. B. The alginate affects the hardness of the surface of stone. To overcome this immerse the impression in a hardening solution for not more than 15 minutes. A 2% solution of potassium sulfate is recommended. (REF. 87-p. 114)

1244. B. The advantages of these materials for preliminary impressions are simplicity of equipment needed, ease of manipulation, little discomfort to the patient, short chair time, and accurate reproduction of undercut areas. The irreversible hydrocolloids are not as accurate in recording detail of hard objects as rubber impression materials. (REF. 87-p. 116)

1245. C. Gelation takes place in approximately five minutes and is accomplished with water-cooled trays. Water temperature below 55°F is not recommended by manufacturers for gelation procedures since too rapid a cooling rate can result in distortion of the agar, however, there is no research to support this theory. Hydrocolloids gel at 100°F. (REF. 87-p. 114)

1246. C. For cast and die procedures, improved die stone is the best. The accuracy and ease of manipulation of stone outweighs its one disadvantage, i. e., friability. Casts may be prepared with removable dies. Margins are accessible for trimming and can be accurately repositioned for soldering relationship and proximal contact. (REF. 87-p. 131)

1247. B. The elastomers consist of the polysulfides (as mercaptans and thiokols), silicones, and polyethers (as epimines). The polysulfides and silicones are supplied in three different viscosities: heavy or Class 1, regular or Class 2, and light (syringe) or Class 3. (REF. 87-p. 134)

1248. D. Polymers of the polysulfide and silicone types of rubber base are mixed with suitable fillers to a paste consistency. In making an impression, this paste is cured to a semisolid rubber by combining it with a suitable catalyst. These rubber bases are used primarily when impressions of hard objects (teeth) are made. The polysulfide base is untidy to handle, and the odor is objectionable. (REF. 87-p. 136)

1249. A. Rubber impression materials remain dimensionally stable for about an hour, do not affect the hardness of the surface of stone, and are easy and tidy to handle. The impression must be poured within 1 hour after removal from the mouth. (REF. 87-p. 138)

1250. E. The powder or polymer of the dental resin is a polymer of methyl methacrylate, and generally it contains benzoyl peroxide as the initiator and pigments, as well as opacifiers for proper shading. The liquid is methyl methacrylate monomer and usually contains hydroquinone as an inhibitor and dimethyl-p-toluidine as an accelerator. Some of the resins contain small amounts of a cross-linking agent. (REF. 87-p. 140)

1251. E. Resin materials have shown conflicting reports in regards to the effects of the restorative resin on the dental pulp. Some investigators report that pulp response is mild and reversible. However, other investigators report severe inflammatory changes, with pulpal abscesses to total pulp necrosis. Resins possess high esthetic qualities, have a low thermal conductivity, and are insoluble in the fluids of the mouth. (REF. 87-p. 141)

1252. C. Radioactive tracer studies show that all restorative resins exhibit marginal leakage. Unfilled restorative resins have a severe drawback due to their high coefficient of thermal expansion, which accounts for a high degree of marginal percolation. It is through the marginal leakage that mouth fluids, microorganisms, and debris gain access to the cavity and cause pulpal irritation and recurrent caries. However, the filled resin restorations are difficult to finish and have poor wear resistance, especially in stress-bearing areas. (REF. 87-p. 142)

1253. B. Conventional acrylic resins processed with the usual dental techniques of compression molding are just as stable in dimension as the special resins and techniques, and reproduce the wax model denture just as accurately. The most accurately fitting dentures are the self-curing type. The heat-cured dentures do not fit as well but are considered good. The processing shrinkage was greatest in the special injection group. The vulcanite dentures are only slightly more accurate in fit than the best of the heat-cured. (REF. 87-p. 220)

1254. B. Manifestations of improper cavity preparation are recurrent decay, fracture of amalgam, periodontal and pulpal involvement. Improper manipulation of amalgam is the second most common cause of amalgam failures. (REF. 101-p. 2)

1255. B. If a cavosurface can be made to avoid an opposing cusp's excursion, the margin will have a better chance of remaining intact. Stress analysis has demonstrated that internal angles should be round not sharp. Stress concentrates in and around sharp line and point angles. (REF. 101-p. 2)

1256. C. One of the matrix alloys or phases is tin-mercury (Sm7Hg). This allowance is gamma-2, which is responsible for early fracture and failure of the older type alloys. Modern efforts have been directed toward eliminating this phase with success. (REF. 101-p. 6)

1257. B. Practically it makes little difference whether or not amalgam slightly contracts or slightly expands. Most of our modern amalgam falls within the ADA limits of ± 0.002 micrometers per centimeter for dimensional change in 5 minutes to 24 hours. (REF. 101-p. 13)

1258. A. Mechanical condensation is useful for amalgam, but it requires a change in the mercury-alloy ratio, i. e., less initial mercury. The vibratory action of the mechanical condenser removes greater quantities of mercury. (REF. 101-p. 18)

1259. A. High copper alloys are not all equal in quality. Because of patents some manufacturers cannot produce high quality materials. The best amalgam alloy is of the admixed variety (as Dispersalloy and Phasealloy). (REF. 101-p. 19)

1260. E. Gold foil has been classified as cohesive or noncohesive. The easy-handling properties of noncohesive gold foil are due to the finding that it does not weld to itself but rather continues to spread and allow itself to be worked into position. (REF. 101-p. 23)

1261. C. Restorative golds are not easy to condense. The latter probably accounts for the vast majority of clinical failures. It is proper compaction which adapts the gold to the surrounding walls and retentive areas of the cavity preparation, sealing the cavo-surface margins. Proper compaction welds and strain-hardens the gold mass and drives out air, welds the gold particles together and reduces porosity, pits and voids. (REF. 101-p. 35)

1262. A. Only the presence of chemical and physical bonds constitutes adhesion. A substance may lack adhesive properties yet be retained by mechanical means. The latter is the case with current acid etch restorative systems. (REF. 101-p. 40)

1263. B. Enamel must undergo conditioning for bonding. A simple method of increasing bond durability utilizes phosphoric acid to modify the enamel physically and chemically, i.e., the acid etch technique. (REF. 16-p. 45)

1264. E. To enhance penetration and improve the esthetic appearance the placement of a chamfer shoulder at the cavo-surface has been recommended. Topical fluoride application before conditioning of enamel is contraindicated. Fluorides should not be applied after enamel conditioning and before resin placement. (REF. 101-p. 62)

1265. A. The bonding of polymerizable resins offers a safe and simple method in experienced hands and should be undertaken only after achieving a thorough understanding of the factors which govern bonding under actual clinical conditions. (REF. 101-p. 69)

1266. E. The most common reason for failure of the acid etch technique is contamination of the etched enamel surface with water, saliva, blood, oil, or other agents prior to placement of the resin coating. The following acids will produce a well-etched tooth surface: lactic acid, citric acid, pyruvic acid, and orthophosphoric acid. (REF. 101-p. 78)

1267. B. Tooth preparation for the pinledge retainer should be undertaken with the following guiding principles: preservation of tooth structure, retention and resistance, structural durability, and marginal integrity. Tooth tissue is conserved by the maintenance of the facial surface and the proximal surface away from the edentulous space. (REF. 101-p. 115)

REFERENCES

REFERENCES

1. B. J. Anson, Morris' Human Anatomy, 12th ed. McGraw-Hill: New York, 1966.

2. B. D. Davis, R. Dulbecco, H. N. Eisen, and H. S. Ginsberg, Microbiology, 3rd ed., Harper & Row: Hagerstown, Maryland, 1980.

3. J. R. Brobeck (ed.), Best and Taylor's Physiological Basis of Medical Pracice, 10th ed. Williams and Wilkins: Baltimore, 1979.

4. D. F. Cappel, and J. R. Anderson (eds.), Muir's Textbook of Pathology, 9th ed. Williams and Wilkins: Baltimore, 1971.

5. H. C. Hopps, Principles of Pathology, 2nd ed. Appleton-Century-Crofts: New York, 1964.

6. S. N. Bhaskar, Synopsis of Oral Histology. C. V. Mosby: St. Louis, Missouri, 1968.

7. "The Metabolism of Oral Tissues," Annals of the New York Academy of Sciences, 85:1-499, 1960.

8. S. N. Bhaskar (ed.), Orban's Oral Histology and Embryology, 9th ed. C. V. Mosby: St. Louis, Missouri, 1980.

9. E. S. West, W. R. Todd, H. S. Mason, and J. T. Van Bruggen. Textbook of Biochemistry, 4th ed. Macmillan: New York, 1966.

10. A. E. Nizel, The Science of Nutrition and Its Application in Clinical Dentistry, 2nd ed. W. B. Saunders: Philadelphia, 1966.

11. H. Sicher, and E. DuBrul, Oral Anatomy, 6th ed. C. V. Mosby: St. Louis, Missouri, 1975.

12. J. H. Scott, The Essentials of Oral Anatomy, E. & S. Livingston: Edinburgh and London, 1967.

13. E. V. Zegarelli, A. H. Kutscher, and G. A. Hyman. Diagnosis of Diseases of the Mouth and Jaws, 2nd ed. Lea and Febiger: Philadelphia, Pennsylvania, 1978.

14. L. Cohen, Oral Diagnosis and Treatment Planning, Charles C Thomas: Springfield, Illinois, 1972.

15. F. I. Jacobson (ed.), Oral Diagnosis and Treatment Planning, Dental Clinics of North America, W. B. Saunders: Philadelphia, Pennsylvania, 1963.

16. A. F. Gardner, Pathology in Dentistry, Charles C Thomas: Springfield, Illinois, 1968.

17. A. F. Gardner, Differential Oral Diagnosis in Systemic Diseases, John Wright and Sons: Bristol, England, 1970.

18. C. M. Goss (ed.), Gray's Anatomy, 29th ed. Lea and Febiger: Philadelphia, 1973.

19. R. E. Buchanan, and N. E. Gibbons (eds.), Bergey's Manual of Determinative Bacteriology, 8th ed. Williams and Wilkins: Baltimore, 1974.

20. D. F. Mitchell, S. M. Standish, and T. B. Fast. Oral Diagnosis/Oral Medicine, 3rd ed. Lea and Febiger: Philadelphia, 1978.

21. W. A. D. Anderson, and T. M. Scotti. Synopsis of Pathology, 10th ed. C. V. Mosby: St. Louis, Missouri, 1980.

22. G. W. Burnett, H. W. Scherp, and G. S. Schuster. Oral Microbiology and Infectious Disease, 4th ed. Williams and Wilkins: Baltimore, 1976.

23. J. M. Dille, Drug Therapy for Dentists, Year Book Medical Publishers: Chicago, Illinois, 1963.

24. L. E. Francis, and D. R. Wood, Dental Pharmacology and Therapeutics, W. B. Saunders: Philadelphia, 1961.

25. C. O. Boucher, Swenson's Complete Dentures, 6th ed. C. V. Mosby: St. Louis, Missouri, 1970.

26. C. M. Heartwell, and A. O. Rahn, Syllabus of Complete Dentures, 3rd ed. Lea & Febiger: Philadelphia, 1980.

27. R. J. Nagle, and V. H. Sears, Denture Prosthetics - Complete Dentures, 2nd ed. C. V. Mosby: St. Louis, Missouri, 1962.

28. C. M. Sturdevant, R. E. Barton, and J. C. Brauer, The Art and Science of Operative Dentistry, McGraw-Hill: New York, 1968.

29. W. H. Wilson, and R. L. Lang, Practical Crown and Bridge Prosthodontics. McGraw-Hill: New York, 1962.

30. J. F. Johnston, R. W. Phillips, and R. W. Dykema, Modern Practice in Crown and Bridge Prosthodontics, 3rd ed. W. B. Saunders: Philadelphia, 1971.

31. W. H. O. McGehee, H. A. True, and E. F. Inskipp, A Textbook of Operative Dentistry, 4th ed. McGraw-Hill: New York, 1956.

32. O. C. Applegate, Essentials of Removable Partial Denture Prosthesis, 3rd ed. W. B. Saunders: Philadelphia, 1965.

33. G. E. Myers, Textbook of Crown and Bridge Prosthodontics. C. V. Mosby: St. Louis, Missouri, 1969.

34. D. Henderson, and V. L. Steffel, McCracken's Removable Partial Prosthodontics, 4th ed. C. V. Mobsy: St. Louis, Missouri, 1973.

35. D. Laskin (ed.), Thoma's Oral Surgery, 6th ed. C. V. Mosby: St. Louis, Missouri, 1982.

36. W. H. Archer, Oral Surgery, 5th ed. W. B. Saunders: Philadelphia, 1975.

37. C. R. Bennett (ed.), Monheim's Local Anesthesia and Pain Control Dental Practice, 6th ed. C. V. Mosby: St. Louis, Missouri, 1978.

38. N. B. Jorgensen, and J. Hayden, Sedation, Local and General Anesthesia in Dentistry, 2nd ed. Lea & Febiger: Philadelphia, 1972.

39. H. W. Gilmore, M. R. Lund, D. J. Bales, and J. P. Vernetti, Operative Dentistry, 4th ed. C. V. Mosby: St. Louis, Missouri, 1982.

40. H. Langa, Relative Analgesia in Dental Practice, 2nd ed. W. B. Saunders: Philadelphia, 1976.

41. J. L. Ingle, Endodontics, 2nd ed. Lea and Febiger: Philadelphia, 1976.

42. D. H. Goose, and R. L. Hartles, Principles of Preventive Dentistry. Macmillan: New York, 1964.

43. N. B. Jorgensen, and J. Hayden, Premedication, Local and General Anesthesia in Dentistry. Lea and Febiger: Philadelphia, 1967.

44. J. Adriani, Fundamentals of General Anesthesia for Students and Practitioners of Dentistry. Charles C Thomas: Springfield, Illinois, 1958.

45. R. H. De Jong, Physiology and Pharmacology of Local Anesthesia. Charles C Thomas: Springfield, Illinois, 1970.

46. L. Baum, Operative Dentistry for the General Practitioner, Charles C Thomas: Springfield, Illinois, 1974.

47. S. R. Spiro, Amnesia - Analgesia Techniques in Dentistry. Charles C Thomas: Springfield, Illinois, 1972.

48. D. E. Beaudreau, Atlas of Fixed Partial Prosthesis. Charles C Thomas: Springfield, Iilinois, 1976.

49. C. O. Dummett, Community Dentistry - Contributions to New Directions. Charles C Thomas: Springfield, Illinois, 1974.

50. O. E. Beder, Fundamentals of Maxillofacial Prosthetics. Charels C Thomas: Springfield, Illinois, 1974.

51. J. R. Hayward, Oral Surgery. Charles C Thomas: Springfield, Illinois, 1976.

52. H. C. Kilpatrick, Work Simplification in Dental Practice, 3rd ed. W. B. Saunders: Philadelphia, 1974.

53. F. A. Castano, and B. A. Alden, Handbook of Expanded Dental Auxiliary Practice. J. B. Lippincott: Philadelphia, 1973.

54. E. Wolfson, Four-Handed Dentistry for Dentists and Assistants, C. V. Mosby: St. Louis, Missouri, 1974.

55. E. J. Green, and N. Kohn, Selection, Hiring, and Training of Dental Auxiliaries. W. B. Saunders: Philadelphia, 1970.

56. M. G. Bounocore, The Use of Adhesives in Dentistry. Charles C Thomas: Springfield, Illinois, 1975.

57. W. E. Brown, Oral Health, Dentistry, and the American Public. University of Oklahoma Press: Norman, Oklahoma, 1974.

58. S. B. Finn, Clinical Pedodontics, 4th ed. W. B. Saunders: Philadelphia, 1973.

59. R. E. Moyers, Handbook of Orthodontics, 3rd ed. Year Book Medical Publishers: Chicago, 1973.

60. R. G. Ellis, and K. W. Davey, Classification and Treatment of Injuries to the Teeth of Children, 5th ed. Year Book Medical Publishers: Chicago, 1970.

61. R. E. McDonald, Dentistry for the Child and Adolescent, 2nd ed. C. V. Mosby: St. Louis, Missouri, 1974.

62. D. H. Goose, and R. L. Hartles, Principles of Preventive Dentistry. Macmillan: New York, 1964.

63. H. Schilder (ed.), Symposium on Endodontics. Dental Clinics of North America, W. B. Saunders: Philadelphia, 1967.

64. A. F. Gardner, Pathology in Dentistry. Charles C Thomas: Springfield, Illinois, 1968.

65. L. I. Grossman, Endodontic Practice, 8th 3d. Lea and Febiger, Philadelphia, 1974.

66. R. F. Sommer, F. D. Ostrander, and M. C. Crowley, Clinical Endodontics, 3rd ed. W. B. Saunders: Philadelphia, 1966.

67. R. W. Tiecke, O. H. Stuteville, and J. C. Calandra, Pathologic Physiology of Oral Disease. C. V. Mosby: St. Louis, Missouri, 1959.

68. W. G. Shafer, M. K. Hine, and B. M. Levy, A Textbook of Oral Pathology, 3rd ed. W. B. Saunders: Philadelphia, 1974.

69. J. L. Bernier, The Management of Oral Disease, 2nd ed. C. V. Mosby: St. Louis, Missouri, 1959.

70. B. J. Orban, and F. M. Wentz, Atlas of Clinical Pathology of the Oral Mucous Membrane, C. V. Mosby: St. Louis, Missouri, 1960.

71. P. E. Boyle, Kronfeld's Histopathology of the Teeth and Their Surrounding Structures, 4th ed. Lea and Febiger: Philadelphia, 1955.

72. R. J. Gorlin, and H. M. Goldman, Thoma's Oral Pathology, 6th ed. C. V. Mosby: St. Louis, Missouri, 1970.

73. S. Bhaskar, Synopsis of Oral Pathology, 5th ed. C. V. Mosby: St. Louis, Missouri, 1980.

74. E. C. Stafne, and J. A. Gibilisco, Oral Roentgenographic Diagnosis, 4th ed. W. B. Saunders: Philadelphia, 1975.

75. L. M. Ennis, H. M. Berry, and J. E. Phillips, Dental Roentgenology, 6th ed. Lea and Febiger: Philadelphia, 1967.

76. S. Blackman, and H. G. Poyton, A Manual of Dental and Oral Radiography. John Wright and Sons: Bristol, England, 1963.

77. J. O. McCall, and S. S. Wald, Clinical Dental Roentgenology, 4th ed. W. B. Saunders: Philadelphia, 1957.

78. F. A. Carranza (ed.), Glickman's Clinical Periodontology, 5th ed. W. B. Saunders: Philadelphia, 1979.

79. D. A. Grant, I. B. Stern, and F. G. Everett, Orban's Periodontics. A Concept-Theory and Practice, 4th ed. C. V. Mosby: St. Louis, Missouri, 1972.

80. R. A. Colby, D. A. Kerr, and H. B. G. Robinson, Color Atlas of Oral Pathology, 3rd ed. J. B. Lippincott: Philadelphia, 1971.

81. H. M. Goldman, and D. W. Cohen, Periodontal Therapy, 6th ed. C. V. Mosby: St. Louis, Missouri, 1980.

82. I. Glickman, and J. B. Smulow, Periodontal Disease. W. B. Saunders: Philadelphia, 1974.

83. H. M. Goldman, and D. W. Cohen, Introduction to Periodontia. C. V. Mosby: St. Louis, Missouri, 1966.

84. W. A. Anderson, and T. M. Scotti, Synopsis of Pathology, 10th ed. C. V. Mosby: St. Louis, Missouri, 1980.

85. L. C. Alexander (ed.), Endodontics, Dental Clinics of North America, W. B. Saunders: Philadelphia, 1963.

86. J. I. Ingle, and E. E. Beveridge, Endodontics, 2nd ed. Lea and Febiger: Philadelphia, 1976.

87. R. W. Phillips, Skinner's Science of Dental Materials, 7th ed. W. B. Saunders: Philadelphia, 1973.

88. A. F. Gardner, Pathology of Oral Manifestations of Systemic Diseases, Hafner Publishing: New York, 1972.

89. A. H. Wuehrmann, and L. R. Manson-Hing, Dental Radiology, 3rd ed. C. V. Mosby: St. Louis, Missouri, 1973.

90. F. J. Orland (ed.), Microbiology in Clinical Dentistry, John Wright-PSG: Bristol, England, 1982.

91. C. E. Crandell (ed.), Comprehensive Care in Dentistry, PSG Publishing: Littleton, Mass., 1979.

92. W. F. P. Malone, and Z. C. Porter, Tissue Management in Restorative Dentistry. John Wright-PSG: Bristol, England, 1982.

93. W. R. Laney, Maxillofacial Prosthetics, PSG Publishing: Littleton, Mass., 1979.

94. H. C. Lundeen, and C. H. Gibbs, Advances in Occlusion, John Wright-PSG: Bristol, England, 1982.

95. G. D. Allen, Dental Analgesia. PSG Publishing: Littleton, Mass., 1979.

96. L. R. Ripa, and J. A. Barenie, Management of Dental Behavior in Children. PSG Publishing: Littleton, Mass., 1979.

97. T. K. Barber, and L. S. Luke, Pediatric Dentistry. John Wright-PSG: Bristol, England, 1982.

98. D. P. DePaola, and H. G. Cheney, Preventive Dentistry, PSG Publishing: Littleton, Mass., 1979.

99. S. J. Chaconas, Orthodontics. PSG Publishing: Littleton, Mass., 1980.

100. A. B. Reiskin, Advances in Oral Radiology. PSG Publishing: Littleton, Mass., 1980.

101. M. H. Reisbick, Dental Materials in Clinical Dentistry. John Wright-PSG: Bristol, England, 1982.